PULMONARY HYPERTENSION

Edited by **Jean M. Elwing**
and **Ralph J. Panos**

Pulmonary Hypertension

http://dx.doi.org/10.5772/45912
Edited by Jean M. Elwing and Ralph J. Panos

Contributors

Ralph Panos, Jean Marie Elwing, Juan C Grignola, Pablo Curbelo, María José Ruiz-Cano, Juan Pablo Salisbury, Gabriela Pascal, Pilar Escribano-Subias, Dimitar Sajkov, Bliegh Mupunga, Jeffrey Bowden, Nikolai Petrovsky, Rajamma Mathew, Mehdi Badidi, M'Barek Nazi, Charles Fox, Philip Kalarickal, Henry Liu, Yiru Tong, Daisuke Inui, Amanda Gelineau, Alan Kaye, Kavitha A Mathew, Michael Yarborough, Aureliano Hernandez, Rafael A. Areiza, Kazuo Maruyama, Junko Maruyama, Ayumu Yokochi, Erquan Zhang, Hirofumi Sawada, Saleem Sharieff

Published by InTech

Janeza Trdine 9, 51000 Rijeka, Croatia

Publishing Process Manager Viktorija Zgela
Typesetting InTech DTP Team
Cover InTech Design Team

Additional hard copies can be obtained from orders@intechopen.com

Pulmonary Hypertension , Edited by Jean M. Elwing and Ralph J. Panos
p. cm.
ISBN 978-953-51-1165-8

For EU product safety concerns:
IN TECH d.o.o., Prolaz Marije Krucifikse Kozulić 3, 51000 Rijeka, Croatia,
info@intechopen.com or visit our website at intechopen.com.

Meet the editors

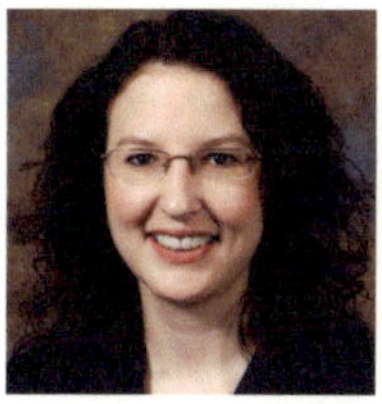

Jean Elwing, M.D. completed her undergraduate and medical education at Saint Louis University in 1997. She remained at Saint Louis University and completed a combined residency in Internal Medicine and Pediatrics in 2001. She received her fellowship training in Pulmonary and Critical Care Medicine at the University of Cincinnati. In January 2007 she joined the faculty in the College of Medicine at the University of Cincinnati. She is currently an Associate Professor of Medicine and the Director of the Pulmonary Hypertension Program in the Division of Pulmonary, Critical Care and Sleep Medicine. Her clinical and research focus is pulmonary vascular disease and pulmonary hypertension.

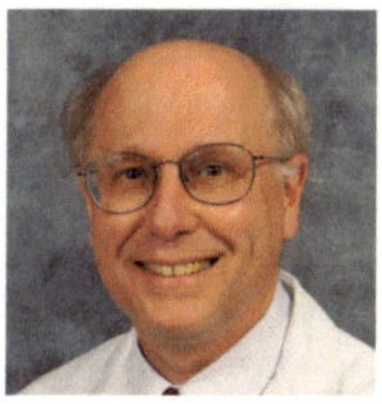

Ralph Panos is Associate Chief of Staff for Research and Development and Medical Director of the VISN 10 TeleICU program at the Cincinnati Veterans Administration Medical Center and Professor of Medicine at the University of Cincinnati College of Medicine. He graduated from the Brown University Program in Medicine, completed his medicine residency and chief residency at the University of Maryland, Baltimore, MD, and his pulmonary fellowship training at the University of Colorado and National Jewish Hospital, Denver, CO. His major research interests are interstitial lung disease and chronic obstructive pulmonary disease.

Contents

Preface

When Viktorija Zgela, Senior Commissioning Editor, InTech, approached us in the spring of 2012 to assist with editing a book about pulmonary hypertension that was already underway, little did we know what we were getting into. The work was already in progress with authors assigned to topics, research and writing started. Indeed, we stepped into fast moving process that had long passed the conceptual stage and was well into realization. We greatly thank Ms. Zgela and her colleagues at InTech for their patience and assistance guiding us through the process to bring this work to publication. Without their assistance, this book would never have made it to the presses.

We are greatly indebted to all the chapter authors who have persevered through multiple revisions, delays, and countless nights and weekends revising and editing. This final work reveals the fruit of all their labor.

In the initial chapter, **Pulmonary Arterial Hypertension: An Overview**, Saleem Sharieff presents a comprehensive synopsis of the epidemiologic, clinical, histopathologic, and therapy of PAH. Next, Dimitar Sajkov, Bliegh Mupunga, Jeffrey J. Bowden, and Nikolai Petrovsky comprehensively review World Health Organization group III PH in **Pulmonary Hypertension in Chronic Lung Diseases and/or Hypoxia**. The focus then shifts to the cellular and biochemical derangements underlying the pathophysiology of PH which are summarized by Rajamma Mathew in the **Pathogenesis of Pulmonary Hypertension**. Specific mechanisms that have been implicated in the pathogenesis of PH are presented by Junko Maruyama, Ayumu Yokochi, Erquan Zhang, Hirohumi Sawada, Kazuo Maruyama in **Nitric Oxide in the Pathophysiology and Treatment of Pulmonary Hypertension**, and Aureliano Hernández and Rafael A. Areiza in **Angiogenesis and Pulmonary Hypertension**. The focus then shifts to PH associated with thromboembolic disease. We discuss PH that occurs in association with acute thromboembolism in **Acute Thromboembolic Pulmonary Hypertension**. Mehdi Badidi and M'Barek Nazi present a comprehensive overview of PH caused by chronic thromboembolic disease in **Chronic Thromboembolic Pulmonary Hypertension**. Juan C.Grignola, María J. Ruiz-Cano, Juan P. Salisbury, Gabriela Pascal, Pablo Curbelo, and Pilar Escribano present a detailed overview of the physiologic assessment of patients with chronic thromboembolic disease prior to surgical pulmonary endarterectomy in **Assessment of Diagnostic Testing to Guide the Surgical Management of Chronic Thromboembolic Pulmonary Hypertension**. Finally, Henry Liu, Philip L. Kalarickal, Yiru Tong, Daisuke Inui, Michael J Yarborough, Kavitha A. Mathew, Amanda Gelineau, and Charles Fox comprehensively review the clinical perioperative evaluation and management of patients with PH in **Perioperative Considerations of Patients with Pulmonary Hypertension.**

We thank all the editors at InTech and all the authors for their diligence and effort in producing and writing this text. Most importantly, we thank our spouses for their lenience and sympathetic tolerance of the long weekends and late nights writing, editing, reading, and revising this work to bring it to publication.

Jean M. Elwing
Ralph J. Panos

Chapter 1

Pulmonary Arterial Hypertension: An Overview

Saleem Sharieff

Additional information is available at the end of the chapter

http://dx.doi.org/10.5772/56055

1. Introduction

Pulmonary hypertension (PH) is a hemodynamic state defined by a resting mean pulmonary artery pressure (PAP) at or above 25 mm Hg.[1] with normal left ventricular filling pressure (mean pulmonary wedge pressure) 15 mmHg or less.

Pre-capillary PH is defined as mean PAP ≥25 mm Hg in association with PAOP ≤15 mm Hg and a pulmonary vascular resistance (PVR) >3 Wood units. This include group 1, 3, 4 and 5 (Table 1). [2] Post-capillary PH (group 2 as shown in Table 1) is characterized by a mean PAP ≥25 mm Hg in association with PAOP >15 mm Hg and PVR ≤3 Wood units.[3] This differentiation in pre- and post-capillary PH is important as it narrows the differential diagnosis and also has treatment implications.

1. Pulmonary arterial hypertension (PAH)
1.1. Idiopathic PAH
1.2. Heritable
1.2.1. BMPR2
1.2.2. ALK1, endoglin (with or without hereditary hemorrhagic telangiectasia)
1.2.3. Unknown
1.3. Drug- and toxin-induced
1.4. Associated with
1.4.1. Connective tissue diseases
1.4.2. HIV infection
1.4.3. Portal hypertension
1.4.4. Congenital heart diseases
1.4.5. Schistosomiasis
1.4.6. Chronic hemolytic anemia

1.5 Persistent pulmonary hypertension of the newborn
1=. Pulmonary veno-occlusive disease (PVOD) and/or pulmonary capillary hemangiomatosis (PCH)
2. Pulmonary hypertension owing to left heart disease
2.1. Systolic dysfunction
2.2. Diastolic dysfunction
2.3. Valvular disease
3. Pulmonary hypertension owing to lung diseases and/or hypoxia
3.1. Chronic obstructive pulmonary disease
3.2. Interstitial lung disease
3.3. Other pulmonary diseases with mixed restrictive and obstructive pattern
3.4. Sleep-disordered breathing
3.5. Alveolar hypoventilation disorders
3.6. Chronic exposure to high altitude
3.7. Developmental abnormalities
4. Chronic thromboembolic pulmonary hypertension (CTEPH)
5. Pulmonary hypertension with unclear multifactorial mechanisms
5.1. Hematologic disorders: myeloproliferative disorders, splenectomy
5.2. Systemic disorders: sarcoidosis, pulmonary Langerhans cell histiocytosis: lymphangioleiomyomatosis, neurofibromatosis, vasculitis
5.3. Metabolic disorders: glycogen storage disease, Gaucher disease, thyroid disorders
5.4. Others: tumoral obstruction, fibrosing mediastinitis, chronic renal failure on dialysis.

ALK1 = activin receptor-like kinase type 1; BMPR2 = bone morphogenetic protein receptor type 2; HIV = human immunodeficiency virus.

Adapted from Simonneau et al. Updated clinical Classification of pulmonary hypertension. J Am Coll Cardiol 2009; Vol. 54 (1): S43–54

Adapted with permission from ELSEVIER.(ref 11)

Table 1. Updated Clinical Classification of Pulmonary Hypertension (Dana Point, 2008)

2. Epidemiology

Pulmonary arterial hypertension (PAH) is a rare disease, with an estimated prevalence of 15-50 cases per million.[4] Idiopathic PAH (IPAH) has an annual incidence of 1-2 cases per million people in the US and Europe and is 2-4 times as common in women as in men.[5], [6] The REVEAL Registry demonstrates a 4.1:1 female-to-male ratio among patients with IPAH, and a 3.8:1 ratio among those with associated pulmonary arterial hypertension (APAH). [4] The mean age at diagnosis is around 45 years.[7] IPAH accounts for at least 40% of cases of PAH, with APAH accounting for the majority of the remaining cases. [8]

The REVEAL Registry population tends to be overweight, with a BMI of 29 kg/m[2]; hence, obesity may be a risk factor for the development of PAH. A variety of comorbid conditions

http://dx.doi.org/10.5772/56055

were identified, including systemic hypertension, obstructive lung disease, sleep apnea, and prior venous thrombo-embolism, which were not believed to represent the principal cause for the patients' pulmonary hypertension. [6]

The median interval from symptom onset to diagnosis remains unacceptably high at 1.1 years in current registry data, [6] unchanged from the experience from the 1980's.[9] Overall survival has improved somewhat, with 3-year survival of 48% in the NIH registry [10], compared to 67% in both US [11] and French [12] contemporary registries.

3. Etiology

Pulmonary arterial hypertension (PAH) is comprised of idiopathic, heritable and associated forms. IPAH was previously referred to as primary pulmonary hypertension. During the 4th World Symposium on pulmonary hypertension in 2008 at Dana Point, California, USA, the group updated the Evian –Venice classification of 2003 of pulmonary hypertension based upon mechanism. [2] (Table 1)

4. Pathophysiology

PAH is a proliferative vasculopathy which is histologically characterized by endothelial and smooth muscle cell proliferation, medial hypertrophy, fibrosis and in-situ thrombi of the small pulmonary arteries and arterioles.[13], [14]

Genetic mutations — Predisposition to pulmonary vascular disease may be related to genetic mutations in the bone morphogenetic protein receptor type II (BMPR2), activin-like kinase type 1, and/or 5-hydroxytryptamine (serotonin) transporter (5HTT) genes. Abnormal BMPR2 may play an important role in the pathogenesis of IPAH, with up to 25 percent of patients with IPAH having abnormal BMPR2 structure or function. [15], [16], [17]

5. Pathobiologic basis of therapy

The pathophysiology of IPAH is not fully elucidated An elevated pulmonary vascular resistance seems to result from an imbalance between locally produced vasodilators and vasoconstrictors, in addition to vascular wall remodeling.

Three major pathobiologic pathways (nitric oxide, endothelin, and prostacyclin) play important roles in the development and progression of PAH.

5.1. Nitric Oxide (N.O)

The endothelium-derived relaxing factor nitric oxide (NO), a potent pulmonary vasodilator, is produced in high levels in the upper and lower airways by nitric oxide synthase II (NOSII) and affects the pulmonary vascular tone in concert with the low NO levels that are produced by nitric oxide synthase III (NOSIII) in the vascular endothelium. NO causes smooth muscle relaxation and proliferation, maintaining the normal pulmonary vascular tone. Patients with IPAH have low levels of NO in their exhaled breath, and the severity of the disease inversely correlates with NO reaction products in bronchoalveolar lavage fluid. [18], [19]

5.2. Endothelin-1

Endothelin-1 is a peptide produced by the vascular endothelium that has potent vasoconstrictive and proliferative paracrine actions on the vascular smooth muscle cells. The pulmonary circulation plays an important role in the production and clearance of endothelin-1, and this physiologic balance is reflected in the circulating levels of endothelin-1. Patients with pulmonary hypertension, IPAH in particular, have an increased expression of endothelin-1 in pulmonary vascular endothelial cells, and serum endothelin-1 levels are increased in patients with pulmonary hypertension.[20], [21]

5.3. Prostacyclin

The endothelium also produces prostacyclin (PGI2) by cyclooxygenase metabolism of arachidonic acid. Prostacyclin causes vasodilation throughout the human circulation and is an inhibitor of platelet aggregation by its action on platelet adenylate cyclase. The final enzyme in the production of PGI2 is prostacyclin synthase. The remodeled pulmonary vasculature in lung tissue obtained from patients with severe IPAH expresses lower levels of prostacyclin synthase when compared with normal lung tissue. [22]

5.4. Remodeling

In IPAH, pulmonary vascular smooth muscle cells that normally have a low rate of multiplication undergo proliferation and hypertrophy. Those smooth cell changes arise from the loss of the antimitogenic endothelial substances (e.g., PGI2 and NO) and an increase in mitogenic substances (e.g., endothelin-1). Other stimuli arise from locally activated platelets, which release thromboxane A2 and serotonin; thromboxane A2 and serotonin act as growth-promoting substances on the vascular smooth muscle cells. Both are vasoconstrictors and serotonin also promotes smooth muscle cell hypertrophy and hyperplasia. In addition to the smooth muscle cell proliferation, abnormalities in extracellular matrix contribute to the medial hypertrophy in PAH.[3] These lead to intimal narrowing and increased resistance to blood flow.

An abnormal proliferation of endothelial cells occurs in the irreversible plexogenic lesion. The plexiform lesions in IPAH have been considered an abnormal growth of modified smooth muscle cells. These lesions are glomeruloid structures forming channels in branches of the pulmonary artery. These may result from a deregulated growth of endothelial cells. [23]

Because the plexiform lesions bear some resemblance to the neovascularization induced by malignant gliomas at both the morphological and immunohistochemical level, one might hypothesize that the plexogenic vessels also represent a unique form of active angiogenesis.

Vascular endothelial cell factor (VEGF) promotes endothelial cell proliferation and is identical to the tumor factor responsible for inducing increased vascular permeability. Lung and brain express high levels of VEGF messenger RNA, and hypoxia triggers the production of VEGF. Furthermore, the presence of inflammatory cells in the perimeter of structurally altered vessels suggests that inflammatory cell-derived cytokines and growth factors may participate in the pathogenesis of PPH. Based on these results PPH may also represent a disorder of endothelial cell differentiation and growth. [23]

5.5. Thrombosis

Blood thrombin activity is increased in patients with pulmonary hypertension, indicating activation of intravascular coagulation, whereas soluble thrombomodulin, a cell membrane protein that acts as an important site of thrombin binding and coagulation inactivation, is decreased. In addition, PGI2 and NO, both inhibitors of platelet aggregation, are decreased at the level of the injured endothelial cell. Circulating platelets in patients with PAH seem to be in a continuous state of activation and contribute to the prothrombotic milieu by aggregating at the level of the injured endothelial cells.[3]

5.6. Other Factors contributing to PAH

- Vasoactive intestinal peptide (VIP) (systemic vasodilator, decreases pulmonary artery pressure and pulmonary vascular resistance, inhibits platelet activation and vascular smooth muscle cell proliferation)
- Vascular endothelial growth factor (VEGF) & receptors (participate in angiogenesis, appears to be disordered in PAH)

6. Signs and symptoms

Early symptoms are nonspecific. The most common symptoms include dyspnea, weakness and recurrent syncope. Other symptoms include fatigue, angina, and abdominal distention. Symptoms at rest are reported only in very advanced cases.[1], [24]

The physical signs of pulmonary hypertension include left parasternal lift, loud pulmonary component of the second heart sound (P_2), pansystolic murmur of tricuspid regurgitation, diastolic murmur of pulmonary insufficiency, and right ventricular S_3. Jugular vein distention, hepatomegaly, peripheral edema, ascites, central cyanosis and cool extremities may be seen in patients with advanced disease. [25] The lung examination is usually normal.

7. Investigations

Diagnostic approach is summarized in Figure 1.[25]

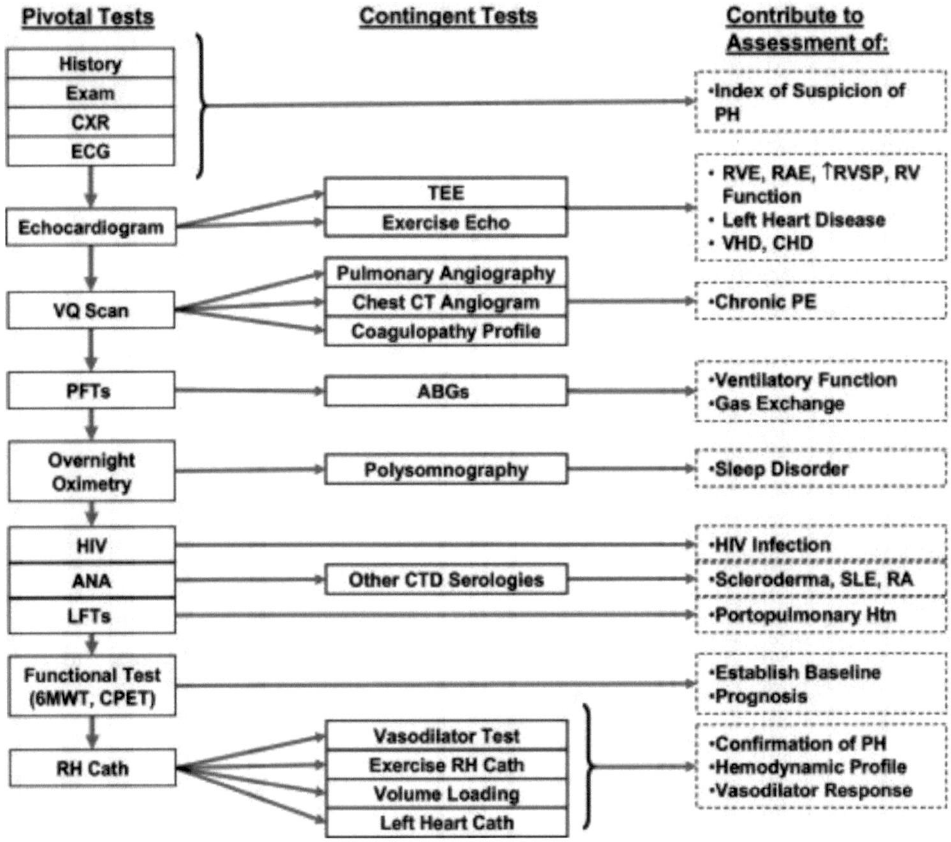

Adapted with permission from ELSEVIER.(ref 25)

Figure 1. Diagnostic Approach to Pulmonary hypertension. 6 MWD indicates 6-minute walk test; ABGs, arterial blood gases; ANA, antinuclear antibody serology; CHD, congenital heart disease; CPET, cardiopulmonary exercise test; CT, computerized tomography; CTD, connective tissue disease; CXR, chest X-ray; ECG, electrocardiogram; HIV, human immunodeficiency virus screening; Htn, hypertension; LFT, liver function test; PE, pulmonary embolism; PFT, pulmonary function test; PH, pulmonary hypertension; RA, rheumatoid arthritis; RAE, right atrial enlargement; RH Cath, right heart catheterization; RVE, right ventricular enlargement; RVSP, right ventricular systolic pressure; SLE, systemic lupus erythematosus; TEE, transesophageal echocardiography; VHD, valvular heart disease; and VQ Scan, ventilation-perfusion scintigram.

7.1. Electrocardiography

ECG results are often abnormal in patients with PAH, revealing right atrial enlargement, right axis deviation, right ventricular hypertrophy, or large P wave and characteristic ST depression and T-wave inversions in the anterior leads. [26] However, a normal ECG does not exclude a diagnosis of PAH.

7.2. Chest radiography

Radiographic signs of pulmonary hypertension include cardiomegaly or prominent central pulmonary arteries. [26]

7.3. Computed tomography and lung scanning

High-resolution chest CT scanning and ventilation-perfusion (V/Q) lung scanning are frequently obtained to help exclude interstitial lung disease and thromboembolic disease.

Radiographically, PH is said to be more likely when the main pulmonary artery diameter (MPAD) is > 29 mm (sensitivity 69%, specificity 100%) [27], [28] and/or the ratio of the main pulmonary artery to ascending aorta diameter is >1 [29]. The most specific CT findings for the presence of PH were both a MPAD > 29 mm and segmental artery-to-bronchus ratio of >1:1 in three or four lobes (specificity 100%) [30]. An additional feature of PH is rapid tapering or "pruning" of the distal pulmonary vessels.

7.4. Echocardiography

Echocardiography is extremely useful for assessing right and left ventricular function, estimating pulmonary systolic arterial pressure, and evaluating for congenital anomalies and valvular disease. [1],[24],[31], [32]

Systolic pulmonary artery pressure is estimated using tricuspid insufficiency jet velocity based on the simplified Bernoulli's equation:

$[4 \times (TRV)^2 + RA \text{ pressure}]$

Normal velocity is 2.0 – 2.5 m/s and a higher velocity indicates pulmonary hypertension, especially if there is associated dilation or dysfunction of the right ventricle.

7.5. Right heart catheterization

Right heart catheterization measures right atrial pressure, mean pulmonary artery pressure (mean PAP), pulmonary artery occlusion pressure (PAOP), cardiac output (CO) by thermodilution / indirect Fick and mixed venous oxygen saturation. Right heart catheterization provides data to calculate the pulmonary vascular resistance (mPAP-PAOP)/CO and transpulmonary gradient (mPAP-PAOP). In addition right heart catheterization evaluates pulmonary vasoreactivity and helps in the diagnosis of left-to-right intracardiac shunts (e.g. ASD, VSD and PDA).

The normal resting mean PAP is 14 ± 3 mm Hg. The normal PAOP is from 6-12 mmHg. The normal pulmonary vascular resistance is 0.3-1.6 Wood Units. Transpulmonary gradient is normally ≤ 12 mmHg. Pulmonary hypertension (PH) is present when mean pulmonary artery pressure (PAP) is greater than 25 mm Hg. The severity of PH is further classified on the basis of mean pulmonary artery pressure as mild (25 to 40 mm Hg), moderate (41 to 55 mm Hg), or severe (> 55 mm Hg) [33] or mild to moderate when PVR is between 2.5 and 4.9 Wood units; and severe when PVR > or =5.0 Wood units. [34]

7.6. Exercise testing

This is very helpful to assess the efficacy of therapy. Severe exercise-induced hypoxemia should cause consideration of a right-to-left shunt. Cardiopulmonary exercise assessment with a widely available 6-minute walk test is commonly used to assess and track functional capacity. [1],[10], [24],[35],[36] However, it lacks specificity in that it cannot be used to discern between several causes of an impaired ability to walk.[10]

Additional Workup: includes:

- Pulmonary function testing with diffusing capacity (DLCO): Elevated pulmonary artery pressure causes restrictive physiology. In patients with PAH, the diffusing lung capacity for carbon monoxide (DLCO) is reduced to approximately 60% to 80% of that predicted.
- Overnight oximetry or polysomnography is useful in detecting obstructive sleep apnea
- Ventilation/perfusion (VQ) scanning Patients with PAH may reveal a relatively normal perfusion pattern or diffuse, patchy perfusion abnormalities
- Pulmonary angiography performed to further evaluate or better define the anatomy in the setting of chronic thromboembolic disease
- Rheumatologic serologies to look for auto-immune diseases.
- Thyroid function testing: There is an increased incidence of thyroid disease in patients with PAH, which can mimic the symptoms of right ventricular failure. Consequently, it is advised that thyroid function tests be monitored serially in all patients.
- B-Type Natriuretic Peptide (BNP): Brain natriuretic peptide (BNP) levels are elevated in patients with pulmonary hypertension and correlate with the pulmonary artery pressure.
- Anti-HIV
- If chronic arterial oxygen desaturation exists, polycythemia should be present. Hypercoagulable states, abnormal platelet function, defects in fibrinolysis, and other abnormalities of coagulation are found in some patients with PAH.

8. Treatment

Despite advances in various treatments, there is no cure for pulmonary hypertension. The goals of treatment for pulmonary hypertension are to treat the underlying cause, to reduce symptoms and improve quality of life, to slow the growth of the smooth muscle cells and the development of blood clots; and to increase the supply of blood and oxygen to the heart, while reducing its workload.

An algorithm for treatment is shown in Figure 2. [37]

http://dx.doi.org/10.5772/56055

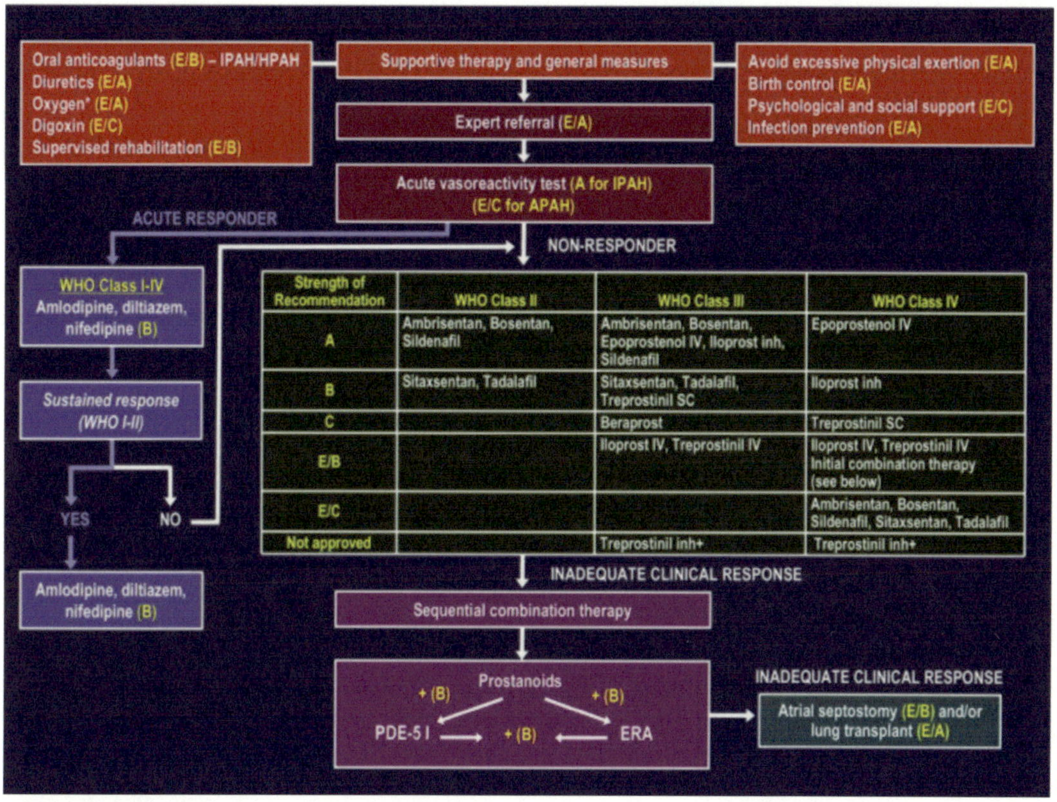

Adapted with permission from ELSEVIER (ref 33)
Barst RJ, Gibbs JS, Ghofrani HA, Hoeper MM, McLaughlin VV, Rubin LJ, Sitbon O, Tapson VF, Galiè N. Updated evidence-based treatment algorithm in pulmonary arterial hypertension. J Am Coll Cardiol. 2009 Jun 30;54(1 Suppl):S78-84.

Figure 2. Evidence-Based Treatment Algorithm. (Drugs within the same grade of evidence are listed in alphabetical order and not order of preference). APAH = associated pulmonary arterial hypertension; ERA = endothelin receptor antagonist; HPAH = heritable pulmonary arterial hypertension; IPAH = idiopathic pulmonary arterial hypertension; IV = intravenous; PAH = pulmonary arterial hypertension; PDE-5 = phosphodiesterase type 5; SC = subcutaneous; WHO = World Health Organization.

8.1. Medical treatment

8.1.1. General measures

- Oral anticoagulation improves survival in IPAH and is recommended in all these patients unless there is a contraindication. [26]
- Supplemental oxygen should be used to maintain oxygen saturation greater than 90%, especially because hypoxemia is a major cause of pulmonary vasoconstriction. Consider supplemental oxygen for PAH patients who are planning air travel, as mild hypobaric hypoxia can start at altitudes between 1500 and 2000 m, and commercial airliners are pressurized to the equivalent of an altitude between 1600 and 2500 m.[31]. Results suggest

travelers with PH, who will be traveling on long flights or those with a history of oxygen use, should be considered for supplemental in-flight oxygen.[32]. A flight simulation test before the flight can help determine oxygen needs at altitude.[24],[35]

- Diuretics are indicated for right ventricular volume overload
- Digoxin is reserved for patients with refractory right ventricular failure and for rate control in atrial flutter or fibrillation. [24],[35],[37]
- No specific diet is recommended; however, a low-sodium and low-fluid diet is recommended in patients with significant volume overload due to right ventricular failure.
- Exercise training is well tolerated and improves quality of life, WHO functional class, peak oxygen consumption, oxygen consumption at the anaerobic threshold, and achieved workload.[38] Patients with pulmonary hypertension and heart failure should perform mild symptom-limited aerobic activity and avoid complete bed rest. Isometric exercises (weight lifting) are contraindicated.
- Vaccination against influenza and pneumococcal pneumonia and avoidance of pregnancy.

9. Pulmonary vascular reactivity testing and vasodilator therapy

Diagnostic catheterization followed by pharmacological testing of vasodilator therapy response is required to test the pulmonary vasoreactivity in patients with IPAH before prescribing a vasodilator. The most commonly used drugs are: iv prostacyclin, iv adenosine, inhaled nitric oxide and inhaled iloprost. Oxygen, nitroprusside, and hydralazine should not be used as pulmonary vasodilator testing agents. A complete right heart catheterization and an invasive monitoring of the systemic pressures are mandatory. The increased pulmonary vascular resistance results from extensive vascular changes and vasoconstriction. Therefore, in pulmonary hypertension true pulmonary vasodilation is only present if, in addition to a decreased pulmonary vascular resistance, reductions in the transpulmonary gradient and the mean pulmonary artery pressure are achieved.

A positive test or 'responder to vasodilator' is defined as a drop in mPAP of ≥ 10 mmHg to an absolute level < 40 mmHg. A positive test is observed in 10-15% of patients with IPAH. However half of these patients will have a long-term response to calcium channel blockers (CCB). [39]

Only patients with an acute vasodilator response to an intravenous or inhaled pulmonary vasodilator challenge (eg, with adenosine, epoprostenol, nitric oxide) derive any long-term benefit from CCBs. Such patients constitute less than 15% of patients with IPAH and probably less than 3% of patients with other forms of PAH. [24], [35], [39]

Patients who do not have an acute vasodilator response to a vasodilator challenge have a worse prognosis on long-term oral vasodilator therapy compared with those who have an initial response. These non-responders are those who have no significant change of the mean pulmonary vascular pressure or symptomatic systemic hypotension and no change or a reduction of cardiac index (by more than 10 %), possibly accompanied by an increase in right atrial pressure (by more than 20 – 25 %). However, the absence of an acute response to intravenous or inhaled vasodilators does not preclude the use of intravenous vasodilator therapy. In fact, continuous intravenous vasodilator therapy is strongly suggested for these patients because CCBs are contraindicated. [40]

10. Calcium Channel Blocker therapy (CCB)

These drugs are thought to act on the vascular smooth muscle to dilate the pulmonary resistance vessels and lower the pulmonary artery pressure. The use of CCBs should be limited to patients without overt evidence of right-sided heart failure. In patients with IPAH (or any other form of PAH), a cardiac index of less than 2 L/min/m^2 or a right atrial pressure above 15 mm Hg is a contraindication to CCB therapy, as these agents may worsen right ventricular failure in such cases.

10.1. Specific vasodilator therapy

These drugs in general work by dilating the pulmonary arteries and, therefore, by reducing the pressure in these blood vessels and some help prevent the excessive overgrowth of tissue in the blood vessels (that decrease remodeling of the vessels). Common side effects include cough, flushing, and headache. Inhaled therapies may be useful as an adjunct to oral therapy.

There are three major classes of drugs used to treat pulmonary arterial hypertension:

10.2. Prostacyclins

Prostacyclin dilates systemic and pulmonary arterial vascular beds. These short acting drugs include epoprostenol [41] (Flolan), treprostinil (Remodulin), iloprost [42] (Ventavis), Treprostinil (Tyvaso). Parenteral vasodilators are used for patients whose IPAH fails to respond to calcium channel blockers or who cannot tolerate these agents and who have New York Heart Association (NYHA) type III or IV right-sided heart failure.

Long-term treatment with intravenous PGI2 improves exercise capacity, hemodynamics, and survival in most patients with PPH in NYHA functional class III or IV. Despite these favorable outcomes, continuous intravenous infusion of PGI2 is not ideal due to its cost and side effects such as flushing, headache, jaw pain, diarrhea and incidence of catheter-related infections. Survival of patients with PPH treated with epoprostenol depends on the severity at baseline, as well as the three-month response to therapy. Lung transplantation should be considered in a subset of patients who remain in NYHA functional class III or IV or in those who cannot achieve a significant hemodynamic improvement after three months of epoprostenol therapy, or both. [40]

10.3. Phosphodiesterase type 5 Inhibitors (PDE5i)

PDE5 inhibitors such as sildenafil [43] (Revatio, Viagra) is an orally active pulmonary vasodilators. (The dosing is much different when these drugs are used for erectile dysfunction). These drugs promote selective smooth muscle relaxation in lung vasculature by inhibiting PDE5 thereby stabilizing cyclic guanosine monophosphate (cGMP, the second messenger of nitric oxide), allowing a more sustained effect of endogenous nitric oxide, an indirect but effective and practical way of using the NO-cGMP pathway. Sildenafil improves exercise capacity, World Health Organization (WHO) functional class, and hemodynamics in patients with symptomatic pulmonary arterial hypertension. The main side effects of Sildenafil include headache, flushing, dyspepsia, nasal congestion, and epistasis Nitrates should be avoided in patients taking PDE5 inhibitors because the additive effects of the drugs may cause severe systemic hypotension. [44]

10.4. Endothelin Receptor Antagonists (ERAs)

Endothelin-1 is a 21–amino acid peptide that plays a key role in the pathobiology of PAH,[45], [46] exerting vasoconstrictor and mitogenic effects by binding to 2 distinct receptor isoforms in the pulmonary vascular smooth muscle cells, endothelin A and B receptors.[47] Endothelin B receptors also are present in endothelial cells, and their activation leads to release of vasodilators and antiproliferative substances such as nitric oxide and prostacyclin that may counterbalance the deleterious effects of endothelin-1.[47]

Bosentan is effective in patients with FC III / IV [48] but more recently bosentan was demonstrated to increase the 6 MWD from baseline in FC II patients as well [49]. Sitaxentan, a selective endothelin (ET)-A receptor antagonist, has negligible inhibition of the beneficial effects of ET_B stimulation, such as nitric oxide production and clearance of ET from circulation. In clinical trials, the efficacy of sitaxentan has been much the same as bosentan with reduced hepatotoxicity. [50] Dosing is once daily, as opposed to twice daily for bosentan.

Ambrisentan is a nonsulfonamide, propanoic acid– based, A-selective endothelin receptor antagonist with a bioavailability and half-life that allow once-daily dosing. In the ARIES study [51], Ambrisentan showed improvements in 6-minute walk distance in patients with WHO functional class II and III symptoms. It is well tolerated and is associated with a low risk of aminotransferase abnormalities. The most frequent side effects of ambrisentan are fluid retention (ranging from swelling of the extremities to heart failure), nasal congestion, sinusitis, flushing, palpitations, nasopharyngitis, abdominal pain and constipation.

ACCP guidelines recommend using the patient's New York Heart Association (NYHA) functional class to guide the choice of vasodilator therapy.[52] Grade A recommendations for vasodilator therapy by functional class from the ACCP are as follows:

- Functional class II - Sildenafil
- Functional class III - Endothelin-receptor antagonists (bosentan), sildenafil, IV epoprostenol, or inhaled iloprost
- Functional class IV - Intravenous epoprostenol.

10.5. Combination therapy

Patients with PAH may experience clinical and hemodynamic deterioration despite treatment with a single agent. This circumstance requires the addition on a second agent to slow disease progression and aid in clinical improvement.[35],[37] Different combinations have been tried, however current guidelines do not favor a particular combination over others. Several studies are on-going to compare the efficacy of single agent versus combination therapy. Failure of combination therapy requires consideration for parenteral therapy and surgical intervention such as lung transplantation.

10.6. Surgery

10.6.1. Atrial septostomy

Atrial septostomy is a palliative procedure that may afford some benefit to patients whose condition is deteriorating in the setting of severe disease with recurrent syncope or right heart failure (or both) despite maximal medical therapy. The procedure can also be used as a bridge to lung transplantation. The rationale for its use is that the controlled creation of an atrial septal defect would allow right-to-left shunting, leading to increased systemic output and systemic oxygen transport despite the accompanying fall in systemic arterial oxygen saturation. The shunt at the atrial level would also allow decompression of the right atrium and right ventricle, alleviating signs and symptoms of right heart failure. Balloon atrial septostomy is a high-risk procedure and should be performed only in experienced centers to reduce the procedural risks. [35],[37]

10.6.2. Lung transplantation

Lung transplantation has been used in treatment for pulmonary hypertension since the 1980s, even before current medical therapies were available. It is indicated in PAH patients with advanced disease that is refractory to available medical therapy. A single- or double-lung transplant is indicated for patients who do not respond to medical therapy. Simultaneous cardiac transplantation may not be necessary even with severe right ventricular dysfunction; however, this depends on the transplant institution. The 3- and 5- year survival rates after lung and heart-lung transplantation are approximately 55% and 45%, respectively. [35],[37]

10.6.3. Pulmonary thromboendarterectomy

Pulmonary thromboendarterectomy provides a potential surgical cure and should be considered in all patients with chronic thromboembolic PAH (CTEPH) affecting central pulmonary arteries. Pulmonary angiography is required to confirm surgical accessibility of chronic thromboemboli. The procedure requires cardiopulmonary bypass and involves dissecting well-organized thromboembolic material as well as part of the intimal layer of the pulmonary arterial bed. Patients with suspected CTEPH should be referred to centers experienced in the procedure for consideration of this procedure. In patients with operable CTEPH, pulmonary thromboendarterectomy is the treatment of choice because it improves hemodynamics, functional status, and survival. [35],[37]

11. Considerations for special populations

11.1. Surgery

Elective surgery involves an increased risk in patients with PAH. The increased risk is proportionate to the severity of the disease. It is not clear which type of anesthesia is advisable, but probably local and regional anesthesia are better tolerated than general anesthesia. Surgery preferably is performed at referral centers with experienced anesthesia and pulmonary hypertension teams that can deal with potential complications.[36],[53] Anticoagulant treatment should be interrupted for as short a period as possible. In patients with CTEPH, bridging with heparin is recommended to minimize the time off anticoagulation.

11.2. Pregnancy

Although successful pregnancies have been reported in PAH patients, pregnancy and delivery in PAH patients are associated with an increased mortality rate of 30% to 50%, and pregnancy should be avoided or terminated. An appropriate method of birth control is highly recommended in all women with pulmonary hypertension who have childbearing potential. Unfortunately, there is no current consensus on the most appropriate birth control method in PAH patients. Because of the increased risk of thrombosis with estrogen-based contraception, some experts suggest the use of estrogen-free products, surgical sterilization, or barrier methods.[24], [35]

12. Natural history and prognosis

PAH has no cure. However, the rate of progression is highly variable and depends upon the type and severity of the PAH. Untreated PAH leads to right-sided heart failure and death.

Prior to the 1990s, therapeutic options were limited. The emergence of prostacyclin analogues, endothelin receptor antagonists, phosphodiesterase-5 inhibitors, and other novel drug therapies has greatly improved the outlook for patients with PAH.

For untreated IPAH, the estimated 3-year survival rate is approximately 41%. In one study of long-term continuous intravenous prostacyclin therapy, 3-year survival increased to approximately 63%. [54] With newer therapies, perhaps in combination, these figures are expected to improve further.

Less symptomatic patients in WHO class II/III, with normal right atrial and ventriclar size and pressure and can walk more than 400 meters on 6 minute walk distance (MWD) are considered lower risk group of patients for morbidity and mortality. While symptomatic patients in WHO class IV with signs of right heart failure, enlarged right atria and ventricle with right ventricular dysfunction and cannot walk more than 300 meters on 6 MWD testing are considered high risk group of pattients with pulmonary hypertension. [25], [55]

The one-year survival of patients with newly diagnosed group 1 PAH can be predicted using a risk score derived from the Registry to Evaluate Early and Long-term PAH Disease Management (i.e. the REVEAL registry). This risk score was validated by a prospective cohort study of 504 patients with a mean 6-minute walk testing (6 MWD) of 308 m and 61.5 percent classified as WHO functional class III, which found that a risk score of 1 to 7, 8, 9, 10 to 11, and ≥ 12 correlated with one-year survival of 95, 92, 89, 72, and 66 percent, respectively. [56]

Severity of PAH – Patients with severe PAH or right heart failure (i.e., cor pulmonale) die sooner without treatment (usually within one year) than patients with mild PAH or no right heart failure. As an example, patients with IPAH and a mean right atrial pressure ≥ 20 mmHg have a median survival of approximately one month.[10]

In conclusion, age, PAH etiology, World Health Organization functional class, pericardial effusion, 6MWT distance, the need for oxygen during the 6MWT, and brain natriuretic peptide are predictors of prognosis in patients PAH receiving specific therapy and might help identify a group that could benefit from aggressive upfront therapy. [57]

Since survival in patients who fall into NYHA classes III or IV is poor (9-18 months), patients with severe symptoms and evidence of impaired cardiac function, which is refractory to conventional therapy or epoprostenol infusion should be considered for lung transplantation.

Author details

Dr Saleem Sharieff MBBS, FCPS, FRCPC[1,2]

1 Grand River Hospital, Kitchener, ON, Canada

2 McMaster University Hospital, Hamilton, ON, Canada

References

[1] Simonneau G, Galiè N, Rubin LJ, et al. Clinical classification of pulmonary hypertension. J Am Coll Cardiol 2004; 43:5S.

[2] Simonneau G, Robbins IM, Beghetti M, et al. Updated clinical classification of pulmonary hypertension. J Am Coll Cardiol 2009; 54:S43-54.

[3] Ghamra ZW, Dweik RA. Primary pulmonary hypertension: an overview of epidemiology and pathogenesis. *Cleve Clin J Med* 2003; 70 Suppl 1:S2-8.

[4] Peacock AJ, Murphy NF, McMurray JJV, et al. An epidemiological study of pulmonary arterial hypertension. *Eur Respir J 2007; 30:104–9.*

[5] Gaine SP, Rubin LJ. Primary pulmonary hypertension. *Lancet 1998; 352:719–25.*

[6] Badesch DB, Raskob GE, Elliott CG, et al. Pulmonary arterial hypertension: baseline characteristics from the REVEAL Registry. *Chest 2010; 137:376–87.*

[7] Frost AE, Badesch DB, Barst RJ, et al. The changing picture of patients with pulmonary arterial hypertension in the United States: how REVEAL differs from historic and non-US Contemporary Registries. *Chest 2011; 139:128–137.*

[8] Humbert M, Sitbon O, Chaouat A, et al. Pulmonary arterial hypertension in France: results from a national registry. Am J Respir Crit Care Med 2006; 173:1023-30.

[9] Rich S, Dantzker DR, Ayres SM, et al. Primary pulmonary hypertension. A national prospective study. *Ann Intern Med* 1987; 107:216-223.

[10] D'Alonzo GE, Barst RJ, Ayres SM, et al. Survival in patients with primary pulmonary hypertension. Results from a national prospective registry. *Ann Intern Med* 1991; 115:343-349.

[11] Thenappan T, Shah SJ, Rich S, et al. A USA-based registry for pulmonary arterial hypertension: 1982-2006. *Eur Respir J* 2007; 30:1103-1110.

[12] Humbert M, Sitbon O, Yaici A, et al. Survival in incident and prevalent cohorts of patients with pulmonary arterial hypertension. *Eur Respir J* 2010; 36:549-555.

[13] Humbert M, Morrell NW, Archer SL, et al. Cellular and molecular pathobiology of pulmonary arterial hypertension. J Am Coll Cardiol 2004; 43:13S.

[14] Pietra GG, Capron F, Stewart S, et al. Pathologic assessment of vasculopathies in pulmonary hypertension. J Am Coll Cardiol 2004; 43:25S.

[15] Deng Z, Morse JH, Slager SL, et al. Familial primary pulmonary hypertension (gene PPH1) is caused by mutations in the bone morphogenetic protein receptor-II gene. Am J Hum Genet 2000; 67:737.

[16] Newman JH, Trembath RC, Morse JA, et al. Genetic basis of pulmonary arterial hypertension: current understanding and future directions. J Am Coll Cardiol 2004; 43:33S.

[17] Kimura N, Matsuo R, Shibuya H, et al. BMP2-induced apoptosis is mediated by activation of the TAK1-p38 kinase pathway that is negatively regulated by Smad6. J Biol Chem 2000; 275:17647.

[18] Kaneko FT, Arroliga AC, Dweik RA, et al. Biochemical reaction products of nitric oxide as quantitative markers of primary pulmonary hypertension. *Am J Respir Crit Care Med* 1998; 158:917-923.

[19] Ozkan M, Dweik RA, Laskowski D, et al. High levels of nitric oxide in individuals with pulmonary hypertension receiving epoprostenol therapy. *Lung* 2001; 179:233-243.

[20] Stewart DJ, Levy RD, Cernacek P, et al. Increased plasma endothelin-1 in pulmonary hypertension: marker or mediator of disease? *Ann Intern Med* 1991; 114:464-469.

[21] Giaid A, Yanagisawa M, Langleben D, et al. Expression of endothelin-1 in the lungs of patients with pulmonary hypertension. *N Engl J Med* 1993; 328:1732-1739.

[22] Tuder RM, Cool CD, Geraci MW, et al. Prostacyclin synthase expression is decreased in lungs from patients with severe pulmonary hypertension. *Am J Respir Crit Care Med* 1999; 159:1925-1932.

[23] Tuder RM, Groves B, Badesch DB, Voelkell NF. Exuberant endothelial cell growth and elements of inflammation are present in plexiform lesions of pulmonary hypertension. Am J Pathol 1994, 144.275-285.

[24] Galie N, Hoeper MM, Humbert M, et al. Guidelines for the diagnosis and treatment of pulmonary hypertension: The Task Force for the Diagnosis and Treatment of Pulmonary Hypertension of the European Society of Cardiology (ESC) and the European Respiratory Society (ERS), endorsed by the International Society of Heart and Lung Transplantation (ISHLT). *Eur Heart J* 2009; 30:2493-2537.

[25] McLaughlin VV, Archer SL, Badesch DB, Barst RJ, Farber HW, Lindner JR, Mathier MA, McGoon MD, Park MH, Rosenson RS, Rubin LJ, Tapson VF, John Varga J. Expert Consensus Document on Pulmonary Hypertension: A Report of the American College of Cardiology Foundation Task Force on Expert Consensus Documents and the American Heart Association. *J Am Coll Cardiol.* 2009; 53(17):1573-1619.

[26] Fuster V, Steele PM, Edwards WD, Gersh BJ, McGoon MD, Frye RL. Primary pulmonary hypertension: natural history and the importance of thrombosis. Circulation. 1984: 70(4):580-7.

[27] Kuriyama K, Gamsu G, Stern RG, Cann CE, Herfkens RJ, Brundage BH. CT-determined pulmonary artery diameters in predicting pulmonary hypertension. *Invest Radiol.* 1984;19:16–22.

[28] Kuo PC, Plotkin JS, Johnson LB, et al. Distinctive clinical features of portopulmonary hypertension. *Chest.* 1997;112:980–986.

[29] Ng CS, Wells AU, Padley SP. A CT sign of chronic pulmonary arterial hypertension: the ratio of main pulmonary artery to aortic diameter. *J Thorac Imaging.* 1999;14:270–278.

[30] Tan RT, Kuzo R, Goodman LR, et al. Utility of CT scan evaluation for predicting pulmonary hypertension in patients with parenchymal lung disease. *Chest.* 1998;113:1250–1256.

[31] Galie N, Hoeper MM, Humbert M, et al. Guidelines for the diagnosis and treatment of pulmonary hypertension. *Eur Respir J* 2009; 34:1219-1263.

[32] McQuillan BM, Picard MH, Leavitt M, et al. Clinical correlates and reference intervals for pulmonary artery systolic pressure among echocardiographically normal subjects. *Circulation* 2001; 104:2797-2802.

[33] Khan MG. Pulmonary hypertension and cor pulmonale. In: Khan MG, Lynch JP III, eds. Pulmonary Disease Diagnosis and Therapy: A Practical Approach. Baltimore: Williams & Wilkins, 1997:603–616.

[34] Chang PP, Longenecker JC, Wang NY, Baughman KL, Conte JV, Hare JM, Kasper EK. Mild vs severe pulmonary hypertension before heart transplantation: different effects on post transplantation pulmonary hypertension and mortality. J Heart Lung Transplant. 2005 (8):998-1007.

[35] McLaughlin VV, Archer SL, Badesch DB, et al. ACCF/AHA 2009 expert consensus document on pulmonary hypertension: a report of the American College of Cardiology Foundation Task Force on Expert Consensus Documents and the American Heart Association: developed in collaboration with the American College of Chest Physicians, American Thoracic Society, Inc., and the Pulmonary Hypertension Association. *Circulation* 2009; 119:2250-2294.

[36] Doyle RL, McCrory D, Channick RN, et al. Surgical treatments/interventions for pulmonary arterial hypertension: ACCP evidence-based clinical practice guidelines. Chest 2004; 126:63S-71S.

[37] Barst RJ, Gibbs JS, Ghofrani HA, et al. Updated evidence-based treatment algorithm in pulmonary arterial hypertension. *J Am Coll Cardiol* 2009; 54:S78-84.

[38] Mereles D, Ehlken N, Kreuscher S, Ghofrani S, Hoeper MM, Halank M, Meyer FJ, Karger G, Buss J, Juenger J, Holzapfel N, Opitz C, Winkler J, Herth FFJ, Wilkens H, Katus HA, Olschewski H, Grunig E. Exercise and respiratory training improve exercise capacity and quality of life in patients with severe chronic pulmonary hypertension. *Circulation.* 2006; 114: 1482–1489.

[39] Tonelli AR, Alnuaimat H, Mubarak K. Pulmonary vasodilator testing and use of calcium channel blockers in pulmonary arterial hypertension. *Respir Med* 2010; 104:481-496.

[40] Sitbon O, Humbert M, Nunes H, et al. Long-term intravenous epoprostenol infusion in primary pulmonary hypertension: prognostic factors and survival. J Am Coll Cardiol 2002; 40:780–788.

[41] Shapiro SM, Oudiz RJ, Cao T, et al. Primary pulmonary hypertension: improved long-term effects and survival with continuous intravenous epoprostenol infusion. J Am Coll Cardiol 1997; 30:343-9.

[42] Olschewski H, Simonneau G, Galiè N, et al. Inhaled iloprost for severe pulmonary hypertension. N Engl J Med 2002; 347:322-9.

[43] Simonneau G, Rubin LJ, Galiè N, et al. Addition of sildenafil to long-term intravenous epoprostenol therapy in patients with pulmonary arterial hypertension: a randomized trial. Ann Intern Med 2008; 149:521-30.

[44] Galiè N, Ghofrani HA, Torbicki A, Barst RJ, Rubin LJ, Badesch D, Fleming T, Parpia T, Burgess G, Branzi A, Grimminger F, Kurzyna M, Simonneau G; Sildenafil Use in Pulmonary Arterial Hypertension (SUPER) Study Group. Sildenafil citrate therapy for pulmonary arterial hypertension. N Engl J Med. 2005; 353(20):2148-57.

[45] Galiè N, Manes A, Branzi A. The endothelin system in pulmonary arterial hypertension. *Cardiovasc Res*. 2004;61:227–237.

[46] Farber HW, Loscalzo J. Pulmonary arterial hypertension. *N Engl J Med*. 2004;351:1655–1665.

[47] Davie N, Haleen S, Upton PD, Polak J, Yacoub M, Morrell N, Wharton J. ET(A) and ET(B) receptors modulate the proliferation of human pulmonary artery smooth muscle cells. *Am J Respir Crit Care Med*. 2002; 165:398–405.

[48] Channick RN, Simonneau G, Sitbon O, et al. Effects of the dual endothelin-receptor antagonist bosentan in patients with pulmonary hypertension: a randomised placebo-controlled study. Lancet 2001; 358:1119–23.

[49] Galiè N, Rubin Lj, Hoeper M, Jansa P, Al-Hiti H, Meyer G, Chiossi E, Kusic-Pajic A, Simonneau G. Treatment of patients with mildly symptomatic pulmonary arterial hypertension with bosentan (EARLY study): a double-blind, randomised controlled trial. Lancet. 2008;371(9630):2093-100.

[50] Barst RJ, Langleben D, Badesch D, Frost A, Clinton Lawrence C, Shapiro S, Naeije R, Galie N. Treatment of Pulmonary Arterial Hypertension With the Selective Endothelin-A Receptor Antagonist Sitaxsentan. J Am Coll Cardiol. 2006;47(10):2049-2056.

[51] Galiè N, Olschewski H, Oudiz RJ, Torres F, Frost A, Ghofrani HA, Badesch DB, McGoon MD, McLaughlin VV, Roecker EB, Gerber MJ, Dufton C, Wiens BL, Rubin LJ. Ambrisentan in Pulmonary Arterial Hypertension, Randomized, Double-Blind, Placebo-Controlled, Multicenter, Efficacy (ARIES) Study 1 and 2. *Circulation*. 2008;117:3010-3019.

[52] Badesch DB, Abman SH, Simonneau G, et al. Medical therapy for pulmonary arterial hypertension: updated ACCP evidence-based clinical practice guidelines. Chest 2007; 131:1917-28.

[53] Kaw R, Pasupuleti V, Deshpande A, et al. Pulmonary hypertension: an important predictor of outcomes in patients undergoing non-cardiac surgery. *Respir Med* 2011; 105:619-624.

[54] Barst RJ, Langleben D, Frost A, Horn EM, Oudiz R, Shapiro S, et al. Sitaxesentan therapy for pulmonary arterial hypertension. Am J Respir Crit Care Med 2004;169 (4):441-7.

[55] McLaughlin VV, McGoon MD. Pulmonary Arterial Hypertension. Circulation. 2006; 114:1417-1431.

[56] Benza RL, Gomberg-Maitland M, Miller DP, et al. The REVEAL Registry risk score calculator in patients newly diagnosed with pulmonary arterial hypertension. Chest 2012; 141:354.

[57] Batal O, Khatib OF, Dweik RA, Hammel JP, McCarthy K, Minai OA. Comparison of baseline predictors of prognosis in pulmonary arterial hypertension in patients surviving ≤2 years and those surviving ≥5 years after baseline right-sided cardiac catheterization. Am J Cardiol. 2012: 15;109(10):1514-20.

Chapter 2

Pulmonary Hypertension in Chronic Lung Diseases and/or Hypoxia

Dimitar Sajkov, Bliegh Mupunga,
Jeffrey J. Bowden and Nikolai Petrovsky

Additional information is available at the end of the chapter

http://dx.doi.org/10.5772/55681

1. Introduction

Pulmonary hypertension is a common complication in lung disease. In the most recent revised classification of pulmonary hypertension (PH), chronic lung diseases or conditions with alveolar hypoxia are included in WHO Group III of PH-related diseases (Table 1) [1,2]. In this classification the structure of this group was for the most part unchanged. The heading has been recently modified to denote cause and effect on PH development. The primary modification was to add a new category of chronic lung disease of a mixed obstructive and restrictive pattern, which includes chronic bronchiectasis, cystic fibrosis and a syndrome characterized by the combination of pulmonary fibrosis (mainly of the lower zones of the lung) and emphysema (mainly of the upper zones of the lung), in which the prevalence of PH is almost 50%.

Alveolar hypoxia and thereby PH may occur in distinct conditions including: parenchymal lung disease, chronic airway diseases, ventilatory control abnormalities, residence at high altitude, progressive neuromuscular diseases and mixed obstructive and restrictive lung diseases [1,3,4]. As both the primary respiratory condition and PH may be associated with dyspnoea, the latter often goes unrecognised. Therefore, data on PH prevalence in each of these conditions is limited [5].

Prevalence of COPD-related PH is influenced by COPD progression, its heterogeneity, co-morbidities and methods of measurement. In a retrospective cohort study of over 4000 patients with advanced COPD awaiting lung transplant, a 30.4% prevalence of PH has been reported [6]. Elevated pulmonary artery pressure (PAP) is common in severe emphysema, although it may be independent of hypoxia [7]. However, the gold standard of measuring PAP by right heart catheterization to define PH has not been applied in the majority of prevalence studies.

In end-stage cystic fibrosis, PH prevalence, defined as mean PAP ≥25 mmHg, has been reported as high as 63% [8].

1. PAH

- 1.1 Idiopathic PAH (IPAH)
- 1.2 Heritable
  - 1.2.1 BMPR2
  - 1.2.2 ALK-1, endoglin (with or without hereditary haemorrhagic telangiectasia)
  - 1.2.3 Unknown
- 1.3 Drugs and toxins induced
- 1.4 Associated with (APAH)
  - 1.4.1 Connective tissue diseases
  - 1.4.2 HIV infection
  - 1.4.3 Portal hypertension
  - 1.4.4 Congenital heart disease
  - 1.4.5 Schistosomiasis
  - 1.4.6 Chronic haemolytic anaemia
- 1.5 Persistent pulmonary hypertension of the newborn

1' Pulmonary veno-occlusive disease and/or pulmonary capillary haemangiomatosis

2. Pulmonary hypertension due to left heart disease

- 2.1 Systolic dysfunction
- 2.2 Diastolic dysfunction
- 2.3 Valvular disease

3. Pulmonary hypertension due to lung diseases and/or hypoxia

- 3.1 Chronic obstructive pulmonary disease
- 3.2 Interstitial lung disease
- 3.3 Other pulmonary diseases with mixed restrictive and obstructive pattern
- 3.4 Sleep-disordered breathing
- 3.5 Alveolar hypoventilation disorders
- 3.6 Chronic exposure to high altitude
- 3.7 Developmental abnormalities

4. Chronic thromboembolic pulmonary hypertension

5. PH with unclear and/or multifactorial mechanisms

- 5.1 Haematological disorders: myeloproliferative disorders, splenectomy
- 5.2 Systemic disorders: sarcoidosis, pulmonary Langerhans cell histiocytosis, lymphangioleiomyomatosis, neurofibromatosis, vasculitis
- 5.3 Metabolic disorders: glycogen storage disease, Gaucher disease, thyroid disorders
- 5.4 Others: tumoural obstruction, fibrosing mediastinitis, chronic renal failure on dialysis

BMPR2: bone morphogenetic protein receptor, type 2; ALK-1: activin receptor-like kinase 1 gene; APAH: associated pulmonary arterial hypertension; PAH: pulmonary arterial hypertension.
From : Simonneau G et al, JACC 2009 [1].

Table 1. Classification of Pulmonary Hypertension

In high altitude residents, PH prevalence is between 8-18% [9,10]. A geographical variation in altitude-related PH prevalence may suggest differences in genetic susceptibility to development of PH in people living above 2000 m [11,12]. Variations have been observed in PAP changes among individuals living in the same regions, with some familial clustering and ethnic differences, although no definite gene polymorphism affecting PAP has been isolated [13].

Until recently there was disagreement whether intermittent hypoxia, such as occurs in obstructive sleep apnoea (OSA), without primary lung or cardiovascular disease can cause sustained PH. Recent studies have resolved this controversy by demonstrating that OSA is associated with PH, with co-prevalence rates varying between 20-40% [14-16]. However, no large population-based studies of PH prevalence in OSA have been reported and management of PH in patients with OSA has been mainly directed to managing the primary condition.

2. Pathophysiology

Alveolar hypoxia is a potent stimulus for pulmonary vasoconstriction. It operates at the endothelial level and is one of the most important pathways leading to PH development in chronic lung diseases. Alveolar hypoventilation precipitates acute pulmonary vasoconstriction in some regions of the lungs, and vasodilation in others, causing physiological shunt. Hypoxia causes pulmonary vasoconstriction leading to an increase in pulmonary vascular resistance. Two mechanisms are postulated to underpin this phenomenon. Vasoconstriction is achieved either through activation of a vasoconstrictor pathway or inactivation of a vasodilator pathway, or alternatively via the effects of hypoxia on the vascular smooth muscle [17]. Studies in rats exposed to hypoxia suggest that hypoxia-exposed arterioles develop smooth muscle in the walls of non-muscular pre-capillary blood vessels, which persists after removal of the stimulus and contributes to ongoing PH [9].

Hypoxic insults can be sustained or intermittent. In sleep-disordered breathing, the presence of intermittent hypoxia has been linked to the development of systemic hypertension with changes in the vasculature similar to the changes in PH. It remains undetermined whether sustained or intermittent hypoxia elicits these changes through similar mechanisms [18]. Studies in mice and rats exposed to intermittent hypoxia, mimicking sleep disordered breathing, showed development of sustained PH and right ventricular hypertrophy [17]. Treatment with CPAP in sleep-disordered breathing results in the reversal of PH, supporting a role for acute hypoxic pulmonary vasoconstriction and endothelial dysfunction in these patients [17,19].

Studies in mouse models of emphysema have suggested alternative mechanisms to the vascular changes associated with PH in COPD patients, as the mice developed pulmonary vascular changes independent of hypoxia indicative of a much more complex mechanism than hypoxia alone [5,20].

The development of PH as a result of hypoxic insults, both intermittent and chronic, is subject to ongoing investigations, with several pathways implicated in hypoxic pulmonary vasoconstriction (HPV). However, neither the oxygen sensing process nor the exact HPV pathways are fully understood [21]. The effector pathway is suggested to include L-type calcium channels, non-specific cation channels and voltage-dependent potassium channels, whereas mitochondria and nicotinamide adenine dinucleotide phosphate oxidases have been described as oxygen sensors (Figure 1). Reactive oxygen species (ROS), redox couples and adenosine monophosphate-activated kinases are also under investigation as mediators of HPV. Moreover, the role of calcium sensitisation, intracellular calcium stores and direction of change of reactive oxygen species is still under debate. Other pathways, such as the endothelin-1 pathway, nitric oxide pathway and ROS may also explain development of sustained PH. Endothelin-1 is an important mediator of systemic hypertension in intermittent hypoxic states [18,22] and ongoing studies suggest a role for endothelin in acute HPV. ROS are highly reactive and unstable free radicals. Intermittent hypoxia stimulates the synthesis and release of ROS through the tyrosine hydroxylase system, leading to the development of systemic hypertension. ROS have also been implicated in the induction of endothelin-1 and in angiotensinogen synthesis with all these agents believed to contribute to the development of PH induced by intermittent hypoxia [18,21,23].

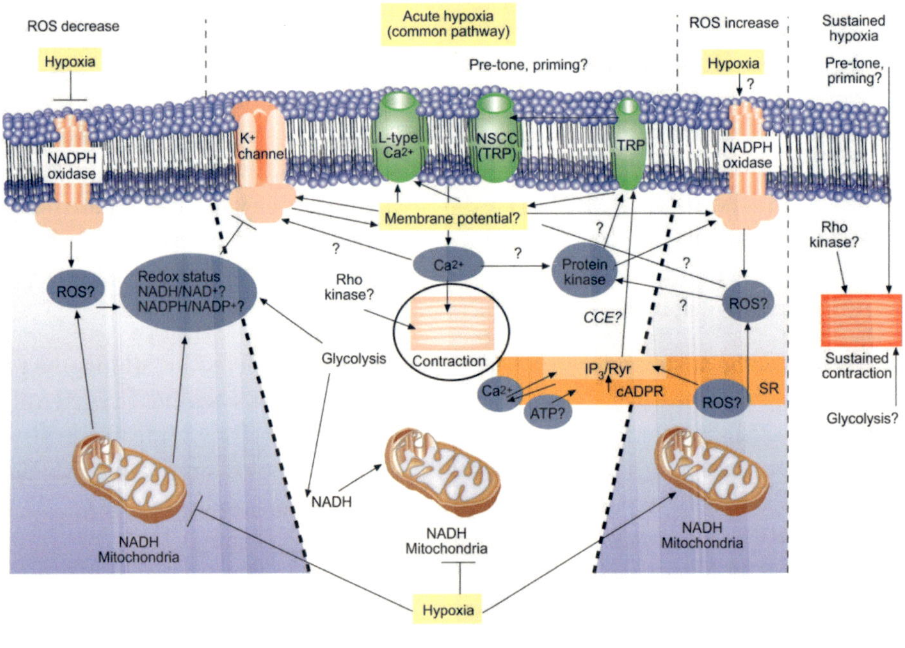

Figure 1. Pathways involved in hypoxic pulmonary vasoconstriction. Acute hypoxia results in an increase of intracellular calcium in pulmonary arterial smooth muscle cells and thus contraction. This increase in calcium is achieved by inflow of extracellular calcium through plasmalemnal calcium channels and release of intracellularly stored calcium. Hypoxic effects could be mediated or modulated by a decrease (left side) or increase (right side) of reactive oxygen species (ROS). NADPH: reduced nicotinamide adenine dinucleotide phosphate; NSCC: nonspecific cation channels; TRP: transient receptor potential; NADH: reduced nicotinamide adenine dinucleotide; NAD: nicotinamide adenine dinulceotide; NADP: nicotinamide adenine dinucleotide phosphate; CCE: capacitative calcium entry; ATP: adenosine triphosphate; IP_3: inositol triphosphate; cADPR: cyclic ADP-ribose; SR: sarcoplasmatic reticulum; *Sommer N et al. Eur Respir J 2008 [21], Reproduced with permission of the European Respiratory Society*

3. Pulmonary vascular remodelling

Studies of the vasculature in hypoxic PH have demonstrated changes including intimal thickening, medial hypertrophy and muscularization of the small arterioles [5]. When the balance between apoptosis and proliferation of endothelial cells in the pre-capillary pulmonary blood vessels, in particular, is altered in favour of proliferation, the overall resistance pattern is increased [24]. As shown in neonatal calves and rodent models, chronic hypoxia triggers endothelial cell proliferation [24,25]. Acute hypoxia triggers adventitial fibroblast proliferation within hours of exposure while medial hypertrophy and hyperplasia takes longer to develop [24,26,27]. Fibroblasts stimulated by chronic hypoxia can transform into smooth muscle cells. Hyperplasia is more prevalent in the less muscular arterioles, while hypertrophy is more common in the muscular arterioles. Chronic hypoxia in rat models results in a doubling of muscular arteries with proliferation into non-muscularized vessels [24]. The response of pulmonary vascular smooth muscle cells to acute hypoxia is still debatable with some studies indicating reduction in proliferation [24,28].

4. Role of systemic inflammation

Inflammation associated with underlying lung disease may be partly responsible for the development of PH in hypoxic states. Inflammatory cells have been detected in local vascular structures in COPD patients, in addition to the evidence of systemic inflammation with raised inflammatory markers, such as CRP and TNF–α [29,30]. In rats exposed to hypoxia, alveolar macrophages play a critical role in the inflammatory process, with inflammation occurring in the presence of reduced alveolar PaO_2 [31]. In alveolar macrophage-depleted conditions, systemic inflammation was not observed [32].

5. COPD and PH

There is a growing body of evidence supporting different phenotypes among patients with COPD. These COPD phenotypes may be useful in defining patients who may benefit from particular therapies or interventions more than others. Potential phenotypes may be defined by symptoms, physiology, radiology and exacerbation history, although the relevant clinical outcomes have not been defined [33].

A PH phenotype in COPD is potentially defined by perceivable effects on functional performance status and mortality [5]. PH is an independent prognostic factor in COPD [34-36]. The current accepted definition of PH in COPD is a mean PAP $\geq$ 25mmHg with underlying hypoxia. PH ideally should be measured by right heart catheterization, which may not be feasible in many cases. As an alternative, Doppler echocardiographic measurements have been used in a number of studies, although Doppler can be technically challenging due to body habitus and poor acoustic windows, precluding detection of a significant left heart pathology, which may also contribute to elevated pulmonary pressures [37]. Scharf et al. in a study of patients with severe COPD, reported over 60% of subjects had elevated pulmonary capillary wedge pressures [7]. The impact of PH on mortality in COPD is independent of age, lung function and blood gas derangements [5].

PH has been associated with exercise limitation in patients with COPD. In a study of 362 pre-transplant patients with COPD, PH (mean PAP ≥25mmHg) was associated with shorter 6-minute walking distance (6MWD) after adjustments for demographics and lung function [38]. In a large retrospective study of COPD patients studied with right heart catheterization, PAP had an inverse relationship with 6MWD [6]. A much smaller study of 29 COPD patients assessed with Doppler echocardiography could not detect statistically significant differences in cardiopulmonary exercise test parameters and 6MWD in patients with or without PH. However, the authors acknowledged that the small sample size and lack of invasive measures could restrict the generalisation of the results [39].

In patients with parenchymal lung disease PH is generally modest (mean PAP 25-35 mmHg). While PAP at rest varies from normal to moderately elevated, it increases significantly during exercise, sleep and acute infective exacerbations. Hilde et al. in a study of 98 patients with COPD undergoing right heart catheterization reported a 27% prevalence of PH. Hemodynamic response to exercise, including mean PAP, was abnormal and similar between the PH and non-PH COPD patients [40].

In some patients with COPD PAP elevations can be more substantial (mean PAP ≥35mmHg). In patients with only moderate pulmonary mechanical impairment, this is considered "out-of-proportion" PH. A subset of COPD patients has been identified where progressive PH has prognostic implications. The term "PH out-of-proportion to COPD" has been applied to this group of patients. An unusual pattern of cardiopulmonary abnormalities has been described in the patients with more severe PH, including mild to moderate airway obstruction, severe hypoxemia, hypocapnia, and a very low diffusing capacity for carbon monoxide. The characteristics of this subset include the presence of obstructive airways disease and presence of fibrosis. A relative preservation of lung function and severe PH in COPD is believed to define this "vascular phenotype" [5]. Thabut et al. in a cluster analysis identified a subgroup of COPD patients with out-of-proportion PH associated with severe hypoxia [41]. Chaouat et al. also identified a similar cluster [42]. The challenge remains, however, to have uniformly applied definition of PH in COPD. As with PH out-of-proportion to left heart disease, large randomized, controlled, studies of medications approved for PAH are not available for PH out-of-proportion for parenchymal lung disease.

6. Treatment of PH in COPD

Although treatment of PH in COPD is conceptually appealing, there are no clear guidelines and no medications currently registered for the treatment of PH secondary to COPD. The primary focus of treatment, therefore, even in the vascular phenotype of COPD involves standard therapy with smoking cessation, bronchodilators, inhaled steroids, long-term oxygen therapy (LTOT) and pulmonary rehabilitation [43]. Symptomatic (non-disease modifying) therapy for COPD-related PH includes LTOT, peripherally-acting calcium channel blockers and non-pharmacological interventions such as activity pacing and relaxation therapies.

6.1. Long-term home oxygen therapy

The only therapy that has demonstrated a survival advantage in people with COPD and co-existent PH is LTOT. Indications for LTOT include patients with severe hypoxemia or those with moderate hypoxemia and cor pulmonale [44-46], as it reduces pulmonary artery pressure [44,47].

LTOT is, however, relatively cumbersome and intrusive, with variable patient adherence. Patients with the most severe COPD have the least reduction in PH with LTOT [44,46]. Patients will often be concerned about the imposition of being physically reliant on a machine [48]. LTOT is also expensive, and may be associated with a small number of very serious adverse events across the community, such as CO_2 retention or burns, particularly where patients continue to smoke [49-51]. Actual adherence rates to LTOT are not precisely known and reports vary between 45 - 70% [52,53].

6.2. Evidence from pulmonary arterial hypertension

PAH includes idiopathic disease and disease secondary to connective tissue disorders such as scleroderma and systemic lupus erythematosus. Current evidence points to the benefits of prostanoids, endothelin antagonists and phosphodiasterase-5 (PDE-5) inhibitors as disease modifying in these people [2].

Given the evidence from PAH, it is plausible that in PH secondary to COPD pulmonary vasodilatation may improve the subjective sensation of dyspnoea and extend exercise endurance. Pulmonary vasodilator treatment (alone or as an adjunct to oxygen supplementation) might be useful to reduce dyspnoea and improve quality of life (QOL) in people with COPD and secondary pulmonary hypertension. Potentially, if these interventions were of benefit, improved physical independence, symptomatic control of dyspnoea and potentially even extended survival could be achieved.

6.3. Prostanoids

Epoprostenol sodium is indicated for patients with idiopathic, heritable or connective tissue disease related PAH (Group 1) as a continuous infusion [54]. Iloprost is a prostacyclin analogue that can be administered orally, intravenously or as an aerosolised formulation [55]. These have been shown to improve exercise tolerance and haemodynamic parameters in patients with PAH.

However, evidence for the use of prostacyclin analogues in COPD-related PH is very limited and current practice does not favour routine use of these medications. The primary concern in using pulmonary vasodilators is related to worsening gas exchange due to ventilation/perfusion (V/Q) inequality [5].

6.4. Endothelin receptor antagonists (ERA)

Bosentan, an oral endothelin-1 receptor antagonist is registered for use in patients with PAH in World Health Organisation (WHO) functional classes (FC) II-IV. It has been shown to reduce pulmonary vascular resistance and moderately improve exercise tolerance in people with mildly symptomatic disease. Hepatotoxicity and teratogenicity are potential toxicities [56]. Ambrisentan has been approved for PAH in WHO FC II-IV and has been shown to delay disease progression and improve exercise tolerance in patients with PAH with lower levels of hepatotoxicity [57].

Trials with endothelin receptor antagonists in patients with COPD and PH have suffered from poor study design and the general trend was worsening gas exchange without improvement in functional capacity.

6.5. Phosphodiesterase-5 (PDE-5) inhibitors

Sildenafil is a selective inhibitor of PDE-5, an enzyme that is specific for both lung and penile vasculature. Although originally developed for treatment of erectile dysfunction, sildenafil is an effective pulmonary vasodilator [58-60]. PDE-5 is found throughout the muscularized pulmonary vascular tree, including in newly muscularized distal pulmonary arteries exposed to hypoxia.

Sildenafil may be preferred to other vasodilator agents, particularly in patients with severe COPD, PH and poor RV function, because hemodynamic effects are likely to be selective on the pulmonary circulation. PDE-5 inhibition with sildenafil attenuates the rise in PAP and vascular remodelling when given before chronic exposure to hypoxia and when administered as a treatment during ongoing hypoxia-induced PH [61].

Previous trials in patients with PAH (primary or associated with scleroderma) showed that sildenafil-induced pulmonary vasodilatation is well tolerated, increased exercise capacity, decreased Borg dyspnoea index and WHO functional class and improved haemodynamics [62,63]. Therefore, it has been proposed to consider the use of this medication in selected patients with COPD-related PH, although clinical trials in this group are limited.

A recent randomized trial in 20 patients with COPD-associated PH demonstrated that sildenafil improved pulmonary haemodynamics both at rest and during exercise, with mild to moderate worsening of gas exchange at rest due to worsening $V/\dot{Q}$ mismatch [64]. A longer duration of 3 months treatment with sildenafil did not significantly alter hemodynamic or functional capacity [65]. A more recent cross-over trial of sildenafil and placebo in COPD-related PH showed significant worsening of gas exchange at rest and quality of life indices with no beneficial effect on exercise capacity [66].

6.6. Calcium channel blockers

The administration of vasodilator drugs has been proposed as an alternative or adjunct to oxygen supplementation in the treatment of PH in COPD for a number of years. However, there remains considerable controversy regarding the likely benefits of non-selective vasodilators [67-69].

Reports of worsening ventilation / perfusion (V/Q) inequality [70,71], a lack of long-term effectiveness (or development of tolerance) [72,73] and the high incidence of side effects [73] have raised doubts about the benefits of a non-selective vasodilator treatment in COPD.

Calcium channel blockers of the dihydropyridine group are the most extensively studied vasodilators in both PAH and PH secondary to COPD [70-85]. However, the non-selective vasodilator properties of these drugs give frequent systemic side effects (e.g. ankle oedema, headache, facial flushing), preventing their wider use in the COPD population. Their use is largely limited to patients who demonstrate acute vasoreactivity testing [73].

In an earlier study by our group, felodipine, a non-selective dihydropyridine calcium channel blocker, significantly improved pulmonary haemodynamics in patients with COPD and PH [83]. Pulmonary vasodilatation in these patients was sustained for 3 months of treatment, without development of tolerance or deterioration in gas exchange, although a high incidence of vasodilator side effects was observed. A subsequent study by our group showed that amlodipine was as effective as felodipine in improving pulmonary haemodynamics in patients with COPD, with fewer side effects than felodipine [84]. One small randomised placebo-controlled trial in patients with COPD and PH reported significant improvement of the dyspnoea score and preserved cardiac output with nifedipine for one year, although there was no significant survival benefit [85]. This supports the hypothesis that pulmonary vasodilatation in patients with severe COPD and PH may improve their functional performance, dyspnoea and QOL, particularly if systemic vasodilatation side effects can be avoided.

An important practice point is that alternative causes of PH in patients with COPD, such as concomitant sleep disordered breathing or chronic thromboembolic disease should be actively investigated, as there are important treatment alternatives in these patients.

7. Sleep disordered breathing and PH

True prevalence of PH in OSA is unknown and ranges from 17 - 52% [86]. In our study of 27 patients with OSA 11 (41%) had mildly elevated PA pressures, mean PAP = 26 mmHg, in the absence of cardiac or pulmonary disease [14].

OSA patients maintain normal daytime oxygenation but experience episodic hypoxic events during sleep. Acute rises in PAP with sleep-disordered breathing have an inverse relationship with the degree of oxygen desaturation. Pulmonary artery pressure is influenced by an obstructive sleep apnoea cycle associated with changes to intra-thoracic pressure with the changes most marked in REM sleep [87]. Three main mechanisms have been proposed including hypoxia, mechanical factors and reflex mechanisms [16]. However, there are conflicting data to support these proposed mechanisms. It has been observed that changes in PA pressure were inversely correlated with the degree of arterial hypoxia [88, 89] while in another study supplemental oxygen did not affect pulmonary artery pressures [90].

Our understanding of the relationship between OSA and PH is evolving following recent studies. Twenty patients with OSA were treated for 4 months with CPAP and a decrease in the mean PAP by 13.9 mmHg was observed for all patients although only five had PH [19]. This reduction of PAP and hypoxic pulmonary vascular reactivity in OSA following CPAP treatment was associated with improved pulmonary endothelial function due to the elimination of intermittent hypoxemia [19]. A randomised controlled cross-over trial using sham and effective CPAP in 23 patients with OSA (AHI = 44 ± 29.3/h) and 10 normal controls concluded that severe OSA was independently associated with PH [86]. The clinical impact of PH in sleep-disordered breathing remains under investigation. PH in OSA patients may lead to dyspnoea and reduction in 6MWD, suggesting functional impairment [91]. In a study of 296 OSA patients (AHI ≥ 20/hr) using nasal CPAP, pulmonary haemodynamics were not independently associated with mortality [42]. There are no consensus guidelines to recommend routine screening for PH in OSA. Although current data suggest improvement in PH when OSA is treated with CPAP therapy, the significance of this improvement in the clinical context remains unclear, particularly with mild to moderate PH observed in most patients with OSA.

8. High altitude PH

High altitude PH (HAPH) prevalence is between 5 and 18% in those living at ≥3000 metres and may be more common in children than adults [9,11,92]. As mentioned previously, the roles of the endothelin-1 and prostaglandin I2 pathways in the pathophysiology in high altitude associated PH have not been clearly defined [9]. Alteration in trans-membrane transport of K^+ and Ca^{2+} has been implicated in the process. Recent work by Beall et al. has suggested a role of free radical-mediated reduction in NO bioavailability [93, 94].

Migration to a lower altitude reverses HAPH. However, due to family, social and economic reasons, migration is not an option for some patients. As an alternative, sildenafil for 3 months has been shown to reduce PAP, improve 6MWD and cardiac index in patients with HAPH [95]. Reduction in mean PAP of up to -6.9 mmHg and improvement in walking distance of up to 45 m was observed and sildenafil was well tolerated [95].

The role of endothelin receptor antagonists in HAPH is yet to be determined. A small randomised cross-over study of 8 patients on bosentan did not improve pulmonary pressures or functional capacity when initiated prior to ascent during high intensity exercise [96]. Acetazolamide was successful in reducing pulmonary pressures and improving cardiac output at 6 months of therapy in patients with excessive erythrocytosis and HAPH [97]. Other drugs under evaluation include angiotensin inhibitors and results of the ongoing studies are pending.

9. PH in Cystic Fibrosis (CF)

PH prevalence in CF population remains uncertain with figures as high as 21-59%. A retrospective study of 179 pre-transplant CF patients revealed that 38.5% had PH with a RHC mean PAP of ≥ 25 mmHg [98]. In a recent series of 57 CF patients with advanced lung disease considered for lung transplant, 36 (63.2%) had PH [99]. Patients with PH were significantly more hypoxaemic than those without PH. A small number of patients (4) had more marked PH with mean PAP ≥40 mmHg [99].

PH develops as a consequence of alveolar hypoxemia and progressive destruction of the lung parenchyma and pulmonary vascular bed. However, other mechanisms may also be involved. An early study of the prevalence and impact of PH in adult patients with CF reported PH in 7 of 17 patients (41%) with stable but severe lung disease. PH correlated with declining FEV_1, diurnal and nocturnal oxygen saturation [4]. However, Doppler echocardiography, although used routinely as an initial screening test to estimate PAP, may frequently be inaccurate and some studies report poor correlation with right heart catheter measures [99]. The clinical impact of PH in most CF patients' management is unclear, although a trend towards worsening mortality has been observed in some small studies.

No properly conducted studies of PH management in CF have been reported.

10. PH in non-CF Bronchiectasis

There are no systematic studies to determine true prevalence of PH in bronchiectasis, which is defined as a progressive and permanent dilatation of predominantly medium and small airways. Bronchiectasis is often accompanied with significant airway obstruction and airflow limitation, and is associated with considerable morbidity but low mortality.

In a recent study of 94 patients with bronchiectasis, 31 patients (32.9%) had PH, defined as systolic PAP of ≥40 mmHg on Doppler echocardiography [100]. Significant correlation was observed between right ventricular dimensions and systolic PAP (r = 0.74) while RV dimensions were inversely related to PaO_2 values (r = - 0.37) suggesting a role for hypoxemia in the development of PH [100].

CT scan-derived measurements of the pulmonary artery have been shown to correlate favourably with the mean PAP derived from right heart catheterization [101-104]. In a study of 91 patients with bronchiectasis, increasing PH as characterised by CT measurements of PA dimensions was found to be an important prognostic marker [104].

As with CF patients, there is lack of data in managing PH in this group of patients.

11. PH in interstitial lung diseases

Interstitial lung diseases (ILD) are characterized by restrictive lung physiology with progressive impairment of gas exchange resulting in alveolar hypoxemia and PH. Mortality in these conditions is predicted by the degree of hypoxemia, spirometry and functional capacity as defined by 6MWD and presence of PH [105-108].

The prevalence of PH in IPF is high and varies between 32 - 85%. PH is mostly of moderate severity although in a few patients pulmonary pressures may approximate systemic levels

[109-111]. In one study of 212 patients with ILD screened by echocardiography and/or right heart catheter 29 (14%) had PH and 13 (6%) had severe PH defined as PAP ≥ 35mmHg [112]. To clinically diagnose PH in ILD is a challenge due to the overlap of symptoms of breathlessness and functional impairment in both conditions.

The pathophysiology of PH due to chronic lung fibrosis is under active investigation (Figure 2). Mechanisms other than alveolar hypoxemia and loss of parenchymal tissue may lead to development of PH in this condition [113-115]. The development of pulmonary fibrosis was closely linked in experimental studies to elevated pulmonary artery pressures [116]. Vascular remodelling in ILDs is heterogeneous with fibrotic areas being less vascularised and normal tissue being hyper-vascularised with the creation of anastomoses between capillaries and pulmonary veins [108]. An imbalance has been observed between pro-angiogenic and anti-angiogeneic factors with reduction of vascular endothelial growth factor (VEGF) and up-regulation of epithelium-derived growth factor (EDGF). In animal models, reduction in VEGF has been linked to endothelial apoptosis and PH [108,117]. Vascular smooth muscle cell growth factors are thought to be released from apoptotic endothelial cells which in turn lead to muscularization of the vasculature which augments PH [116,117]. In addition, endothelial dysfunction with reduced levels nitric oxide and prostacyclins and increased presence of vasoconstrictive mediators, such as endothelin-1 and thromboxanes may contribute to the development of PH [108,116,117].

Recent experimental work focused on the role of adenosine in development of PH in chronic lung disease [118]. Adenosine through G protein linked pathways has been associated with progression of fibrotic lung disease and PH through the adenosine receptor, A2bR [118,119]. Karmouty-Quintana et al. were able to demonstrate that inhibition of the A2bR, by inhibition or genetic removal of the receptor, slowed the progression of the fibrotic process and associated PH in rodents [120].

Vascular remodelling has been observed in other forms of interstitial lung diseases. In systemic sclerosis an autoimmune disorder involving skin fibrosis, respiratory complications are the commonest causes of death [121]. The prevalence of PH in systemic sclerosis is as high as 45% [115]. Autoantibodies, including anti-fibrillin and anti-EC antibodies, have been implicated in endothelial apoptosis and endothelial injury with the resultant inflammatory reaction. Advanced systemic sclerosis is associated with reduced capillary density which could contribute to PH [108,122,123].

In sarcoid, granulomatous involvement of the pulmonary arteries with occlusion and peri-vascular inflammation, invasion of pulmonary veins with inflammatory cells, and direct compression of the arteries by lymph nodes are thought to contribute to the development of PH. Endothelin-1 has an important role in PH in sarcoid with high levels reported in the broncho-alveolar fluid of affected patients [124]. Currently there is no clear evidence to suggest a role for angiogenesis or endothelial injury in sarcoid-related PH [107,125].

Few small studies have suggested a possible role of vasodilators in attenuating the progression of PH in ILD [126,127]. The development of PH in ILD is associated with high mortality, hazard ratio for death of 8.5 (95%CI: 4-17) [128]. However, most guidelines do not recommend use of PAH-specific treatments in patients with ILD [2,129].

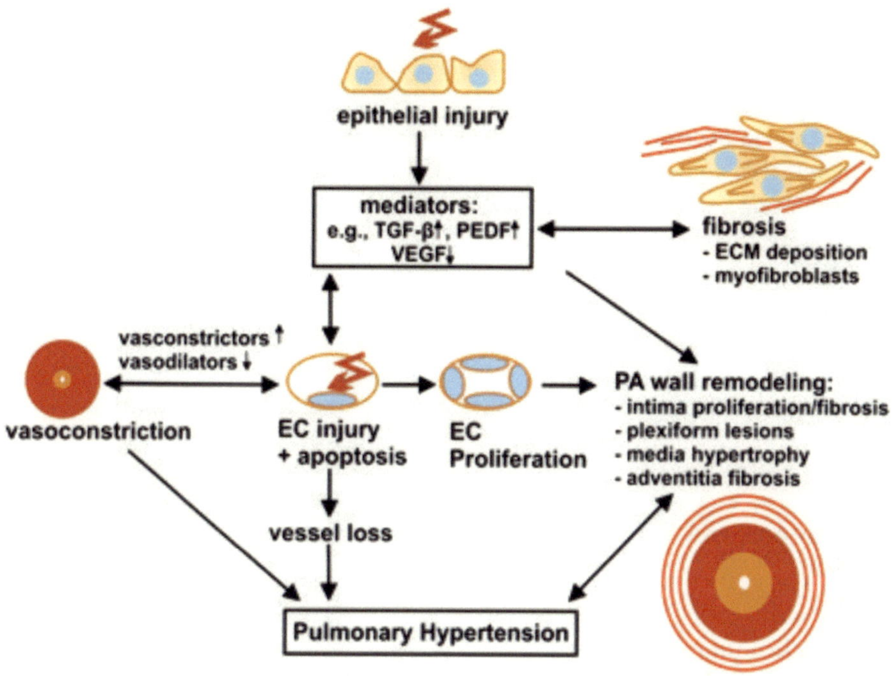

Figure 2. Concept for the development of pulmonary hypertension (PH) in IPF/UIP. Epithelial injury with subsequent production of different mediators is the hallmark of fibrosis induction. These mediators induce fibroblast activation with extracellular matrix (ECM) deposition, which leads to fibrosis. Some of these mediators (e.g., TGF-β) also activate ECs and, as a result of a shift in favor of increased angiostatic (e.g., pigment epithelium–derived factor [PEDF]) and reduced angiogenic factors (e.g., vascular endothelial growth factor [VEGF]), EC apoptosis results. Apoptotic ECs produce less vasodilators, but more vasoconstrictors, which leads to augmented vasoconstriction of smooth muscle cells (SMCs). At the same time, EC apoptosis gives rise to a reduction in vascular density, but also to enhanced production of vascular SMC (VSMC) growth factors, which is important for remodeling of mesenchymal cells in the PA wall. However, EC apoptosis also results in proliferation of apoptosis-resistant ECs or endothelial progenitors, with the consequence of angioproliferative lesions, including plexiform lesions. Another component of PA wall remodeling is the release of additional factors generated in the fibrotic tissue, which contribute to PA wall remodeling from the outside of the vessel; *Farkas L et al., AJRCMB 2011 [107], Reprinted with permission of the American Thoracic Society.*

12. Developmental abnormalities and PH

In the largest registry to date, 42 (12%) of 362 children (< 18 years) with confirmed PH (defined as mean PAP of ≥25mmHg) had associated respiratory diseases or hypoxemia [130]. Bronchopulmonary dysplasia (BPD) was the commonest condition; other disorders included congenital diaphragmatic hernia, congenital pulmonary hypoplasia and kyphoscoliosis [130]. BPD traditionally was defined by the presence of persistent respiratory distress, abnormal chest radiography and requirement for oxygen supplementation [131]. With improvements in neonatal care, persistent lung disease after prematurity is no longer characterised by florid fibro-proliferative lung disease, but reduced vascular development and enlargement of distal airspaces associated with impaired gas exchange and development of PH [132]. Congenital diaphragmatic hernia presents similarly and is associated with variable lung growth leading to persistent PH [133]. Specific drug treatments for PH in this group of disorders have not been studied.

13. Conclusions

Pulmonary hypertension in chronic lung disease and/or hypoxia is a relatively common complication caused by complex pathophysiologic processes. Alveolar hypoxia, either sustained or repetitively intermittent, triggers the development of PH, although other mechanisms are also important. Development of PH is associated with worsening dyspnoea with the long-term prognosis dependant on the underlying disease process. Treatment of PH is largely defined by the underlying lung pathology. Therefore, etiological diagnosis and assessment of PH by WHO functional class is critical for management. Different classes of drug therapies have been developed as a result of our current understanding of the pathophysiology of PH. Although the treatments have had some impact on the progression of PH, further research is required to more fully understand the condition and develop better therapeutic approaches.

Acknowledgements

Supported by a research grant from Foundation Daw Park Inc., Australian Respiratory and Sleep Medicine Institute and Flinders Medical Centre Professional Development Fund.

Author details

Dimitar Sajkov*, Bliegh Mupunga, Jeffrey J. Bowden and Nikolai Petrovsky

*Address all correspondence to: Dimitar.Sajkov@health.sa.gov.au

Australian Respiratory and Sleep Medicine Institute (ARASMI), Flinders Medical Centre and Flinders University, Flinders Drive, Bedford Park, Adelaide, Australia

References

[1] Simonneau, G, Robbins, I. M, Beghetti, M, Channick, R. N, Delcroix, M, Denton, C. P, et al. Updated clinical classification of pulmonary hypertension. J Am Coll Cardiol (2009). Suppl S): S, 43-54.

[2] Galie, N, Hoeper, M. M, Humbert, M, Torbicki, A, Vachiery, J. L, Barbera, J. A, et al. Guidelines for the diagnosis and treatment of pulmonary hypertension: the Task Force for the Diagnosis and Treatment of Pulmonary Hypertension of the European Society of Cardiology (ESC) and the European Respiratory Society (ERS), endorsed by the International Society of Heart and Lung Transplantation (ISHLT). Eur Heart J (2009). , 30, 2493-2537.

[3] Cottin, V, Nunes, H, Brillet, P. Y, Delaval, P, Devouassoux, G, Tillie-leblond, I, et al. Combined pulmonary fibrosis and emphysema: a distinct underrecognised entity. Eur Respir J (2005). , 26, 586-593.

[4] Fraser, K. L, Tullis, D. E, Sasson, Z, Hyland, R. H, Thornley, K. S, & Hanly, P. J. Pulmonary hypertension and cardiac function in adult cystic fibrosis: role of hypoxemia. Chest (1999). , 115(5), 1321-1328.

[5] Orr, R, Smith, L. J, & Cuttica, M. J. Pulmonary hypertension in advanced chronic obstructive pulmonary disease. Curr Opin Pulm Med (2012). , 18(2), 138-143.

[6] Cuttica, M. J, Kalhan, R, Shlobin, O. A, Ahmad, S, Gladwin, M, Machado, R. F, et al. Categorization and impact of pulmonary hypertension in patients with advanced COPD. Respir Med (2010). , 104, 1877-1882.

[7] Scharf, S. M, Iqbal, M, Keller, C, Criner, G, Lee, S, & Fessler, H. E. Hemodynamic characteristics of patients with severe emphysema. Am J Respir Crit Care Med (2002). , 166, 314-322.

[8] Tonnelli, A. R, Fernandez-bussy, S, Lodhi, S, Akindipe, O. A, Carrie, R. D, Hamilton, K, et al. Prevalence of pulmonary hypertension in end-stage cystic fibrosis and correlation with survival. J Heart Lung Transplant (2010). , 29(8), 865-872.

[9] Xu, X-Q, & Jing, Z-C. High-altitude pulmonary hypertension. Eur Respir Rev (2009). , 18(111), 13-17.

[10] Leon-velarde, F, Maggiorini, M, Reeves, J. T, Aldashev, A, Asmus, I, Bernardi, L, et al. Consensus statement on chronic and subacute high altitude diseases. High Alt Med Biol (2005). , 6, 147-157.

[11] Aldashev, A. A, Sarybaev, A. S, Sydykov, A. S, Kalmyrzaev, B. B, Kim, E. V, Mamanova, L. B, et al. Characterization of high-altitude pulmonary hypertension in the Kyrgyz: association with angiotensin-converting enzyme genotype. Am J Respir Crit Care Med (2002). , 166(10), 1396-1402.

[12] Wu, T. Y, & Ge, R. L. An investigation on high-altitude heart disease. Natl Med J China (1983). , 63, 90-92.

[13] Leon-velarde, F, & Mejia, O. Gene expression in chronic high altitude diseases. High Alt med Biol (2008). , 9, 130-139.

[14] Sajkov, D, Cowie, R. J, Thornton, A. T, Espinoza, H. A, & Mcevoy, R. D. Pulmonary hypertension and hypoxemia in obstructive sleep apnea syndrome. Am J Respir Crit Care Med (1994). , 144, 416-422.

[15] Sajkov, D, Wang, T, Saunders, N. A, Bune, A. J, & Neill, A. M. Douglas McEvoy RD. Daytime pulmonary hemodynamics in patients with obstructive sleep apnea patients without lung disease. Am J Respir Crit Care Med (1999). , 159, 1518-1526.

[16] Sajkov, D, & Mcevoy, R. D. Obstructive sleep apnea and pulmonary hypertension. Progress in cardiovascular diseases (2009). , 51(5), 363-370.

[17] Sylvester, J. T, Shimoda, L. A, Aaronson, P. I, & Ward, J. P. Hypoxic pulmonary vasoconstriction Physiol Rev (2012). , 92(1), 367-520.

[18] Bosc, L. V, Resta, T, Walker, B, & Kanagy, N. L. Mechanisms of intermittent hypoxia induced hypertension. J Cell Mol Med (2010).

[19] Sajkov, D, Wang, T, Saunders, N. A, Bune, A. J, & Mcevoy, R. D. Continous positive airway pressure treatment improves pulmonary hemodynamics in patients with obstructive sleep apnea. Am J Respir Crit Care Med (2002). , 165, 152-158.

[20] Wrobel, J. P, Thompson, B. R, & Williams, T. J. Mechanisms of pulmonary hypertension in chronic obstructive pulmonary disease: a pathophysiologic review. J Heart Lung Transplant (2012). , 31(6), 557-564.

[21] Sommer, N, Dietrich, A, Schermuly, R. T, Ghofrani, H. A, Gudermann, T, Schulz, R, et al. Regulation of hypoxic pulmonary vasoconstriction: Basic mechanisms. Eur Respir J (2008). , 32(6), 1639-1651.

[22] Kanagy, N. L, Walker, B. R, & Nelin, L. D. Role of endothelin in intermittent hypoxia-induced hypertension. Hypertension (2001). , 37, 511-515.

[23] Liu, J. Q, Zelko, I. N, Erbynn, E. M, Sham, J. S, & Folz, R. J. Hypoxic pulmonary hypertension: role of superoxide and NADPH oxidase (gp91phox). Am J Physiol Lung Cell Mol Physiol (2006). L, 2-10.

[24] Pak, O, Aldashev, A, Welsh, D, & Peacock, A. The effects of hypoxia on the cells of the pulmonary vasculature. Eur Respir J (2007). , 30, 364-372.

[25] Stiebellehner, L, Beknap, J. K, Ensley, B, Tucker, A, Orton, E. C, Reeves, J. T, et al. Lung endothelial cell proliferation in normal and pulmonary hypertensive neonatal calves. Am J Physio (1998). LL600., 593.

[26] Reid, L. M, & Davies, P. Pulmonary vascular physiology and pathophysiology. In: Weir EK. Reeves JF. (ed.)Lung Biology in Health and Disease. New York, Marcel Dekker, (1989). , 541-611.

[27] Hunter, C, Barer, G. R, Shaw, J. W, & Clegg, E. J. Growth of the heart and lungs in hypoxic rodents: a model of human hypoxic disease. Clin Sci Mol Med (1974). , 46, 375-391.

[28] Stiebellehner, L, Frid, M, Reeves, J, Low, R. B, Gnanasekharan, M, & Stenmark, K. R. Bovine distal pulmonary arterial media is composed of a uniform population of well-differentiated smooth muscle cells with low proliferation capabilities. Am J physio Lung Cell Mol Physiol (2003). LL828., 819.

[29] Joppa, P, Petrasova, D, Stancak, B, & Tkacova, R. Systemic inflammation in patients with COPD and pulmonary hypertension. Chest (2006). , 130(2), 326-233.

[30] Kwon, Y. S, Chi, S. Y, Shin, H. J, Kim, E. Y, Yoon, B. K, Ban, H. J, et al. Plasma C-reactive protein and endothelin-1 level in patients with chronic obstructive pulmonary disease and pulmonary hypertension. J Korean Med Sci (2010). , 25(10), 1487-1491.

[31] Chao, J, Wood, J. G, & Gonzalez, N. C. Alveolar hypoxia, alveolar macrophages, and systemic inflammation. Respir Res (2009).

[32] Chao, J, Wood, J. G, Blanco, V. G, & Gonzalez, N. C. The systemic inflammation of alveolar hypoxia is initiated by alveolar macrophage-borne mediator(s). Am J Respir Cell Mol Biol (2009). , 41(5), 573-582.

[33] Han, M. K, Bartholmai, B, Liu, L. X, Murray, S, Curtis, J. L, Sciurba, F. C, et al. Clinical significance of radiological characterizations in COPD. COPD (2009). , 6(6), 459-467.

[34] Skwarski, K. MacNee W, Wraith PK, Sliwinski P, Zielinski J. Predictors of survival in patients with chronic obstructive pulmonary disease treated with long-term oxygen therapy. Chest (1991). , 100(6), 1522-1527.

[35] Oswald-mammosser, M, Weitzenblum, E, Quoix, E, Moser, G, Chaouat, A, Charpentier, C, et al. Prognostic factors in COPD patients receiving long-term oxygen therapy; importance of pulmonary artery pressure. Chest (1995). , 107, 1193-1198.

[36] Stone, A. C, & Machan, J. T. Mazer J Casserly B, Klinger JR. Echocardiographic evidence of pulmonary hypertension is associated with increased 1-year mortality in patients admitted with chronic obstructive pulmonary disease. Lung (2011). , 189, 207-212.

[37] Sajkov, D, Cowie, R. J, Bradley, J. A, Mahar, L, & Mcevoy, R. D. Validation of new pulsed Doppler echocardiographic techniques for assessment of pulmonary hemodynamics. Chest (1993). , 103(5), 1348-1353.

[38] Sims, M. W, Margolis, D. J, Localio, A. R, Panettieri, R. A, Kawut, S. M, & Christie, J. D. Impact of pulmonary artery pressure on exercise function in severe COPD. Chest (2009). , 136, 412-419.

[39] Pynnaert, C, Lamotte, M, & Naeije, R. Aerobic exercise capacity in COPD patients with and without pulmonary hypertension. Respir Med (2010). , 104(1), 121-126.

[40] Mykland Hilde J, Skjørten I, Hansteen V, Nissen Melsom M, Hisdal J, Humerfelt S, Steine K.Hemodynamic responses to exercise in patients with COPD. Eur Respir J (2012). Epub ahead of print doi:

[41] Thabut, G, Dauriat, G, Stern, J. B, Logeart, D, Lévy, A, Marrash-chahla, R, et al. Pulmonary hemodynamics in advanced COPD candidates for lung volume reduction surgery or lung transplantation. Chest (2005). , 127, 1531-1536.

[42] Chaouat, A, Bugnet, A. S, Kadaoui, N, Schott, R, Enache, I, Ducoloné, A, et al. Severe pulmonary hypertension and chronic obstructive pulmonary disease. Am J Respir Crit Care Med (2005). , 172, 189-194.

[43] Qaseem, A, Wilt, T. J, Weinberger, S. E, Hanania, N. A, Criner, G, Van Der Molen, T, et al. Diagnosis and management of stable chronic obstructive pulmonary disease: a clinical practice guideline update from the American college of physicians, American college of chest physicians, American thoracic society, and European respiratory society. Ann Intern Med (2011). , 155, 179-191.

[44] Timms, R. M, Khaja, F. U, & Williams, G. W. Hemodynamic response to oxygen therapy in chronic obstructive pulmonary disease. Ann Intern Med (1985). , 102, 29-36.

[45] MRC Working PartyLong term domiciliary oxygen therapy in chronic hypoxic cor pulmonale complicating chronic bronchitis and emphysema. Report of the Medical Research Council Working Party. Lancet (1981). , 1(8222), 681-686.

[46] NOTT groupContinuous or nocturnal oxygen therapy in hypoxemic chronic obstructive lung disease: a clinical trial. Nocturnal Oxygen Therapy Trial Group. Ann Intern Med (1980). , 93(3), 391-398.

[47] Ashutosh, K, & Dunsky, M. Noninvasive tests for responsiveness of pulmonary hypertension to oxygen. Prediction of survival in patients with chronic obstructive lung disease and cor pulmonale. Chest (1987). , 92(3), 393-399.

[48] Currow, D. C, Fazekas, B, & Abernethy, A. P. Oxygen use-patients define symptomatic benefit discerningly. J Pain Symptom Manage (2007). , 34, 113-114.

[49] Mcdonald, C. F, Crockett, A. J, & Young, I. H. Adult domiciliary oxygen therapy. Position statement of the Thoracic Society of Australia and New Zealand. Med J Aust (2005). , 182(12), 621-626.

[50] Robinson, T. D, Freiberg, D. B, Regnis, J. A, & Young, I. H. The role of hypoventilation and ventilation-perfusion redistribution in oxygen-induced hypercapnia during acute exacerbations of chronic obstructive pulmonary disease. Am J Respir Crit Care Med (2000). , 161, 1524-1529.

[51] Bone, R. C, & Pierce, A. K. Johnson RL Jr. Controlled oxygen therapy in acute respiratory failure in chronic obstructive pulmonary disease. Am J Med (1978). , 65, 896-902.

[52] Katsenos, S, & Constantopoulos, S. H. Long-term oxygen therapy in COPD: factors affecting and ways of improving patient compliance. Pulm Med 2011; (2011).

[53] Neri, M, Melani, A. S, Miorelli, A. M, Zanchetta, D, Bertocco, E, Cinti, C, et al. Long-term oxygen therapy in chronic respiratory failure: a multicenter Italian study on oxygen therapy adherence (MISOTA). Respir Med (2006). , 100(5), 795-806.

[54] Barst, R. J, Rubin, L. J, Long, W. A, Mcgoon, M. D, Rich, S, Badesch, D. B, et al. A Comparison of continuous intravenous epoprostenol (Prostacyclin) with conventional therapy for primary pulmonary hypertension. N Engl J Med (1996). , 334, 296-301.

[55] Krug, S, Sablotzki, A, Hammerschmidt, S, Wirtz, H, & Seyfarth, H. J. Inhaled iloprost for the control of pulmonary hypertension. Vasc Health Risk Manag (2009). , 5(1), 465-474.

[56] Dhillon, S, & Keating, G. M. Bosentan: a review of its use in the management of mildly symptomatic pulmonary arterial hypertension. Am J Cardiovasc Drugs (2009). , 9(5), 331-350.

[57] Kingman, M, Ruggiero, R, & Torres, F. Ambrisentan, an endothelin receptor type A-selective endothelin receptor antagonist, for the treatment of pulmonary arterial hypertension. Expert Opin Pharmacother (2009). , 10(11), 1847-1858.

[58] Ichinose, F, Erana-garcia, J, Hromi, J, Raveh, Y, Jones, R, Krim, L, et al. Nebulized sildenafil is a selective pulmonary vasodilator in lambs with acute pulmonary hypertension. Crit Care Med (2001). , 29(5), 1000-1005.

[59] Kleinsasser, A, Loeckinger, A, Hoermann, C, Puehringer, F, Mutz, N, Bartsch, G, et al. Sildenafil modulates hemodynamics and pulmonary gas exchange. Am J Respir Crit Care Med (2001). , 163(2), 339-343.

[60] Weimann, J, Ullrich, R, Hromi, J, Fujino, Y, Clark, M. W, Bloch, K. D, et al. Sildenafil is a pulmonary vasodilator in awake lambs with acute pulmonary hypertension. Anesthesiology (2000). , 92(6), 1702-1712.

[61] Sebkhi, A, Strange, J. W, Phillips, S. C, Wharton, J, & Wilkins, M. R. Phosphodiesterase type 5 as a target for the treatment of hypoxia-induced pulmonary hypertension. Circulation (2003). , 107(25), 3230-3235.

[62] Bharani, A, Mathew, V, Sahu, A, & Lunia, B. The efficacy and tolerability of sildenafil in patients with moderate-to-severe pulmonary hypertension. Indian Heart J (2003). , 55(1), 55-59.

[63] Michelakis, E. D, Tymchak, W, Noga, M, Webster, L, Wu, X. C, Lien, D, et al. Long-term treatment with oral sildenafil is safe and improves functional capacity and hemodynamics in patients with pulmonary arterial hypertension. Circulation (2003). , 108, 2066-2069.

[64] Blanco, I, Gimeno, E, Mundoz, P. A, Pizarro, S, Gistau, C, Rodriguez-roisin, R, et al. Hemodynamic and gas exchange effects of sildenafil in patients with chronic obstructive pulmonary disease and pulmonary hypertension. Am J Respir Crit Care Med (2010). , 181(3), 270-278.

[65] Rietema, H, Holverda, S, Bogaard, H. J, Marcus, J. T, Smit, H. J, Westerhof, N, et al. Sildenafil treatment in COPD does not affect stroke volume or exercise capacity. Eur Respir J (2008). , 31, 759-764.

[66] Lederer, D. J, Bartels, M. N, Schluger, N. W, Brogan, F, Jellen, P, Thomashow, B. M, et al. Sildenafil for chronic obstructive pulmonary disease: a randomized crossover trial. COPD (2012). , 9(3), 268-275.

[67] Weitzenblum, E, Kessler, R, Oswald, M, & Fraisse, P. Medical treatment of pulmonary hypertension in chronic lung disease. Eur Respir J, (1994). , 7, 148-152.

[68] MacNee WPathophysiology of Cor Pulmonale in Chronic Obstructive Pulmonary Disease: Part one. Am J Respir Crit Care Med (1994). , 150(3), 833-852.

[69] Salvaterra, C. G. Investigation and management of pulmonary hypertension in chronic obstructive pulmonary disease. Am Rev Respir Dis (1993).

[70] Karla, L, & Bone, M. F. Effect of nifedipine on physiological shunting and oxygenation in chronic obstructive pulmonary disease. Am J Med (1993). , 94, 419-423.

[71] Melot, C, Naeije, R, Mols, P, Vandenbossche, J. L, & Denolin, H. Effects of nifedipine on ventilation/perfusion matching in primary pulmonary hypertension. Chest (1983). , 83(2), 203-207.

[72] Agustoni, P, Doria, E, Galli, C, Tamborini, G, & Guazzi, M. D. Nifedipine reduces pulmonary pressure and vasodilator tone during short- but not long-term treatment of pulmonary hypertension in patients with chronic obstructive pulmonary disease. Am Rev Respir Dis (1989). , 139, 120-125.

[73] Mookherjee, S, Ashutosh, K, Dunsky, M, Hill, N, Vardan, S, Smulyan, H, et al. Nifedipine in chronic cor pulmonale: acute and relatively long-term effects. Clin Pharmacol Ther (1988). , 44, 289-296.

[74] Kennedy, T, Michael, J, Huang, C, Kallman, C. H, Zahka, K, Schlott, W, et al. Nifedipine inhibits hypoxic pulmonary vasoconstriction during rest and exercise in patients with chronic obstructive pulmonary disease. Am Rev Respir Dis (1984). , 129, 544-551.

[75] Morley, T, Zappasodi, S, Belli, A, Belli, A, & Giudice, J. C. Pulmonary vasodilator therapy for chronic obstructive pulmonary disease and cor pulmonale: treatment with nifedipine, nitroglycerin, and oxygen. Chest (1987). , 92, 71-76.

[76] Rich, S, & Brundage, B. H. High-dose calcium channel-blocking therapy for primary pulmonary hypertension: evidence for long-term reduction in pulmonary arterial pressure and regression of right ventricular hypertrophy. Circulation (1987). , 76, 135-141.

[77] Rich, S, Kaufmann, E, & Levy, P. S. The effect of high doses of calcium-channel blockers on survival in primary pulmonary hypertension. N Engl J Med (1992). , 327, 76-81.

[78] Saadjian, A, Philip-joet, F, & Arnaud, A. Hemodynamic and oxygen delivery: responses to nifedipine in pulmonary hypertension secondary to chronic obstructive lung diseases. Cardiology (1987). , 74, 196-204.

[79] Saadjian, A. Y, Philip-joet, F. F, Vestri, R, & Arnaud, A. G. Long-term treatment of chronic obstructive lung disease by nifedipine: an 18 month hemodynamic study. Eur Respir J (1988). , 1, 716-720.

[80] Bratel, T, Hedenstierna, G, Lundquist, H, Nyquist, O, & Ripe, E. Cardiac function and central hemodynamics in severe chronic obstructive lung disease: acute and long-term effects of felodipine. Eur Respir J (1988). , 1, 262-268.

[81] Bratel, T, Hedenstierna, G, Nyquist, O, & Ripe, E. The use of vasodilator, felodipine, as an adjuvant to long-term oxygen treatment in COLD patients. Eur J Respir Dis (1990). , 3, 46-54.

[82] Rubin, L. J, & Moser, K. Long-term effects of nifedipine on hemodynamics and oxygen transport in patients with cor pulmonale. Chest (1986). , 89, 141-145.

[83] Sajkov, D, Mcevoy, R. D, Cowie, R. J, Bradley, J. A, Antic, R, Morris, R. G, et al. Felodipine improves pulmonary hemodynamics in chronic obstructive pulmonary disease. Chest (1993). , 103(5), 1354-1361.

[84] Sajkov, D, Wang, T, Frith, P. A, Bune, A. J, Alpers, J. A, & Mcevoy, R. D. A comparison of two long acting vasoselective calcium antagonists in pulmonary hypertension secondary to COPD. Chest (1997). , 111(6), 1622-1630.

[85] Vestri, R, Philip-joet, F, Surpas, P, Arnaud, A, & Saadjian, A. One-year clinical study on nifedipine in the treatment of pulmonary hypertension in chronic obstructive lung disease. Respiration (1988). , 54(2), 139-144.

[86] Arias, M. A, Garcia-rio, F, Alonso-fernandez, A, Martínez, I, & Villamor, J. Pulmonary hypertension in obstructive sleep apnoea: effects of continuous positive airway pressure: a randomized, controlled cross-over study. Eur heart J (2006). , 27, 1106-1113.

[87] Stoohs, R, & Guilleminault, C. Cardiovascular changes associated with obstructive sleep apnea syndrome. J Appl Physiol (1992). , 72(2), 583-589.

[88] Schafer, H, Hasper, E, Ewig, S, Koehler, U, Latzelsberger, J, Tasci, S, et al. Pulmonary haemodynamics in obstructive sleep apnoea: time course and associated factors. Eur Respir J (1998). , 12, 679-684.

[89] Marrone, O, Bellia, V, Ferrara, G, Milone, F, Romano, L, Salvaggio, A, et al. Transmural pressure measurements. Importance in the assessment of pulmonary hypertension in obstructive sleep apneas. Chest (1989). , 95, 338-342.

[90] Marrone, O, Bellia, V, Pieri, D, Salvaggio, A, & Bonsignore, G. Acute effects of oxygen administration on transmural pulmonary artery pressure in obstructive sleep apnoea. Chest (1992). , 101, 1023-1027.

[91] Minai, O. A, Ricaurte, B, Kaw, R, Hammel, J, Mansour, M, Mccarthy, K, et al. Frequency and impact of pulmonary hypertension in patients with obstructive sleep apnea syndrome. Am J Cardiol (2009). , 104, 1300-1306.

[92] Chen, Y. C. An analysis of 300 cases of adult high-altitude heart disease. Zhonghua Xin Xue Guan Bing Za Zhi (1982). , 10, 256-258.

[93] Beall, C. M, Laskowski, D, Strohl, K. P, Soria, R, Villena, M, Vargas, E, et al. Pulmonary nitiric oxide in mountain dwellers. Nature (2001). , 414(6862), 411-412.

[94] Beall, C. M, Laskowski, D, & Erzurum, S. C. Nitric oxide in adaptation to altitude. Free Radic Biol Med (2012). , 52(7), 1123-1134.

[95] Aldashev, A. A, Kojonazarov, B. K, Amatov, T. A, Sooronbaev, T. M, Mirrakhimov, M. M, Morrell, N. W, et al. Phosphodiesterase type 5 and high-altitude pulmonary hypertension. Thorax (2005). , 60, 683-687.

[96] Seheult, R. D, Ruh, K, Foster, G. P, & Anholm, J. D. Prophylactic bosentan does not improve exercise capacity or lower pulmonary artery systolic pressure at high altitude. Respir Physiol Neurobiol (2009).

[97] Richalet, J. P, Rivera-ch, M, Maignan, M, Privat, C, Pham, I, Macarlupu, J. L, et al. Acetazolamide for Monge's disease: efficiency and tolerance of 6-month treatment. Am J Respir Crit Care Med (2008). , 177, 1370-1376.

[98] Venuta, F, Tonelli, A. R, Anile, M, Diso, D, De Giacomo, T, Ruberto, F, et al. Pulmonary hypertension is associated with higher mortality in cystic fibrosis patients awaitning lung transplantation. J Cardiovasc Surg (Torino). (2012). May 28. [Epub ahead of print]

[99] Tonelli, A. R, Fernandez-bussy, S, Lodhi, S, Akindipe, O. A, Carrie, R. D, Hamilton, K, et al. Prevalence of pulmonary hypertension in end stage cystic fibrosis and correlation with survival. J Heart Lung Transplant (2010). , 29(8), 865-872.

[100] Alzeer, A. H, Al-mobeirek, A. F, Al-otair, H. A, Elzamzamy, U. A, Joherjy, I. A, & Shaffi, A. S. Right and left ventricular function and pulmonary artery pressure in patients with bronchiectasis. Chest (2008). , 133, 464-473.

[101] Haimovici, J. B, Trotman-dickienson, B, Halpern, E. F, Dec, G. W, Ginns, L. C, Shepard, J. A, et al. Relationship between pulmonary artery diameter at computed tomography and pulmonary artery pressures at right-sided heart catheterization. Massachusetts General Hospital Lung Transplantation Program. Acad Radiol (1997). , 4, 327-334.

[102] Ng, C. S, & Wells, A. U. Padley SPA. CT sign of chornic pulmonary arterial hypertension: the ratio of main pulmonary artery to aortic diameter. J Thorac Imaging (1999)., 14, 270-278.

[103] Kuriyama, K, Gamsu, G, Stern, R. G, Cann, C. E, & Herfkens, R. J. Brundage BHCT-determined pulmonary artery diameters in predicting pulmonary hypertension. Invest Radiol (1984)., 19, 16-22.

[104] Devaraj, A, Wells, A. U, Meister, M. G, Loebinger, M. R, Wilson, R, & Hansell, D. M. Pulmonary hypertension in patients with bronchiectasis: prognostic significance of CT signs. AJR (2011)., 196, 1300-1304.

[105] Flaherty, K. R, Mumford, J. A, Murray, S, Kazerooni, E. A, Gross, B. H, Colby, T. V, et al. Prognostic implications of physiologic and radiographic changes in idiopathic interstitial pneumonia. Am J Respir Crit Care Med (2003)., 168, 543-548.

[106] Kawut, S. M, Shea, O, Bartels, M. K, Wilt, M. N, Sonett, J. S, & Arcasoy, J. R. SM. Exercise testing determines survival in patients with diffuse parenchymal lung disease evaluated for lung transplantation. Respir Med (2005)., 99, 1431-1439.

[107] Farkas, L, Gauldie, J, Voelkel, N. F, & Kolb, M. Pulmonary hypertension and idiopathic pulmonary fibrosis: a tale of angiogenesis, apoptosis, and growth factors. Am J Respir Cell Mol Biol (2011)., 45(1), 1-15.

[108] Lettieri, C. J, Nathan, S. D, Barnett, S. D, Ahmad, S, & Shorr, A. F. Prevalence and outcomes of pulmonary arterial hypertension in advanced idiopathic pulmonary fibrosis. Chest (2006)., 129, 746-752.

[109] Patel, N. M, Lederer, D. J, Borczuk, A. C, & Kawut, S. M. Pulmonary hypertension in idiopathic pulmonary fibrosis. Chest (2007)., 132, 998-1006.

[110] Nathan, S. D, Noble, P. W, & Tuder, R. M. Idiopathic pulmonary fibrosis and pulmonary hypertension: connecting the dots. Am J Respir Crit Care Med (2007)., 175, 875-880.

[111] Nadrous, H. F, Pellikka, P. A, Krowka, M. J, Swanson, K. L, Chaowalit, N, Decker, P. A, et al. Pulmonary hypertension in patients with idiopathic pulmonary fibrosis. Chest (2005)., 128, 2393-2399.

[112] Andersen, C. U, Mellemkjær, S, Hilberg, O, Nielsen-kudsk, J. E, Simonsen, U, & Bendstrup, E. Pulmonary hypertension in interstitial lung disease: prevalence, prognosis and 6 min walk test. Respir Med. (2012)., 106(6), 875-82.

[113] Strange, C, & Highland, K. B. Pulmonary hypertension in interstitial lung disease. Curr Opin Pulm Med (2005)., 11, 452-455.

[114] Ryu, J. H, Krowka, M. J, Pellikka, P. A, & Swanson, K. L. McGoon MD, Pulmonary hypertension in patients with interstitial lung diseases. Mayo Clin Proc (2007)., 82, 342-350.

[115] Farkas, L, Farkas, D, Ask, K, Möller, A, Gauldie, J, Margetts, P, et al. VEGF ameliorates pulmonary hypertension through inhibition of endothelial apoptosis in experimental lung fibrosis in rats. J Clin Invest (2009)., 119, 1298-1311.

[116] Strieter, R. M, Gomperts, B. N, & Keane, M. P. The role of CXC chemokines in pulmonary fibrosis. J Clin Invest (2007)., 117, 549-556.

[117] Sakao, S, Taraseviciene-stewart, L, Wood, K, Cool, C. D, & Voelkel, N. F. Apoptosis of pulmonary microvascular endothelial cells stimulates vascular smooth muscle growth. Am J Physio Lung Cell Mol Physiol (2006). LL368., 362.

[118] Zhou, Y, Schneider, D. J, & Blackburn, M. R. Adenosine signaling and the regulation of chronic lung disease. Pharmacol Ther (2009)., 123(1), 105-116.

[119] Zhou, Y, Murthy, J. N, Zeng, D, Belardinelli, L, & Blackburn, M. R. Alterations in adenosine metabolism and signaling in patients with chronic obstructive pulmonary disease and idiopathic pulmonary fibrosis. PLoS One (2010). Feb 16;5(2):e9224.

[120] Karmouty-quintana, H, Zhong, H, Acero, L, Weng, T, Melicoff, E, West, J. D, et al. The A2B adenosine receptor modulates pulmonary hypertension associated with interstitial lung disease. FASEB J (2012)., 26(6), 2546-2557.

[121] Antoniou, K. M, & Wells, A. U. Scleroderma lung disease: evolving understanding in light of newer studies. Curr Opin Rheumatol (2008)., 20, 686-691.

[122] Guiducci, S, Distler, O, Distler, J. H, & Matucci-cerinic, M. Mechanisms of vascular damage in SSc- implications for vascular treatment strategies. Rheumatology (2008). suppl 5):, 18-v20

[123] Renzoni, E. A, Walsh, D. A, Salmon, M, Wells, A. U, Sestini, P, Nicholson, A. G, et al. Interstitial vascularity in fibrosing alveolitis. Am J Respir Crit Care Med (2003)., 167, 438-443.

[124] Reichenberger, F, Schauer, J, Kellner, K, Sack, U, Stiehl, P, & Winkler, J. Different expression of endothelin in the bronchoalveolar lavage in patients with pulmonary diseases. Lung (2001)., 179, 163-174.

[125] Koyama, S, Sato, E, Haniuda, M, Numanami, H, Nagai, S, & Izumi, T. Decreased level of vascular endothelial growth factor in bronchoalveolar lavage fluid of normal smokers and patients with pulmonary fibrosis. Am J Respir Crit Care Med (2002)., 166(3), 382-385.

[126] Ghofrani, H. A, Wiedemann, R, Rose, F, Schermuly, R. T, Olschewski, H, Weissmann, N, et al. Sildenafil for treatment of lung fibrosis and pulmonary hypertension: a randomised controlled trial. Lancet (2002)., 360(9337), 895-900.

[127] Olschewski, H, Ghofrani, H. A, Walmrath, D, Schermuly, R, Temmesfeld-wollbruck, B, Grimminger, F, et al. Inhaled prostacyclin and iloprost in severe pulmonary hy-

pertension secondary to lung fibrosis. Am J Respir Crit Care Med (1999). , 160(2), 600-607.

[128] Andersen, C. U, Mellemkjær, S, Hilberg, O, Nielsen-kudsk, J. E, Simonsen, U, & Bendstrup, E. Pulmonary hypertension in interstitial lung disease: prevalence, prognosis and 6 min walk test. Respir Med (2012). , 106(6), 875-882.

[129] Pitsiou, G, Papakosta, D, & Bouros, D. Pulmonary hypertension in idiopathic pulmonary fibrosis: a review. Respiration (2011). , 82(3), 294-304.

[130] Berger, R. M, Beghetti, M, Humpl, T, Raskob, G. E, Ivy, D. D, Jing, Z. C, et al. Clinical features of paediatric pulmonary hypertension: a registry study. Lancet (2012). , 379(9815), 537-46.

[131] Northway WH Jr, Rosan RC, Porter DY. Pulmonary disease following respirator therapy of hyaline-membrane disease. Bronchopulmonary dysplasia. N Engl J Med (1967). , 276(7), 357-368.

[132] Stenmark, K. R, & Abman, S. H. Lung vascular development: implications for the pathogenesis of bronchopulmonary dysplasia. Annu Rev Physiol (2005). , 67, 623-661.

[133] Pennaforte, T, Rakza, T, Sfeir, R, Aubry, E, Bonnevalle, M, Fayoux, P, et al. Congenital diaphragmatic hernia: respiratory and vascular outcomes [Article in French]. Rev Mal Respir (2012). , 29(2), 337-46.

Chapter 3

Pathogenesis of Pulmonary Hypertension

Rajamma Mathew

Additional information is available at the end of the chapter

http://dx.doi.org/10.5772/56179

1. Introduction

Pulmonary arterial hypertension (PAH), although rare, is a progressive disease with a high morbidity and mortality rate. In 1981, Ernst von Romberg, a German physician described pulmonary vascular lesions as "pulmonary vascular sclerosis", the first description of histological changes in PAH [Fishman 2004]. The average survival time for untreated patient is around 2.8 yrs [D'Alonzo 1991]. Despite remarkable progress made since then, the pathogenesis of PAH, however, is not yet well understood; because a large number of cardiopulmonary and systemic diseases can lead to PAH, and in addition, multiple signaling pathways have been implicated. Current advances in therapy, have improved the quality of life and delayed the progression of the disease, but have not provided a cure. Lack of cure in PAH is further underscored by a recent study showing persistent large plexiform lesions and inflammatory infiltrates in patients despite having been on a long term prostacyclin therapy [Pogoriler 2012]. One of the main reasons for the failure of therapy is that the diagnosis is often made late because of vague symptoms; and by the time the diagnosis is made extensive pathologic changes have already taken place in pulmonary vasculature. From experimental studies, it is clear that pathological changes in the vasculature occur before the onset of PAH [Huang 2010]. Another problem is that a large number of signaling molecules implicated in PAH may not be relevant in all patients; and the activation of some of these molecules may depend on the stage of the disease.

The current clinical classification updated in 2008 maintains five major groups [Simonneau 2009]. *Group 1*: Pulmonary arterial hypertension (PAH): Included in this group are idiopathic (IPAH) and heritable PAH (HPAH), PAH associated with congenital heart defects (CHD), connective tissue diseases, portal hypertension, infection, chronic hemolytic anemia, drug toxicity and persistent pulmonary hypertension of the newborn (PPHN). Pulmonary veno-occlusive disease and pulmonary capillary hemangiomatosis are included in this group as a subcategory. Approximately 70% of HPAH and 26% IPAH exhibit heterozygous germline mutations in BMPRII, a member of TGFβ superfamily; however, only about 20% of people with BMPRII mutation develop PAH. The incidence of HPAH is reported to be 3.9% of IPAH. [Thompson 2000, Machado 2006, Cogan 2006, Sztrymf 2007, Humbert 2006]. It has recently been shown that in BMPRII+/- mice, a "second hit" such as inflammation or serotonin increases the susceptibility to develop PAH [Song 2008, Long 2006]. In addition, altered metabolism of estrogen resulting in low production of 2 methylestradiol is also thought to be a "second hit" for the development of PAH in females with BMPRII mutation [Austin 2009]. Interestingly, a short exposure to fenfluramine, a diet suppressant, is enough to induce PAH in patients with a BMPRII mutation [Humbert 2002]. Thus, the "second hit" is almost a requirement for the development of PAH in patients with BMPRII mutations. Approximately 6% of adults and children with congenital heart defect CHD and PAH also exhibit BMPRII mutations [Roberts 2004]. In addition, mutations of activin-like receptor kinase 1 (ALK1) and endoglin, both belonging to the TGFβ superfamily have been reported in patients with hereditary hemorrhagic telangiectasia, and some of these patients develop PAH [Trembath 2001]. Recently mutation of SMAD 8, belonging to another member of the TGF-β family, and thrombospondin-1 (TSP-1) were found in patients with PAH and HPAH respectively. Interestingly, TSP-1 is known to regulate the activation of TGF-β [Shintani 2009, Maloney 2012]. Thus, the TGF-β/BMP signaling pathway has an important role in pulmonary vascular health and disease. Polymorphisms of other genes have been described in PH such as serotonin (LL allele), TRPC6 gene promoter, and Norrie disease with deficiency of monoamine oxidases, which degrades serotonin have been reported in patients with PH [*reviewed in* Mathew 2011]. In addition, polymorphism of the *KCNA5* gene with altered expression and function of Kv1.5 channels has been observed in pulmonary vascular smooth muscle cells (SMC) from IPAH patients [Remillard 2007].

Among adults, PAH occurs more frequently in women than men. The French national registry revealed female to male ratio to be 1.9:1 and in a recent report from the US registry the ratio was reported to be around 4:1 with better survival rate among the females. The higher incidence of PAH in females in the US was thought to be related to the higher incidence of obesity [Humbert 2006, Shapiro 2012]. In HIV-PAH, however, there is higher incidence in males (M:F 1.5:1), because more male patients have HIV infection [Cicalini 2011]. PAH is the leading cause of death in patients with scleroderma, and the estimated prevalence of PAH in this group is 8-12% [Mathai 2011]. *Group 2*: PH due to left heart diseases such as mitral valve disease, systemic hypertension, ischemic heart disease and cardiomyopathy are included in this group. These diseases lead to LV diastolic overload, impaired function and passive congestion in capillaries. Sustained elevated pressure in pulmonary venous circulation results in structural and functional damage of pulmonary arteries, and endothelial dysfunction leading to PH. Heart failure with preserved ejection fraction (HFpEF) is recognized as the major cause of PH associated with left heart disease. In one study, female preponderance (58%) was observed in HFpEF + PH group. These patients have higher LV end-diastolic pressure. It is important to distinguish this group from PAH (group 1), because the therapy used in PAH is not effective in patients in this group [Guazzi 2010, Thenappan 2011, Hill 2011]. *Group 3*: This group encompasses PH due to chronic obstructive pulmonary disease (COPD) and other parenchymal lung diseases associated with hypoxia. Major components in this group are vasoconstriction and vascular remodeling. Inflammation plays a significant role in the pathobiology of lung diseases. Recent studies suggest that the pathological changes seen in COPD and idiopathic pulmonary fibrosis are related to oxidative stress and aging as evidenced by increased expression of senescence markers in lungs and enhanced tissue destruction [MacNee 2009, Faner 2012]. Furthermore, senescent pulmonary artery SMC exhibit telomere shortening and increased production of cytokines, thus, contributing to the progression of the disease [Noureddine 2011]. *Group 4*: Included in this group is PH resulting from an incomplete resolution of chronic pulmonary thromboembolism. The incidence of PH in this group is reported to be approximately 4% at 2 yrs. About 10% of patients develop PH even after satisfactory thrombo-endarterectomy. Worsening of the disease is thought to occur because of recurrent thromboembolism, or in situ thrombosis and pulmonary vascular remodeling. Reduction in the expression of eNOS and impaired endothelium-dependent, NO-mediated relaxation response in pulmonary arteries distal to ligation was recently reported in a porcine pulmonary artery ligation model. Importantly, histological features include pulmonary vascular remodeling and plexiform lesions indistinguishable from PAH [Moser 1993, Pengo 2004, Dartevelle 2004, Fadel 2000]. *Group 5*: This group includes a large number of miscellaneous diseases such as PH secondary to other systemic diseases such as sarcoidosis, myeloproliferative diseases, metabolic and hematological disorders, Thyroid diseases, Gaucher's disease and chronic renal failure requiring dialysis.

1.1. PH in pediatric age group

PH in pediatric age group has several different features compared with the adult patients. In children, medial hypertrophy is the main feature; with increasing age other pathological features such as intimal proliferation, concentric fibrosis and subsequently dilatation and plexiform lesions appear [Wagenvoort 1970]. A recent study revealed that females comprised 46% of all PH and 51% of all PAH group patients [van Loon 2011]. The major causes of PH in children are CHD, PPHN, lung diseases such as respiratory distress syndrome (RDS), bronchopulmonary dysplasia (BPD), and congenital defects associated with hypoplasia of the lungs [Mathew 2000]. Antenatal and perinatal problems have adverse effects on vascular and alveolar development. Preterm delivery disrupts normal pulmonary vascular and broncho-alveolar development which leads to reduced cross sectional area of the pulmonary vasculature resulting in increased pulmonary vascular resistance and PH [Farquhar 2010]. Another interesting difference from the adult group is that >80% of pediatric patients have transient PH. These include resolution of PPHN and in the majority of the cases after surgical correction of CHD [van Loon 2012]. However, poor outcome has been reported in children with IPAH or HPAH associated with BMPRII mutation [Chida 2012]. A new classification for pediatric PH has been proposed that is comprised of 10 major groups and includes prenatal and developmental anomalies. The main categories are: 1. Prenatal or developmental pulmonary hypertensive vascular disease, 2. Prenatal pulmonary vascular maladaptation, 3. Pediatric cardiovascular disease, 4. Bronchopulmonary dysplasia, 5. Isolated pediatric PAH, 6. Pulmonary hypertensive vascular disease in congenital malformation syndrome, 7. Pediatric lung disease, 8. Pediatric thromboembolic disease, pediatric hypobaric hypoxic exposure, 10. Pediatric pulmonary vascular disease associated with other systemic disorders [del Cerro 2011]. Irrespective of the underlying pathology, patients usually present with similar changes in the lungs including endothelial dysfunction, impaired vascular reactivity, activation of inflammatory processes, vascular remodeling, with subsequent neointima formation and eventually right heart failure.

2. Pulmonary vascular physiology

Monolayer formed by endothelial cells (EC) is a critical interface between the circulating blood and underlying SMC and provides a non-thrombogenic barrier. EC transform mechanical stimuli into biological responses and depending on the stimuli, EC secrete several transducing molecules that participate in a number of biological functions such as vascular tone, cell proliferation, apoptosis, inflammation and thrombosis. EC maintain vascular tone by activating cGMP and cAMP pathways. Nitric oxide (NO) is synthesized from L-arginine through the catalytic activity of endothelial NO synthase (eNOS). NO activates soluble guanylate cyclase (sGC) that catalyzes guanylate triphosphate (GTP) to cyclic guanosine monophosphate (cGMP), which via cGMP-dependent protein kinase (PKG) induces vascular relaxation, inhibits cell proliferation and modulates inflammation. Subsequently cGMP is metabolized and inactivated by Phosphodiesterase 5. Prostacyclin (PGI_2), an arachidonic acid metabolite is produced by the enzymatic activity of cyclooxygenase and PGI_2 synthase. The prostacyclin receptor found on EC and platelets belongs to the family of G-protein coupled receptors. PGI_2 binds to the receptor and stimulates adenylyl cyclase which catalyzes the conversion of ATP to second messenger cAMP. In addition, the cAMP/PKA pathway activates NO production via phosphorylation of eNOS. Both cGMP and cAMP mechanisms induce vascular relaxation and inhibit platelet aggregation and DNA synthesis. Juxtaposition of EC and SMC facilitates crosstalk, and EC maintain SMC in a quiescent state. [Mathew 2011a]. SMC inhibits flow-mediated activation of the mammalian target of rapamycin (mTOR) in EC, and SMC also participate in altering the expression of the factors involved in coagulation and fibrinolysis [Balcells 2010].

Caveolae, a subset of specialized microdomains (omega shaped invaginations, 50-100 nm) are found on a variety of cells including EC, SMC, fibroblasts and epithelial cells. They serve as a platform and compartmentalize a number of signaling molecules that reside in or are recruited to caveolae. They are also involved in transcytosis, endocytosis and potocytosis. Caveolin-1 (22kD) is the major scaffolding protein that supports and maintains the structure of caveolae. It interacts and regulates a number of proteins including Src family of kinases, G-proteins (α subunits), G protein-coupled receptors, H-Ras, PKC, eNOS, integrins and growth factor receptors such as vascular endothelial growth factor-receptor (VEGF-R), and epidermal growth factor-receptor (EGF-R). Caveolin-1 stabilizes these signaling proteins, and negatively regulates the target proteins within caveolae, through caveolin-1-scaffolding domain (CSD, residue 82-101). For optimal activation, eNOS is targeted to caveolae. Although it is negatively regulated by caveolin-1, caveolin-1 is essential for NO-mediated angiogenesis. In addition, the downstream effector of NO, sGC has been shown to compartmentalize in caveolae to facilitate its activation. In caveolin-1 knockout mice, the loss of caveolin-1 is associated with the hyper-activation of eNOS, and increased cGMP production. The hyper-activation of eNOS subsequently leading to PKG nitration-induced stress is considered responsible for PH in these mice; and re-expression of endothelial caveolin-1 restores vascular and cardiac abnormalities [*reviewed in* Mathew 2011b]. Caveolin-1 functions as an antiproliferative molecule; it negatively regulates proliferative pathways such as mitogen-activated protein kinase/extracellular signal-regulated kinase (MAPK/ERK), tyrosine- phosphorylated signal transducer and activator of transcription (PY-STAT) 3, EGF and platelet-derived growth factor (PDGF). Caveolin-1 also regulates cell cycle and apoptosis. In addition, caveolin-1 interacts with major ion channels such as Ca^{2+} -dependent potassium channels, voltage-dependent K^+ channels (Kv1.5), and a number of molecules responsible for Ca^{2+} handling such as inositol triphosphate receptor (IP_3R), heterodimeric GTP binding protein, Ca^{2+} ATPase and several transient receptor potential channels in caveolae. Through these interactions, caveolin-1 modulates cell proliferation and cell cycle progression. In SMC, caveolin-1 regulates Ca^{2+} entry and enables vasoconstriction. The localization of Ca^{2+} regulating proteins in caveolae and the proximity to the sarcoplasmic reticulum suggests an important role for caveolae/caveolin-1 for Ca^{2+} homeostasis [*reviewed in* Mathew 2011b]. RhoA interacts directly with caveolin-1, and the translocation of RhoA to caveolae is essential for myogenic tone. The CSD peptide of caveolin-1 has been shown to inhibit the agonist-induced redistribution of RhoA and PKC-α. Caveolin-1 blockage results in impaired formation of capillary tubes, and the overexpression of caveolin-1 accelerates EC differentiation and tube formation [Santibanz 2008, Liu 2002]. Furthermore, caveolin-1 modulates inflammation. It has recently been shown that caveolin-1 inhibits HIV replication through NF-κB [Wang 2011].

BMPRII is predominantly expressed in EC, and a part of BMPRII colocalizes with caveolin-1 in caveolae and also in golgi bodies. BMPRII signaling, essential for BMP-mediated regulation of vascular SMC growth and differentiation also protects EC from apoptosis [Yu 2008, Teichert-Kuliszewska 2006]. BMPRII directly modulates proteins involved in cytoskeletal organization, possibly through Mas1 (G-protein-coupled receptor) interaction with Rho GTPase. Recently discovered angiotensin converting enzyme (ACE) 2, an endogenous inhibitor of ACE, is endothelium-bound. ACE2 cleaves angiotensin (Ang) I to Ang 1-9 which is an inactive compound. ACE2 metabolizes Ang I to produce Ang 1-7 which is a physiological antagonist of Ang II. ACE2/Ang (1-7) pathway antagonizes Ang II acting through Mas1, increases NO production via the Akt-dependent pathway, releases PGI2 and it inhibits Ang II-induced reactive oxygen species (ROS) formation within the cell nucleus. Loss of ACE2 causes increased vascular permeability, pulmonary edema and worsening lung function. The over-expression of Ang-(1-7) has a protective effect on MCT-induced PH and bleomycin-induced lung fibrosis. Interestingly, inhibition of Rho kinase has been shown to activate the ACE2/Ang-(1-9) pathway resulting in increased eNOS expression and amelioration of hypertension [Johnson 2012, Burton 2011, Lovern 2008, Mathew 2011, Ocaranza 2011, Shenoy 2010]. Thus, under normal conditions EC maintain homeostasis by producing cell protective factors and inhibiting inflammation and cell proliferation.

3. Pathobiology of pulmonary hypertension

Endothelial dysfunction associated with an impaired endothelium-dependent vascular relaxation response is an important feature of clinical and experimental models of PH. It is the EC that bear the major brunt of injury regardless of the underlying disease, and the loss of the vascular dilatation mechanism associated with the activation of proliferative and anti-apoptotic pathways are the hallmarks of PH [*reviewed in* Mathew 2011]. Genetic susceptibility may make the effects of injury to occur earlier and to be more severe. It is becoming clear that epigenetics has a significant role in the pathogenesis of PH. Epigenetics is the study of changes in phenotype or gene expression not caused by any alterations in the underlying DNA sequence. Epigenetic mechanisms include 1) DNA methylation, 2) modification of histone proteins and 3) microRNAs [Kim 2011].

3.1. Loss of vasodilatation mechanisms

Impaired endothelium-dependent, NO-mediated relaxation and reduced cGMP levels are well documented in PH. Monocrotaline (MCT)-induced PH is associated with progressive disruption and loss of endothelial proteins. At 2 weeks post-MCT, the expression of eNOS is not significantly lower compared with the controls, but is associated with the loss of the eNOS activating molecules, HSP90 and Akt, thus leading to uncoupling of eNOS, and ROS generation. ROS generation returns to normal by 3-4 wks as the eNOS levels diminish. In PH patients, the expression of eNOS in the lungs is reported to be either low or increased. This is not surprising because the disease does not progress uniformly; thus, the expression of eNOS may depend on the stage of disease in a given lung section. Increased eNOS expression and PKG nitration have been shown in caveolin-1 null mice and also in the lungs of patients with IPAH, contributing to worsening of PH. In PH, the initial loss of EC is followed by the appearance of apoptosis resistant EC. These neointimal EC have increased expression of eNOS and reduced expression of caveolin-1, leading to uncoupling of eNOS and oxidant and nitration injury. The expression of PGI_2 synthase is reduced in the lungs of patients with PH, and the release of PGI_2 is decreased in these patients. Interestingly, mice with over-expression of PGI_2 synthase are protected from hypoxia-induced PH. In addition, PGI_2 synthase expression is reduced in the lungs of patients with PH, and the release of PGI_2 is decreased in these patients. Interestingly, overexpression of PGI_2 synthase protects mice from hypoxia-induced PH [*reviewed in* Mathew 2011 and Mathew 2011a]. Loss of cGMP and cAMP mechanisms leads to loss of endothelium-dependent vasodilatation, elevation of pulmonary artery pressure, platelet aggregation, increased mitogenic activity and negative modulation of inflammation.

3.2. Activation of proliferative pathways

During the development of PH, several proliferative and antiapoptotic pathways are activated. Endothelin-1 (ET-1) was discovered in 1980s as a potent vasoconstrictor predominantly produced by vascular endothelial cells from the inactive big endothelin-1 by catalytic activity of endothelin-converting enzyme (ECE)-1. ET1 is involved in several physiological and pathological processes such as vascular contraction, wound healing, cancer and vascular diseases [Khimji 2010]. ET-1 has mitogenic and inflammatory properties; and it acts in paracrine and autocrine fashion. The effects of ET-1 are mediated through ETA and ETB receptors. Endothelial cells possess ET-B receptors which induce NO upon stimulation. ETA and a subpopulation of ETB receptors cause vasoconstriction in SMC. Increased levels of ET-1 have been reported in the lungs of patients with PH and in pulmonary arteries in the MCT-model of PH. Interestingly, higher levels of ET-1 and both its receptors have been reported in pulmonary arteries of the patients with irreversible PAH associated with CHD compared with the reversible ones. The reversible PAH had higher expression of ET-1 and ET receptors compared with the controls [Huang 2011, Mathew 2011].

Platelet-derived growth factor (PDGF) was identified in 1970s as a serum growth factor for cells including fibroblasts and SMC; it induces proliferation of SMC and fibroblasts. PDGF is synthesized by a variety of cells including SMC and EC, and functions in both paracrine and autocrine manners. PDGF receptors are more pronounced in SMC compared with EC. Increased expression of PDGF receptor β (PDGFR β) has been reported in patients with IPAH and also in MCT and hypoxia models of PH. Furthermore, inhibition of PDGF receptor with imatinib, a tyrosine kinase inhibitor, reverses MCT and hypoxia-induced PH [Schermuly 2005, Perros 2008]. Both PDGF and VEGF belong to the same superfamily of signaling molecules. Interestingly, VEGF-A can stimulate both PDGF α and β receptors, and both receptors mediate VEGF-A and PDGF signaling; inhibition of either receptor significantly attenuates VEGF-A-induced cell migration. Thus, both participate in promoting recruitment and proliferation of vascular SMC both under physiological and pathological conditions [Mathew 2012]. After vascular injury, increased expression of PDGF ligand and its receptor occur. PDGF down regulates SMC genes, altering SMC phenotype from a contractile to an undifferentiated synthetic type, which is required for vascular repair. After repair, SMC revert to a contractile phenotype; whereas the deregulated synthetic phenotype leads to vascular disease. Micro (mi) RNA-221 is considered essential for PDGF-induced cell migration. MiRNA-221 is thought to promote proliferation through binding to the 3'-untranslated region of cell cycle inhibitor, and inhibiting p27/kip1 expression. Importantly, miRNA-221 reduces c-Kit mRNA. The inhibition of c-Kit leads to PDGF-mediated downregulation of SMC gene expression resulting in an undifferentiated synthetic phenotype and leading to cell proliferation. In several cell systems, activation of STAT3 is required for PDGF-induced cell proliferation; furthermore, inhibition of the PDGF receptor suppresses cell proliferation via inactivation of PY-STAT3 signaling [Mathew 2012].

STAT3 belongs to a family of cytoplasmic proteins that functions as extracellular effectors of cytokines and growth factors, and plays a role in a number of biological processes. Phosphorylation of STAT3 at tyrosine 705 residue leads to dimerization, nuclear translocation to nucleus, DNA synthesis and transcription of genes that mediate survival and cell proliferation. PY-STAT3 plays a critical role in cell growth, anti-apoptosis, survival, and immune function and inflammation; and it is a downstream effector of cytokines such as IL-6 and also growth factors. PY-STAT3 is activated by the JAK family of receptor–associated tyrosine kinases, and also by non-receptor tyrosine kinases such as Src, EGF and PDGF. Persistent phosphorylation of STAT3 associated with a number of primary tumors confers resistance to apoptosis. A role for STAT3 in vascular diseases including PH is emerging. Inhibition of the activated PY-STAT3 in the carotid arterial injury model prevents neointima formation. In addition, progressive activation of PY-STAT3 has been reported in several forms of experimental PH including MCT and hypoxia models, and in EC obtained from patients with IPAH. The downstream effectors of PY-STAT3 are cyclin D1 (cell cycle regulator), survivin and Bcl-xL (anti-apoptotic factors), and they are upregulated in PH. Inhibition of PY-STAT3 reduces the expression of cyclin D1, survivin and Bcl-xL, and attenuates PH. STAT3 also plays a significant role in stabilizing hypoxia inducible factor (HIF) 1α, a pivotal event in hypoxia-induced PH, and its interaction with HIF1α mediates transcriptional activation of VEGF promoter. Abundant expression of HIF1α and VEGF has been reported in plexiform lesions in the lungs of the patient with PH [*reviewed in* Mathew 2010].

Rho kinase (ROCK), an effector of small GTPase binding proteins was identified in 1990s. The RhoA/ROCK pathway plays pivotal role in the organization of actin-cytoskeletons, cell cycle progression, cell proliferation and migration. ROCK isoforms (I and II) are expressed in vascular tissue. Rho/ROCK signaling modulates a number of cellular functions such as inflammation, vascular tone, barrier function, vascular remodeling, atherogenesis and cell transformation. Furthermore, it promotes endothelial repair and maintains SMC differentiation [Rolfe 2005]. Interestingly, Rho is required for STAT3 activation; and Rho-mediated cell proliferation and migration occur via STAT3. In some cell systems, IL-6 increases the expression of active RhoA in a time and dose-dependent manner, and promotes cell migration and invasiveness. Rho activation is well established in PH, and inhibition of Rho kinase has been shown to attenuate PH in experimental models, such as hypoxia, bleomycin and MCT, and in a shunt model of PH with increased pulmonary blood flow. Furthermore, inhibition of STAT3 or Rho-associated kinase suppresses neointima formation in balloon-injured arteries [Mathew 2010, Mathew 2011].

Serotonin or 5 hydroxytryptamine (5HT) is synthesized in enterochromaffin cells and stored in platelets and is also synthesized in pulmonary artery EC. Serotonin through 5HT transporter (5HTT) is involved in pulmonary artery SMC and fibroblasts proliferation. Interestingly, 5HT-induced ROCK activation is essential for 5HT-induced SMC proliferation. Serotonin through 5HT transporter (5HTT) is internalized in pulmonary artery SMC and is linked to RhoA by intracellular type 2 transglutaminase leading to constitutive RhoA activation also known as RhoA serotonylation. Enhanced RhoA serotonylation associated with increased RhoA and Rho kinase activity has been observed in IPAH. In addition, EC from patients with PH exhibit increased expression of tryptophan hydroxylase, a rate limiting enzyme responsible for the synthesis of 5HT and increased production of 5HT. These patients have increased plasma levels of 5HT. Both 5HT transporter (5HTT) and 5HT receptors promote pulmonary artery SMC proliferation and migration, vasoconstriction and local microthrombi, considered to be dependent on RhoA/ROCK. In hypoxia-induced PH, 5HT receptors are thought to contribute to RhoA/ROCK-mediated Ca^{2+} sensitization. In addition, 5HTT transactivates PDGF β receptors in pulmonary artery SMC, indicating crosstalk between 5HT and PDGF pathways, both of which are implicated in the pathogenesis of PH. Mice with over-expression of 5HTT develop PH spontaneously and on exposure to hypoxia or MCT, they exhibit a significantly increased pulmonary artery pressure compared with the wild type mice. The MCT model of PH revealed an early and sustained increase in the expression of 5HTT in the rat lungs, and the inhibition of 5HTT but not the inhibition of 5HT receptors significantly attenuated MCT-induced PH. The 5HT pathway is thought to have played an important role in anorexigen drugs-induced PAH; these drugs have been shown to be 5HTT substrates [Mathew 2011, Guilluy 2009]. Prenatal exposure to selective serotonin uptake inhibitors has been shown to increase the risk of developing PPHN in infancy [Chambers 2006]. Thus, serotonin alone or in interaction with other mitogens participates in the pathogenesis of PH.

Evidence is emerging to suggest that Notch and mTOR signaling pathways may have a role in the pathogenesis of PH. Notch3 in SMC regulates cell proliferation and antiapoptotic activity and interestingly, increased expression of Notch3 is reported in the lungs of patients with non-familial PAH, and in the MCT and hypoxia-induced PH [Li 2009]. mTOR, a signaling protein for cell proliferation via the Akt pathway is well studied in cancer and interestingly, mTOR/Akt pathway may play a key role in hypoxia-induced adventitial fibroblast proliferation [Gerasimoskaya 2005]. Furthermore, ET1, 5HT and PDGF are known to enhance mTOR activation. Inhibition of mTOR significantly reduces 5HT-induced cell proliferation; and in PASMC from CTEPH patients, mTOR inhibition attenuates store-operated Ca^{2+} entry into cells [Ogawa 2009, Liu 2006]. Huang et al in 2011 reported increased expression of mTOR in the pulmonary artery medial layer in the reversible form of PAH associated with CHD, but increased expression in both medial and intimal layers in the irreversible form, further supporting a role for mTOR in PAH..

3.3. TGF-β/BMP signaling pathway

TGF-β is a large family with 3 isoforms, activins and BMPs. They play an important role during embryogenesis and are involved in vasculogenesis and cardiac development. TGF-β participates in cell proliferation, transformation, apoptosis and matrix deposition, and it maintains homeostasis. TGF-β is stored in the extracellular matrix (ECM) in an inactive form. Several mediators including plasmin, TSP1 and integrins are known to cause stromal release of TGF-β. TGF-β binds to its receptor TβRII leading to the formation of a complex with ALK5 or ALK1. BMPs (2, 4, 6 and 7) stimulate heterodimerization and the activation of BMP receptors (I and II) and initiate phosphorylation of Smad proteins (1, 5 and 8) which combines with Smad4, translocates to the nucleus and binds to genes to activate or repress their transcription. Similarly, TGF-β/ TβRII /ALK5 complex initiates phosphorylation of Smad2/3 which combines with Smad4 and translocates to nucleus to affect gene transcription. BMP2 has been shown to inhibit SMC proliferation after balloon-induced arterial injury in rats and also to attenuate hypoxia-induced PH. BMP-mediated regulation of vascular SMC growth and differentiation occur via BMPRII signaling [Goumans 2009, Eickelberg 2007, Davies 2012].

TGF- β, also referred to as fibrotic cytokine, decreases caveolin-1 expression in fibroblasts. Caveolin-1 suppresses TGF- β-mediated fibrosis, and regulates TGF- β/SMAD signaling through an interaction with the receptor TβRI [Wang 2006, Razani 2001]. Interestingly, TGF-β inhibits proliferation of pulmonary artery (PA) SMC from normal and patients with PAH; however, it has no antiproliferative effects on PASMC harvested from patients with IPAH or HPAH. BMPRII maintains vascular integrity and dampens inflammatory signals and its dysfunction results in TGF- β-induced secretion of pro-inflammatory cytokines such as IL-6 and IL-8, and the loss of TGF- β-mediated antiproliferative effects [Morrell 2001, Davies 2012]. Furthermore, loss of BMPRII has been shown to increase the expression of CXCR1/2 endothelial receptor for a proinflammatory cytokine IL-8. Mice with specific endothelial loss of BMPRII exhibit increased expression of CXCR1/2, leukocyte migration and PH; and the blockade of CXCR1/2 receptor attenuates PH [Burton 2011].

There is a significant interaction and crosstalk between the BMP system and IL-6/STAT3 pathway; therefore, a reduction in the expression of BMPRII may exacerbate the inflammatory response in PH. Furthermore, persistent activation of PY-STAT3 leads to a reduction in the BMPRII protein expression, and BMP2 induces apoptosis by inhibiting PY-STAT3 activation and down-regulating Bcl-xL. Interestingly, persistent activation of STAT3 leads to a strong upregulation of mature miR-20a, a microRNA that reduces the expression of BMPRII [Hagen 2007, Brock 2009, Kawamura 2000]. In addition to the association of BMPRII mutation and PAH, reduction in the expression of BMPRII has been reported in patients with IPAH without BMPRII mutation, and to a lesser extent in patients with secondary PH [Atkinson 2002]. Both MCT and hypoxia models of PH have been reported to be associated with the reduction in the expression of BMPRII. Both these models exhibit PY-STAT3 activation [Murakami 2010, Mathew 2011b]; therefore, it is likely that the STAT3 activation by itself may have a negative effect on BMPRII expression. In addition, BMPRII mutation may lead to PAH through the loss of its normal inhibition of inflammation

Recent studies have drawn attention to the role of gremlin in PH. Gremlin; a glycoprotein constitutively expressed in EC has been identified as an antagonist of BMP2, BMP4 and BMP7. It also functions as an angiogenesis factor independent of its action on BMPs. Increased expression of gremlin confined to EC has been reported in the lungs of patients with IPAH and HPAH. In hypoxia-induced PH, there is an increased expression of gremlin, and haplo-deficiency of gremlin attenuates PH [Costello 2010, Cahill 2012], further underscoring the importance of a balance between TGF-β/BMP and the antagonist, gremlin in maintaining vascular health.

TGF-β1 is also an immunomodulator; it plays an important role in the mechanism of regulatory T cells (CD4+CD25+). Regulatory T cells (Treg) are thought to be a primary source of TGF-β1 and it maintains self tolerance and prevents autoimmune diseases. It is further suggested that IL-6 counteracts TGF-β1 effect on Treg generation [Bommireddy 2007, Redstake 2009]. In scleroderma, Treg function has been shown to be compromised. Interestingly, Treg levels were low in mice prone to develop autoimmune diseases. In IPAH, several T cell subset abnormalities were noted, however, Treg levels were increased in this group compared with the controls. All these patients were on PH therapy. It is not certain whether the increased levels of Treg reflect an attempt to control inflammation or whether their function is impaired [Austin 2010].

3.4. Inflammation

As seen in the preceding sections, loss of cGMP/cAMP mechanisms, deregulated TGF-β and activation of multiple growth factors significantly affect and exacerbate the inflammatory response in PH. The importance of inflammation in PH is further strengthened by the fact that patients suffering from systemic inflammatory and autoimmune diseases, and infectious diseases such as scleroderma [Mathai 2011], sarcoidosis [Nunes 2006], POEMS syndrome [Lesprit 1998] acquired immuno-deficiency syndrome [Cicalini 2011] and schistosomiasis [Kolosionek 2011] develop PH. Furthermore, these patients are shown to have perivascular inflammatory cells, regulated upon activation normal T-cell expressed and secreted

http://dx.doi.org/10.5772/56179

(RANTES), dendritic cells, anti-fibroblast and anti-endothelial antibodies [Tuder 1994, Dorfüller 2002, Perros 2007, Terrier 2008, Tamby 2005]. Elevated plasma levels of proinflammatory cytokines and chemokines such as interleukin (IL)-1, IL-6, IL-8, fractalkine and CC chemokine ligand 2 (CCL2) have been documented in patients with IPAH. Interestingly, IL-6 also contributes to PH in patients with COPD. IL-6 is produced by a variety of cells including EC, SMC, fibroblasts and macrophages. In the MCT model of PH, increased levels and the activity of IL-6 and PY-STAT3 activation occur before the onset of PH, and early treatment with dexamethasone inhibits IL-6 activation and attenuates PH. IL-6 augments hypoxia-induced PH, and not surprisingly, IL-6 knockout mice exhibit less inflammation and attenuated PH in response to hypoxia [*reviewed in* Mathew 2010]. Importantly, dysregulated cytokines in IPAH and HPAH are associated with negative effects on survival [Soon 2012].

Recent studies have shown the presence of lymphoid neogenesis in IPAH. These are highly organized tertiary lymphoid tissue occurring throughout the pulmonary vasculature possibly sustaining chronic inflammation and contributing to autoimmunity. In addition, expression of CD44, a cell adhesion molecule is reported in the plexiform lesions in the patients with IPAH. Importantly, neither the lymphoid neogenesis nor CD44 expression has been observed in the controls as well as in PAH associated with CHD (Eisenmenger syndrome) [Perros 2012, Ohta-Ogo 2012]. Persistent inflammation observed in IPAH through lymphoid neogenesis may contribute to autoimmunity in IPAH. These differences between IPAH and Eisenmenger syndrome may in part be responsible for the observed better survival in the latter group.

3.5. Caveolin-1

a. Loss/Dysfunction of Caveolin-1: Loss of endothelial caveolin-1 has been reported in several clinical and experimental forms of PH. The MCT model of PH has been extensively studied to understand the pathogenesis of PH. Disruption of endothelial caveolae associated with progressive loss of caveolin-1 accompanied by the activation of PY-STAT3 and increased expression of Bcl-xL occurs as early as 48 hrs post-MCT, before the onset of PH. The downstream effectors of PY-STAT3, survivin, Bcl-xL and cyclin D1 are upregulated in PH. Caveolin-1 functions as a suppressor of cytokine signaling-3, and inhibits PY-STAT3 activation. Importantly, rescue of endothelial caveolin-1 inhibits the activation of proliferative pathways and attenuates MCT-induced PH [*reviewed in* Mathew R 2011b].

Similar to the MCT model, in hypoxia-induced PH, impaired endothelium-dependent, NO-mediated pulmonary vascular relaxation and low basal and agonist-induced cGMP are present. However, in contrast to the MCT model, there is no reduction in caveolin-1 expression in hypoxia-induced PH. During hypoxia, eNOS forms a tight complex with caveolin-1 and remains dissociated from HSP90 and calmodulin, resulting in eNOS dysfunction. Furthermore, hypoxia-induced PH and pulmonary endothelial cells exposed to hypoxia exhibit hyperactivation of PY-STAT3. PY-STAT3 activation in hypoxia-induced PH despite the unaltered expression of caveolin-1 protein strongly suggests that caveolin-1 is dysfunctional and has lost its inhibitory function. Thus, the disruption of EC membrane and ensuing caveolin-1 loss, or perturbation of EC membrane with mislocalization of caveolin-1 leads to its dysfunction resulting in the initiation and progression of PH [Mathew 2011b].

Caveolin-1 in fibroblasts regulates ECM production. Low levels of caveolin-1 have been reported in fibroblasts from patients with scleroderma and idiopathic pulmonary fibrosis. Loss of caveolin-1 in fibroblasts leads to hyperactivation of MEK, ERK, Akt signaling pathways resulting in enhanced expression of collagen type I and III, tenascin C, reduction in ECM degradation and fibrosis; these processes are inhibited with the re-expression of caveolin-1. In addition, loss of caveolin-1 results in the activation of TGF- β signaling and upregulation of CXCR4 in monocytes resulting in their migration to damaged tissue where CXCL12, its ligand is produced [del Galdo 2008, Tourkina 2012].

b. Enhanced Expression of Caveolin-1 in SMC: Vascular SMC play an important role in the pathobiology of PH. During the progression of PH, SMC change from contractile to synthetic phenotype. These cells then can proliferate and migrate leading to neointima formation. Caveolin-1 functions as an antiproliferative factor in SMC; it keeps mitogens inactive and regulates Ca^{2+} entry in SMC. Recent studies have shown loss of endothelial caveolin-1 and enhanced expression of caveolin-1 in SMC in clinical and experimental PH. Pulmonary vascular SMC from IPAH revealed enhanced caveolin-1 expression, altered Ca^{2+} handling, increased capacitative Ca^{2+} entry and increased $[Ca^{2+}]_i$, and augmented DNA synthesis. Silencing caveolin-1 mRNA in these SMC has an inhibitory effect on capacitance Ca^{2+} entry and DNA synthesis [Patel 2007]. The enhanced caveolin-1 expression in SMC was reported in a recent case report of a child who presented with severe PH two years after a complete clinical recovery from acute respiratory distress syndrome. Lung biopsy revealed marked endothelial caveolin-1 loss, and the arteries with additional loss of von Willebrand Factor (vWF) exhibited robust expression of caveolin-1 in SMC, ultimately leading to neointima formation and a loss of response to therapy [Mathew 2011c]. Increased expression of caveolin-1 in SMC is also reported in patients with PH and associated COPD [Huber 2009]. MCT-induced PH is associated with progressive disruption of EC and loss of endothelial caveolin-1. During the progression of the disease at 4 wks, 29% of the arteries exhibited loss of vWF, in addition to a further loss of endothelial caveolin-1. Importantly, 70% of the arteries with vWF exhibited enhanced expression of caveolin-1 in SMC. Loss of vWF is indicative of extensive endothelial damage. It is worth noting here that an increased circulating level of vWF or EC is associated with poor prognosis in PH [Huang 2012].

Matrix metalloproteinase (MMP) 2 degrades ECM, and facilitates cell proliferation and migration. Caveolin-1 is known to inhibit MMP2 expression and activity. In the MCT model at 4 wks, despite enhanced expression of caveolin-1 in SMC, MMP2 expression and activity are reported to be increased. This indicates that caveolin-1 has lost its inhibitory function. In cultured SMC, caveolin-1 translocates from caveolae to non-caveolar sites within the plasma membrane in response to cyclic strain; the translocated caveolin-1 facilitates cell cycle progression and cell proliferation. Caveolin-1 blockade abolishes the stretch-induced cell proliferation, indicating that caveolin-1 plays a pivotal role in stretch-induced cell proliferation. It is likely that the extensive damage and/or loss of endothelial cells observed in PH may impose wall strain induced by elevated pressure directly on to SMC leading to translocation of caveolin-1 from caveolae and increased expression in SMC, which may cooperate with MMP2 to facilitate further proliferation and cell migration, and, thus, contribute to the worsening of the disease. Enhanced expression of caveolin-1 and possibly translocation from caveolar sites to non-caveolar sites, switches caveolin-1 from being an anti-proliferative to a pro-proliferative molecule, and thus, may contribute to SMC change from a contractile to a synthetic phenotype [Huang 2012]. Thus, caveolin-1 plays an important role in the pathogenesis of PH and its function depends on the cell context and the disease stage.

3.6. Micro RNAs (miRNAs, MiRs)

MiRNAs are recently discovered small (~22 nucleotides) non-coding RNAs that play a key role in post-translational regulation of a number of genes. Since 1993, close to 1000 miRNAs have been identified in the human genome which regulate one third of all mRNAs. Maturation of miRNA is mediated by RNase III endonucleases, Drosha and Dicer. MiRNAs negatively regulate gene transcription by interacting with the 3' untranslated region of specific mRNA target to repress translation and enhance mRNA degradation. Interestingly, one miRNA can influence several mRNAs and one mRNA is influenced by several miRNAs. They participate in a variety of physiological and pathological functions such as development, cell proliferation, apoptosis, differentiation and inflammation; and they can act as oncogenes or tumor suppressors [Urbich 2008, Zhang 2007].

A number of miRNAs have been reported to participate in cardiovascular pathobiology. Smooth muscle-specific miRNAs miR-143/145, miR-221, miR-222 and mir-26A play a significant role in the regulation of VSMC phenotype. MiR 143 and miR-145 are well expressed in contractile VSMC and are deficient in the synthetic phenotype. In contrast, miR-221 and miR-222, transcriptionally induced by PDGF signaling are over-expressed during neointima formation. Over-expression of miR-221 represses SMC markers via downregulation of c-Kit, and promotes cell proliferation by inhibiting p27Kip1 [Cordes 2009, Song 2010, Bockmeyer 2012]. In addition, miR-26a has been shown to play a significant role in vascular SMC proliferation, inhibit differentiation and apoptosis, and alter TGF-β signaling [Leeper 2011]. Furthermore, induction of miR-1 in SMC inhibits cell proliferation and miR-100 functions as an inhibitor of mTOR and attenuates cell proliferation of EC and SMC [*reviewed in* Mathew 2011]. Over-expression of miR-17/92 cluster has been shown to reduce BMPRII expression. IL-6 activates 17/92 miR cluster via STAT3 activation, furthermore, it inactivates the TGF-β pathway by inhibiting p21 and BIM (Bcl2 interacting mediator of cell death) [Brock 2009, Petrocca 2008]. The importance of miR-17 and miR-20 in PH is supported by recent studies showing upregulation of p21 and attenuation of MCT-induced PH by antagomiR-17, and restoration of BMPRII function and attenuation of hypoxia-induced pulmonary vascular remodeling and RVH by antagomiR-20a [Pullamsetti 2012, Brock 2012]. IL-6 and PY-STAT3 play a significant role in PH, furthermore, STAT3 activation is thought to suppress the expression of miR-204, which is significantly down-regulated in SMC from PH patients and from experimental models; and treatment with miR-204 significantly inhibits STAT3 activation and attenuates MCT-induced PH [Courboulin 2011].

In cancer, miR-21 induction by IL-6 is dependent on STAT3, and miR-21 is thought to contribute to STAT3-mediated proliferative activity and immune responses [Löffler 2007, Kumaraswamy 2011]. MiR-21 is abundantly expressed in EC, and it modulates eNOS activity and apoptosis. Over-expression of miR-21 in EC inhibits cell proliferation, cell migration and angiogenesis [Weber 2010, Sabatel 2011]. However, aberrantly expressed miR-21 participates in cell proliferation and neointima formation. Furthermore, there is an increased expression of miR-21 in undifferentiated vascular SMC compared with the differentiated ones [Ji 2007]. In addition to STAT3, TGF-β and BMP4 upregulate miR-21, and it is suggested that it may have a role in profibrotic effects [Kumaraswamy 2011]. Interestingly, downregulation of miR-21 has been reported in the lungs and serum of the patients with IPAH, and also in *SMAD9* mutation-associated HPAH suggesting a role for Smad8 in the processing of miR-21. Interestingly, miR-21 was down-regulated in the MCT-induced PH, but not in the hypoxia model [Caruso 2010, Drake 2011]. Another endothelial-specific miR-126 is thought to activate VEGF signaling and facilitate angiogenesis [Nicoli 2010].

Significant differences in the miRNAs expression in the concentric and plexiform lesions in the lungs of patients with PAH have been reported. Interestingly, the expression of miR-126, which enhances the VEGF-A signaling pathway for angiogenesis was significantly higher in plexiform lesions compared with the concentric lesions. In contrast, the expression of miR 143/145, which maintains the contractile SMC phenotype, was significantly lower in plexiform lesions, thus, underscoring the presence of deregulated angiogenesis in plexiform lesions [Bockmeyer 2012]. Although, miRNAs are known to play an important role in cancer; the field of miRNAs, however, is in its nascent stage in PH. It is already becoming clear that miRNAs do play an important role in PH.

3.7. Deregulated angiogenesis

The term angiogenesis is applied to the process of new vessels sprouting from the preexisting vessels. Angiogenesis is a tightly controlled process involving a number of signaling pathways including VEGF, bFGF, PDGF-B, TGF-β, BMPs, angiopoietin1/Tie2 and Notch etc. to produce a number of coordinated signals leading to a proper and mature vascular network. Angiogenesis is very active during the embryonic stage, and it becomes active again during adulthood when new vessel formation is required such as during pregnancy and wound healing, and also under various pathological conditions. VEGF is essential for the initiation of angiogenic sprouting [Folkman 1996, Holderfield 2008]. The TGF-β superfamily of proteins plays a significant role in angiogenesis by regulating VEGF expression in a coordinated fashion. TGF-β modulates activities of VEGF and bFGF during wound healing. It is thought TGF- β via Alk5/BMPRII/Smad2 enhances VEGF activity and facilitates angiogenesis, whereas BMP9 via Alk1/BMPRII/Smad1 suppresses angiogenesis. Interestingly, in plexiform lesions, loss of TGF- β family signaling is associated with increased expression of VEGF, highlighting deregulated angiogenesis. The importance of the TGF- β superfamily in angiogenesis is further supported by the observation of the mutation of endoglin as well as Alk1 in hemorrhagic hereditary telengiectasia [David 2009, Shao 2009, Richter 2004, Tuder 2001, Hirose 2000]. RhoA/ROCK signaling is also required for VEGF-mediated angiogenesis; and thrombospondin-1 (TSP1), an endogenous anti-angiogenic factor regulates VEGF signaling by controlling the activation of VEGF-R2 [Bryan 2010]. In plexiform lesions, in addition to increased VEGF expression, increased expression of other signaling molecules such as HIF-1α, HIF-1β, MMP9, Notch4 and

TSP-1has been reported. HIF-1α and HIF-1β are hypoxia-inducible factors facilitating hypoxia-induced induction of VEGF. Notch 4 is thought to be involved in reshaping of the local vasculature, via cross-talk with VEGF and TGF- β in EC. MMP9 participates in basement membrane remodeling [Jonigk 2011, Tuder 2001]. Interestingly, increased expression of ET-1 receptors observed in patients with PAH and CHD is also thought to play a role in neointima formation and neo-angiogenesis [Huang 2011]. Thus, the altered expression of several signaling molecules leads to deregulated angiogenesis, a hallmark of plexiform lesion, which facilitates in sustaining the disease and its progression.

3.8. Right Ventricular Failure (RVF)

Becuase of increased pulmonary vascular resistance, right ventricular hypertrophy (RVH) occurs as an adaptive measure to maintain cardiac output. Right ventricular (RV) contractility is impaired during the progression of the disease, leading to RVF characterized by RV dysfunction, increased filling pressure and low cardiac output. RVF is the major cause of deterioration in PH leading to death. In a recent study, a mortality rate of 41% was found in patients with PH admitted to the intensive care unit with acute right heart failure. Interestingly, patients with Eisenmenger syndrome develop RVF at a much later time compared with IPAH patients with comparable RV afterload. The experimental models of RV pressure overload reveal more cardiac fibrosis, capillary rarefaction, diminished antioxidant protection and oxidative damage. Furthermore, pressure-induced reversal of cardiomyocyte phenotype to fetal stage in chronic PH results in relocation of critical cytoskeletal stress proteins leading to progressive deterioration of RV function; and in PH, these alterations are limited to the RV. Therefore, it is thought that the pressure overload itself may not be sufficient for the RVF in PH [Sztrymf 2010, Bogaard 2009]. Oxidant injury has been thought to play a key role in RVF associated with PH. ROS have a direct effect on cellular structure and function; and can lead to inflammation and apoptosis. Increased generation of ROS can induce mitochondrial DNA damage leading to a reduction in mitochondrial function, thus, facilitating further ROS generation and cellular injury, worsening heart failure. Impaired mitochondrial glucose oxidation and reduction in glucose-based oxygen consumption of RV myocardium have been reported in experimental models of RV pressure overload (MCT-induced PH, and pulmonary artery band-induced RVH). In the MCT model of PH, both NADPH oxidase and mitochondrial ROS generation were shown to be increased associated with reduction in the mRNA expression of both superoxide dismutase (SOD) 1 (cytosolic) and SOD2 (mitochondrial). Treatment with EUK-134, an SOD and catalase mimetic when given at 10 days post-MCT significantly improved RV function and prevented cardiac fibrosis without altering the lung weight [Piao 2010, Redoute 2010]. Thus, oxidant injury may be a key determinant of RV function in PH-associated RVH.

3.9. Reversibility vs irreversibility of PH

Under most circumstances, PH is a progressive disease, ultimately becoming irreversible with a negative impact on survival. Reversibility of PH is seen especially in infants and children with PPHN, PH associated with RDS/BPD or CHD. In the former cases, as the lung vascular/

alveolar development improves, PH is reversed barring associated co-morbidities, which can have a negative influence. In the latter cases (PH associated with CHD), closure of the defect in a timely fashion is effective. However, in some instances PH may progress despite the correction of the underlying defect. Most clinical and experimental studies suggest that the status of EC may determine the reversibility or irreversibility. In MCT-induced PH, progressive disruption of endothelial caveolin-1 is accompanied by the activation of proliferative and anti-apoptotic pathways. At 2 wks post-MCT, PH is accompanied by the loss of cytosolic proteins indicating further EC damage. Loss of vWF which is stored in Weibel Palade bodies within the EC occurs at 4 wks post-MCT, indicative of extensive EC damage or loss. This is accompanied by enhanced expression of caveolin-1 in SMC and increased expression and activity of MMP2. These changes can lead to further cell proliferation, cell migration and possible neointima formation. Interestingly, EC apoptosis is reported to be followed by exuberant apoptotic resistant EC [Huang 2010, Huang 2012, Sakao 2005]. This view is supported by a recent case report showing loss of endothelial caveolin-1 and vWF; and associated enhanced expression of caveolin-1 in SMC, followed by neointima formation [Mathew 2011c].

Loss of miR-21, which is abundant in EC, occurs in patients with IPAH and HPAH, and in MCT-induced PH but not in hypoxia-induced PH [Caruso 2010, Drake 2011]. This is a significant observation, because unlike MCT, hypoxia-induced PH does not lead to endothelial disruption [Mathew 2011b] and PH reverses when hypoxia is discontinued [Sluiter 2012]. These observed differences in miR-21 expression, therefore, are very likely dependent on the underlying status of EC. These observations support the view that the EC integrity may determine the eventual outcome of the disease as shown in the proposed model (Figure 1).

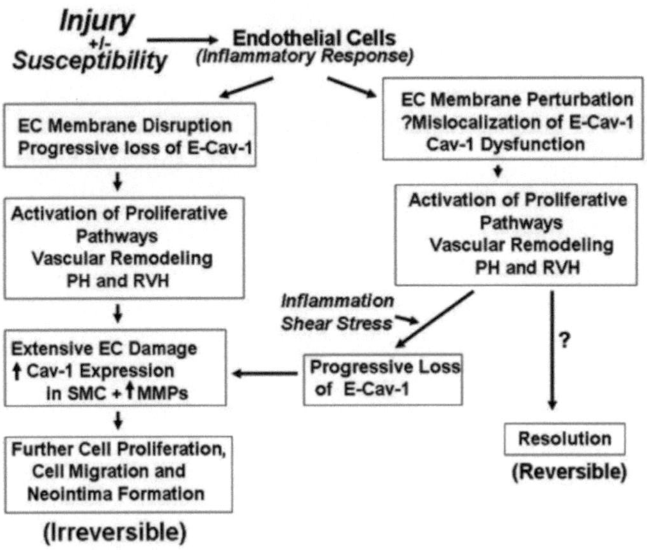

Figure 1. This figure depicts proposed pathways in PH. Injury in patients with or without susceptibility evokes an inflammatory response resulting in disruption or perturbation of endothelial cell membrane leading to the activation of proliferative and antiapoptotic pathways and PH. The status of endothelial cell membrane may determine the reversibility or irreversibility of PH.

4. Summary

PH is the result of an imbalance between vasoconstriction and vasodilatation, cell proliferation and apoptosis, and between pro-angiogenesis and anti-angiogenesis. Intricate and delicate intermeshing of a large number of signaling molecules in pulmonary vasculature cooperate to preserve the balance between the opposing signaling and activities, thus, maintain vascular health. Loss or increased expression of a molecule secondary to an injury can derail the delicate network of signaling pathways resulting in deregulated inflammatory response, cell proliferation, cell migration and angiogenesis leading to the initiation and progression of PH. Some of these changes occur before PH becomes clinically manifest, thus, impacting the response to therapy and survival. Genetics, epigenetics, severity of injury and the associated inflammatory response further influence the outcome.

Author details

Rajamma Mathew*

Address all correspondence to: rajamma_mathew@NYMC.edu

Departments of Pediatrics and Physiology, New York Medical College, Valhalla, NY, USA

References

[1] Atkinson C, Stewart S, Upton PD, Machado R, Thomson JR et al. Primary pulmonary artery hypertension is associated with reduced pulmonary vascular expression of type II bone morphogenetic protein receptor. Circulation 2002; 105:1672-1678

[2] Austin ED, Cogan JD, West JD, Hedges LK, Hamid R et al. Alterations in oestrogen metabolism: Implications for higher penetrance of familial pulmonary arterial hypertension in females. *Eur Respir J*. 2009; 34:1093-1099

[3] Austin ED, Rock MT, Mosse CA, Vnencak-Jones CL, Yoder SM et al. T-lymphocyte subset abnormalities in the blood and lung in pulmonary arterial hypertension. *Respir Med* 2010; 104:454-462

[4] Balcells M, Martorell J, Olivé C, Santacana M, Chitalia V et al. Smooth muscle cells orchestrate the endothelial cells response to flow and injury. *Circulation* 2010; 121:2192-2199

[5] Bockmeyer CL, Maegel L, Janciauskiene S, Rische J, Lehmann U et al. Plexiform vasculopathy of severe pulmonary arterial hypertension and microRNA expression. *J Heart Lung Transplant* 2012; 31:764-772

[6] Bogaard HJ, Natarajan R, Henderson SC, Long C, Kraskauskas D et al. Chronic pulmonary artery pressure elevation is insufficient to explain right heart failure. *Circulation* 2009, 120: 1951-1960

[7] Bommireddy R, Doetschman T. TGF-β1 and Treg cells: alliance for tolerance. *Trends Mol Med* 2007; 13:492-501

[8] Brock M, Trenkmann M, Gay RE, Michel BA, Gay S et al. Interkleukin-6 modulates the expression of the bone morphogenic protein receptor type II through a novel STAT3-microRNA cluster 17/92 pathway. *Circ Res* 2009; 104:1184-1191

[9] Brock M, Samillan VJ, Trenkmann M, Schwarzwald C, Uirich S et al. AntagomiR directed against miR-20a restores functional BMPR2 signalling and prevents vascular remodeling in hypoxia-induced pulmonary hypertension. *Eur Heart J* 2012; doi: 10.1093/eurheartj/ehs060

[10] Bryan BA, Dennstedt E, Mitchell DC, Walshe TE, Noma K et al. RhoA/ROCK signaling is essential for multiple aspects of VEGF-mediated angiogenesis. *FASEB J* 2010; 24:3186-3195

[11] Burton VJ, Ciulan LI, Holmes AM, Rodman DM, Walker C, Budd DC. Bone morphogenetic protein receptor-II regulates pulmonary artery endothelial cell barrier function. *Blood* 2011; 117:333-341

[12] Burton VJ, Holmes AM, Cuiclan LI, Robinson A, Roger JS et al. Attenuation of leukocyte recruitment via CXCR1/2 inhibition stops progression of pulmonary arterial hypertension in mice with genetic ablation of endothelial BMPRII. *Blood* 2011a; 118:4750-4758

[13] Cahill E, Costello CM, Rowan SC, Harkin S, Howell K et al. Gremlin plays a key role in the pathogenesis of pulmonary hypertension. Circulation 2012; 125:920-930

[14] Caruso P, MacLean M.R, Khanin R, McClure J, Soon, E et al. Dynamic changes in lung microRNA profiles during the development of pulmonary hypertension due to chronic hypoxia and monocrotaline. *Arterioscler. Thromb. Vasc. Biol.* 2010, 30:716-723

[15] Chambers CD, Hernandez-Diaz S, van Marter LJ, Werler MM, et al. Selective serotonin-reuptake inhibitors and risk of persistent pulmonary hypertension of the newborn. *N Eng J Med* 2006; 354:579-587.

[16] Chida A, Shintani M, Yagi H, Fujiwara M, Kojima Y et al. Outcome of childhood pulmonary arterial hypertension in BMPR2 and ALK1 mutation carriers. *Am J Cardiol* 2012; 110:586-593

[17] Cicalini S, Almodovar S, Grilli E, Flores S. Pulmonary hypertension and human immunodeficiency virus infection: epidemiology, pathogenesis and clinical approach. *Clin Microbiol Infect* 2011; 17:25-33

[18] Cogan JD, Pauciulo MW, Batchman AP, Prince MA, Robbins IM et al. High frequency of BMPR2 exonic deletions/duplications in familial pulmonary arterial hypertension. *Am. J. Respir. Crit. Care Med.* 2006, 174(5), 590-598

[19] Cordes KR, Sheehy NT, White MP, Berry EC, Morton SU et al. miR-145 and miR-143 regulate smooth muscle cell fate and plasticity. *Nature* 2009; 460:705-710

[20] Costello CM, Cahill E, Martin F, Gaine S, McLaughlin P. Role of gremlin in the lung development and desease. *Am J respir Cell Mol Biol* 2010; 42:517-523

[21] Courboulin A, Paulin R, Giguère N, Saksouk N, Perreault T et al. Role for miR-204 in human pulmonary arterial hypertension. *J. Exp. Med.* 2011, 208(3), 535-548

[22] D'Alonzo GE, Barst RJ, Ayers SM, Bergofsky EH, Brundage BH et al. Survival in patients with primary pulmonary hypertension: results from a national prospective registry. *Ann Intern Med* 1991; 115:343-349

[23] Dartevelle P, Fadel E, Mussot S, Chapelier A, Hervé P et al. Chronic thromboembolic pulmonary hypertension. *Eur Respir J* 2004; 23:637-648

[24] David L, Feige JJ, Bailly S. Emerging role of bone morphogenic proteins in angiogenesis. *Cytokine Growth Factor Rev.* 2009; 20:203-212

[25] Davies RJ, Holmes AM, Deighton J, Long L, Yang X et al. BMP type II receptor deficiency confers resistance to growth inhibition by TGF-β in pulmonary artery smooth muscle cells: Role of proinflammatory cytokines. *Am J Physiol* 2012; 302:L604-L615

[26] del Cerro MJ, Abman S, Diaz G, Freundenthal AH, Freundenthal F, Harikrishnan S et al. A consensus approach to the classification of pediatric pulmonary hypertensive vascular disease: Report from the PVRI pediatric taskforce, Panama 2011. *Pulm. Circ.* 2011; 1:286-298

[27] del Galdo F, Lisanti MP, Jimenez S. Caveolin-1, TGF- β receptor internalization, and the pathogenesis of systemic sclerosis. *Curr Opin Rheumatol* 2008; 20:713-719

[28] Dorfmüller P, Zarka V, Durand-Gasselin J, Monti G, Balbanian K et al. Cytokine RANTES in severe pulmonary arterial hypertension. *Am J Respir Crit Care Med* 2002;165:534-539

[29] Drake KM, Zygmunt D, Mavrakis l, Harbor P, Wang L et al. Altered microRNA processing in heritable pulmonary arterial hypertension: An important role of Smad-8. *Am J Crit Care Med* 2011; 184:1400-1408

[30] Eickelberg O, Morty RE. Transforming growth factor beta/bone morhogenic protein signaling in pulmonary arterial hypertension: remodeling revisited. *Trends Cardiovac Med* 2007; 17:263-269

[31] Fadel E, Mazmanian GM, Baudet B, Detruit H, Verhoye JP et al. Endothelial nitric oxide function in pig lung after chronic pulmonary artery obstruction. *Am J Respir Crit Care Med* 2000; 162:1429-1434

[32] Faner R, Rojas M, MacNee W, Agusti A. Abnormal lung aging in chronic obstructive pulmonary disease and idiopathic fibrosis. *Am J Respir Crit Care Med* 2012; 186:306-313

[33] Farquhar M, Fitzgerald DA. Pulmonary hypertension in chronic neonatal lung disease. *Pediatr Respir Rev* 2010; 11:149-153

[34] Fishman AP. Primary pulmonary hypertension: a look back. *J Amer Coll Cardiol* 2004; 43:2S-4S

[35] Folkman J, D'Amore PA. Blood vessel formation: what is its molecular basis? *Cell* 1996; 87:1153-1155

[36] Gerasimovskaya EV, Tucker DA, Stenmark KR. Activation of phosphatidylinositol3 kinase, Akt, and mammalian target of rapamycin is necessary for hypoxia-induced pulmonary arterial adventitial fibroblast proliferation. *J Appl Physiol* 2005; 98:722-731

[37] Goumans MJ, Liu Z, ten Dijke P. TGF-beta signaling in vascular biology and dysfunction. *Cell Res* 2009: 19:116-127

[38] Guazzi M, Arena R. Pulmonary hypertension with left-sided heart disease. *Nature Reviews/Cardiology* 2010; 7:648-659

[39] Guilluy C, Eddahibi S, Agard C, Guignabert C, Izziki M et al. RhoA and Rho kinase activation in human pulmonary hypertension. *Am J Respir Crit Care Med* 2009; 179:1151-1158

[40] Hagen M, Fagan K, Steudel W, Carr M, Lane K et al. Interaction of interleukin-6 and BMP pathway in pulmonary smooth muscle. *Am J Physiol* 2007; 292:L1473-L1479

[41] Hill NS, Preston I, Roberts K. Defining the phenotypes for pulmonary hypertension associated with diastolic heart failure. *Circ Heart Failure* 2011; 4:238-240

[42] Hirose S, Hosoda Y, Furuya S, Otsuki T, Ikeda E. Expression of vascular endothelia growth factor and its receptors correlates closely with formation of the plexiform lesion in human PH. *Pathol Int* 2000; 50:472-479.

[43] Holderfield MT, Hughes CC. Crosstalk between vascular endothelial growth factor, notch, transforming growth factor-β in vascular morphogenesis. *Circ Res* 2008; 102:637-652

[44] Huang H. Zhang P, Wang Z, Tang F. Jiang Z. Activation of endothelin-1 receptor signaling pathways is associated with neointima formation, neoangiogenesis and irreversible pulmonary arterial hypertension in patients with congenital heart disease. Circ J 2011; 75:1463-1471

[45] Huang J, Wolk J, Gewitz MH, Mathew R. Progressive Endothelial Cell Damage in an Inflammatory Model of Pulmonary Hypertension. *Expt. Lung Res* 2010; 36:57-66

[46] Huang J, Wolk JH, Gewitz MH. Mathew R. Caveolin-1 expression during the progression of pulmonary hypertension. *Exp Biol Med* 2012; 237:956-965

[47] Huber LC, Soltermann A, Fischler M, Gay S, Weder W et al.Caveolin-1 expression and hemodynamics in COPD patients. *Open Respir Med J* 2009; 3:73-78

[48] Humbert M, Deng Z, Simonneau G, Barst RJ, Sitbon O et al. BMPR2 germline mutations in pulmonary hypertension associated with fenfluramine derivatives. *Eur Resp J* 2002; 20:518-523

[49] Humbert M, Sitbon O, Chaouat A, Bertocchi M, Habib G et al. Pulmonary arterial hypertension in France: results from national registry. *Am J Respir Critical Care Med* 2006; 173:1023-1030

[50] Ji R, Cheng Y, Yue J, Yang J, Liu X et al. MicroRNA expression signature and antisense mediated depletion reveal an essential role of microRNA in vascular neointimal lesion formation, Circ Res 2007; 100:1579-1588

[51] ohnson JA, Hemnes AR, Perrien DS, Schuster M, Robinson LJ et al. Cytskeletal defect in Bmpr2-associated pulmonary arterial hypertension. *Am J Physiol* 2012; 302: L474-L484

[52] Jonigk D, Golpon H, Bockmeyer CL, Maegel L, Hoeper MM et al. Plexiform lesions in pulmonary arterial hypertension: composition, architecture and microenvironment. *Am J Pathol* 2011; 179:167-179

[53] Kawamura C, Kizaki m, Yamato K, Uchida H, Fukuchi Y et al. Bone morphogenetic protein-2 induces apoptosis in human myeloma cells with modulation of STAT3. *Blood* 2000; 96:2005-2011

[54] Khimji AK, Rockey DC. Endothelin: Biology and disease. *Cell Signal* 2010; 22:1615-1625

[55] Kim GH, Ryan JJ, Marsboom G, Archer SL. Epigenetic mechanisms of pulmonary hypertension. *Pulm Circ* 2001; 1:347-356

[56] Kolosionek E, Graham BB, Tuder RM, Butrous G. Pulmonary vascular disease associated with parasitic infection: the role of schistosomiasis. *Clin Microbiol Infect* 2011; 17:15-24

[57] Kumarswamy R, Volkmann I, Thum T. Regulation and function of miR-21 in health and disease. *RNA Biol* 2011; 8:706-713

[58] Leeper NJ, Raiesdana A, Kojima Y, Chun HJ, Azuma J et al. MicroRNA-26a is a novel regulator of vascular smooth muscle cell function. *J cell Physiol* 2011; 226:1035-1043.

[59] Lesprit P, Godeau B, Authier FJ, Soubrier M, Zuber M et al. Pulmonary hypertension in POEMS syndrome: a new feature mediated by cytokines. Am J Respir Crit Care Med 1998; 157:907-911

[60] Li X, Zhang X, Leathers R, Makino A, Huang C et al. Notch3 signaling is required for the development of pulmonary arterial hypertension. *Nat Med* 2009; 15:1289-1297

[61] Liu J, Wang XB, Park DS, Lisanti MP. Caveolin-1 expression enhances endothelial capillary tube formation. J Biol Chem 2002; 277:10661-10668

[62] Liu Y, Fanburg BL. Serotonin-induced growth of pulmonary arterial smooth muscle requires activation of phosphatidylinositol3-kinase/serine-threonine protein kinase B/mammalian target of rapamycin/p70 ribosomal S6 kinase-1. *Am J Respir Crit Care Med* 2006; 34:182-191

[63] Löffler D, Brocke-Heidrich K, Pfeifer G, Stocsits C, Hackermüller et al. Interleukin-6-dependent survival of multiple myeloma cells involves the Stat3-mediated induction of microRNA-21 through a highly conerved enhancer. *Blood* 2007; 110:1330-1333

[64] Long L, MacLean MR, Jeffery TK, Morecroft I, Yang X et al. Serotonin increases susceptibility to pulmonary hypertension in BMPR2-deficeint mice. *Circ Res* 2006, 98(6), 818-827

[65] Lovern F, Pan Y, Quan A, Teoh H, Wang G et al. Angiotensin converting enzyme-2 confers endothelial protection and attenuates atherosclerosis. *Am J Physiol* 2008; 295:H1377-H1384

[66] Machado R, Aldred MA, James V, Harrison RE, Patel B et al. Mutations of the TGF-β type II receptor BMPR2 in pulmonary arterial hypertension. *Hum. Mutation* 2006, 27(2), 121-132.

[67] MacNee W, Tuder RM. New paradigms in the pathogenesis of chronic obstructive pulmonary disease. *Proc Am Thorac Soc* 2009; 6:527-531

[68] Maloney JP, Stearman RS, Bull TM, Calabreses DW, Tripp-Addison ML et al. Loss-of-function thrombospondin-1 mutations in familial pulmonary hypertension. *Am J Physiol* 2012; 302:L541-L554

[69] Mathai S, Hassoun PM. Pulmonary arterial hypertension associated with systemic sclerosis. *Expert Rev Respir Med* 2011; 5:267-279

[70] Mathew R, Gewitz MH. Pulmonary hypertension in infancy and childhood. *Heart Dis* 2000; 2:362-368.

[71] Mathew R. Inflammation and Pulmonary Hypertension. *Cardiol Rev* 2010; 18:67-7272.

[72] Mathew R. Pulmonary hypertension: current therapy and future prospects. *Cardiovasc Hematol Agents Medicinal Chem* 2011; 9:165-182

[73] Mathew R. Pulmonary Hypertension: Endothelial cell Function 2011a, pp 3-24. *In* Pulmonary hypertension: From Bench Research to Clinical Challenge. Eds Sulica R, Preston I. Publishers-INTECH. ISBN 978-953-307-835-9

[74] Mathew R. Cell-specific dual role of caveolin-1 in pulmonary hypertension. *Pulm Med* 2011; 2011b:573432

[75] Mathew R, Huang J, Katta UD, Krishnan U, Sandoval C, Gewitz MH. Immunosuppressant- induced endothelial damage and pulmonary arterial hypertension. *J Ped Hem Onc* 2011c; 33:55-58

[76] Mathew R. PDGF Receptor Blocker for Pulmonary Hypertension: A New Agent in Therapeutic Arsenal. Expert Opin Invest Drugs. 2012; 21:139-142

[77] Morrell NW, Yang X, Upton PD, Jourdan KB, Morgan N et al. Altered growth responses of pulmonary artery smooth muscle cells from patients with primary pulmonary hypertension to transforming growth factor –beta (1) and bone morphogenetic proteins. Circulation 2001; 104:790-795

[78] Moser KM, Bloor CM. Pulmonary vascular lesions occurring in patients with chronic major vessel thromboembolic pulmonary hypertension. Chest 1993; 103:685-692

[79] Murakami K, Mathew R, Huang J, Farahami R, Peng H et al Smurf-1 ubiquitin ligase causes downregulation of BMP receptors and is induced in monocrotaline and hypoxia models of pulmonary arterial hypertension. *Exp Biol Med* 2010; 235:805-813

[80] Nicoli S, Standley C, Walker P, Hurlstone A, Fogarty KE, Lawson ND. MicroRNA-mediated integration of hemodynamics and Vegf signaling during angiogenesis. *Nature* 2010; 464:1196-1200

[81] Nunes H, Humbert M, Capron F, Brauner M, Sitbon O et al. Pulmonary hypertension associated with sarcoidosis: mechanisms, hemodynamics and prognosis. *Thorax* 2006; 61:68-74

[82] Noureddine H, Gary-Bobo G, Alifano M, Marcos E, Saker M et al. Pulmonary artery smooth muscle cell senescence is a pathogenic mechanism for pulmonary hypertension in chronic lung disease. *Circ Res* 2011; 109:543-553

[83] Ocaranza MP, Rivera P, Novoa U, Pinto M, González L et al. Rho kinase inhibition activates the homologous angiotensin-converting enzyme-angiotensin-(1-9) axis in experimental hypertension, J Hypertens 2011; 29:706-715

[84] Ogawa A, Firth AL, Yao W, Madani MM, Kerr KM et al. Inhibition of mTOR attenuates store-operated Ca^{2+} entry in cells from endarterectomized tissues of patients with chronic thromboembolic pulmonary hypertension. *Am J Physiol* 2009; 297:L666-L676

[85] Ohta-Ogo K, Hao H, Ishibashi-Ueda H, Hirota S, Nakamura K et al. CD44 expression in plexiform lesions of idiopathic pulmonary arterial hypertension. *Path Int* 2012; 62:219-225

[86] Patel HH, Zhang S, Murray F, Suda RY, Head BP et al. Increased smooth muscle cell expression of caveolin-1 and caveolae contribute to the pathophysiology of idiopathic pulmonary arterial hypertension. *FASEB J.* 2007; 21:2970-2979

[87] Pengo V, Lensing AW, Prins MH, Marchiori A, Davidson Bl et al. Incidence of chronic thromboembolic pulmonary hypertension after pulmonary embolism. *New Eng J Med* 2004:350:2257-2264

[88] Perros F, Dorfmüller P, Souza R, Durand-Gasselin I, Mussot s et al. Dendritic recruitment in lesions of human and experimental pulmonary hypertension. *Eur Respir J* 2007; 29:462-468

[89] Perros F, Montani D, Dorfmuller P, Durand-Gasselin I, Tcherakian C et al. Platelet-derived growth factor expression and function in idiopathic pulmonary arterial hypertension. *Am J Respir Crit Care Med* 2008; 176:81-88

[90] Perros F, Dorfmüller P, Montani D, Hammad H, Waelput W et al. Pulmonary lymphoid neogenesis in idiopathic pulmonary arterial hypertension. *Am J Respir Crit Care Med* 2012; 185:311-321.

[91] Petrocca F, Vecchione A, Croce CM. Emerging role of miR-106b-25/miR-17-92 clusters in the control of transforming growth factor β signaling. *Cancer Res* 2008; 68:8191-8194

[92] Piao L, Marsboom G, Archer S L. Mitochondrial metabolic adaptation in right ventricular hypertrophy and failure. *J. Mol. Med.* 2010, 88:1011-1020

[93] Pogoriler JE, Rich S, Archer SL, Hussain AN. Persistence of complex vascular lesions despite prolonged prostacyclin therapy of pulmonary arterial hypertension. *Histopathology* 2012: PMID 22748137

[94] Pullamsetti SS, Doebele C, Fischer A, Savai R, Kojonazarov B et al. Inhibition of microRNA-17 improves lung and heart function in experimental pulmonary hypertension. *Am J Respir Crit Care Med* 2012; 185:409-419

[95] Radstake TR, van Bon L, Broen J, Weink M, Santigoets K et al. Increased frequency and compromised function of T regulatory cells in systemic sclerosis (SSc) is related diminished CD69 and TGF-β expression. *PLoS ONE* 2009; 4:e5981

[96] Razani B, Zhang XL, Bitzer M, von Gersdof G, Bottinger EP, Lisanti MP. Caveolin-1 regulates transforming growth factor (TGF) - β/SMAD signaling through an interaction with the TGF- β type 1 receptor. *J Biol Chem* 2001; 276:6727-6738

[97] Redoute EM, van der Toorn A, Zuidwijk MJ, van der Kolk CW, van Echteld CJ et al. Antioxidant treatment attenuates pulmonary arterial hypertension-induced heart failure. *Am. J. Physiol.* 2010, 298: H1038-H1047

[98] Remillard CV, Tigno DD, Platoshyn O, Burg ED, Brevnova EE, Conger D et al. Function of Kv1.5 channels and genetic variations of *KCNA5* in patients with idiopathic pulmonary arterial hypertension. *Am J Physiol* 2007; 292:C1837-C1853

[99] Richter A, Yeager ME, Zaiman A, Cool CD, Voelkel NF, Tuder RM. Impaired transforming growth factor – β signaling in idiopathic pulmonary arterial hypertension. *Am J Respir Crit Care Med* 2004; 170:1340-1348

[100] Rolfe BE, Worth NF, World CJ, Campbell JH, Campbell GR. Rho and vascular disease. *Atherosclerosis* 2005; 183:1-16.

[101] Roberts KE, McElroy JJ, Wang WP, Yen E, Widlitz A et al. BMPR2 mutations in pulmonary arterial hypertension with congenital heart disease. *Eur Respir J* 2004; 24:371-374

[102] Sabatel C, Malvaux L, Bovy N, Deroanne C, Lambert V et al. MicroRNA-21 exhibits antiangiogenic function by targeting RhoB expression in endothelial cells. *PLoS* One 2011; 6:e16979

[103] Sakao S, Taraseviciene-Stewart L, Lee JD, Wood K, Cool CD, Voelkel NF. Initial apoptosis is followed by increased proliferation of apoptosis-resistant endothelial cells. FASEB J 2005; 19:1178-1180

[104] Santibaniz JF, Blanco FJ, Garrido-Martin EM, Sanz-Rodriguez F, del Pozza MA, Bernabeu C. Caveolin-1 interacts and cooperates with transforming growth factor- β type 1 receptor ALK1 in endothelial caveolae. Cardivasc Res 2008; 77:791-799

[105] Schermuly RT, Dony E, Ghofrani HA, Pullamsetti S, Savai R et al. Reversal of experimental pulmonary hypertension by PDGF inhibition. *J Clin Invest* 2005; 115:2811-2821

[106] Shao ES, Lin L, Yao Y, Boström KI. Expression of vascular endothelial growth factor is coordinately regulated by the activin-like kinase receptors 1 and 5 in endothelial cells. *Blood* 2009; 114:2197-2206

[107] Shapiro S, Traiger GL, Turner M, McGoon MD, Wason P, Barst RJ. Sex differences in the diagnosis, treatment, and outcome of patients with pulmonary arterial hypertension enrolled in the registry to evaluate early and long-term pulmonary arterial hypertension disease management. *Chest* 2012; 141:363-373

[108] Shenoy V, Ferreira AJ, Qi Y, Fraga-Silva RA, Diez-Freire C, Dooies A et al. The angiotensin converting enzyme-2/angiogenesis-(1-7)/Mas axis confers cardiopulmonary protection against lung fibrosis and pulmonary hypertension. *Am J Respir Crit Care Med* 2010; 182:1065-1072

[109] Shintani M, Yagi H, Nakayama T, Saji T, Matsuoka R. A new nonsense mutation of SMAD8 associated with pulmonary arterial hypertension. *J Med Genet* 2009; 46:331-337

[110] Simonneau G, Robbins IM, Beghetti M, Channick RN, Delcroix M et al. Updated classification of pulmonary hypertension. *J Am Coll Cardiol* 2009; 54:S43-S54

[111] Sluiter I, van Heijst A, Hassdijk R, Kempen MB, Boerema-de Munck MA et al. Reversal of pulmonary vascular remodeling in pulmonary hypertensive rats. *Exp Pulm Pathol* 2012; 93:66-73.

[112] Song Y, Coleman L, Shi J, Beppu H, Sato K, Waksh K et al. Inflammation, endothelial injury and persistent pulmonary hypertension in heterozygous BMPR2 mutant mice. *Am. J. Physiol.* 2008, 295: H677-H690

[113] Song Z, Li G. Role of specific microRNAs in regulation of vascular smooth muscle cell differentiation and the response of injury. *J Cardiovasc Transl Res* 2010: 3:246-250

[114] Soon E, Holmes AM, Trearcy CM, Doughty NJ, Southgate L et al. Elevated levels of inflammatory cytokines predict survival in idiopathic and familial pulmonary arterial hypertension. *Circulation* 2010; 122:920-927.

[115] Sztrymf B, Yaïci A, Girerd B, Humbert M. Genes and pulmonary arterial hypertension. *Respiration* 2007:74:123-132

[116] Sztrymf B, Souza R, Bertoletti L, Jaïs X, Sitbon O e al Prognostic factors of acute heart failure in patients with pulmonary arterial hypertension. *Eur. Respir. J.* 2010; 35: 1286-1293

[117] Tamby MC, Chanseaud Y, Humbert M, Fermanian J Guilpain P et al. Anti endothelial cell antibodies in idiopathic and systemic-sclerosis associated pulmonary arterial hypertension. *Thorax* 2005; 60:765-772

[118] Terrier B, Tamby MC, Camoin L, Guilpain P, Broussard C et al. Identification of target antigens in antifibroblasts antibodies in pulmonary arterial hypertension. *Am J Respir Crit Care Med* 2008; 177:1128-1134

[119] Thenappan T, Shah SJ, Gomberg-Maitland M, Collander B, Vallakati A et al. Clinical characteristics of pulmonary hypertension in patients with heart failure and preserved ejection fraction. *Circ Heart Failure* 2011; 4:257-265

[120] Thomson JR, Machado RD, Pauciulo MW, Morgan NW, Humbert M et al. Sporadic primary pulmonary hypertension is associated with germline mutations of the gene encoding BMPR-II, a receptor member of the TGF-beta family. *J. Med. Genet.* 2000, 37(10), 741-745

[121] Tiechert-Kuliszewska-K, Kutryk MJ, Kuliszewski MA, Karoubi G et al. Bone morphogenetic protein receptor-2 signaling promotes pulmonary arterial endothelial cell survival: Implications for loss-of-function mutations in the pathogenesis of pulmonary hypertension. *Circ Res* 2006; 98:209-217

[122] Tourkina E, Hoffman S. Caveolin-1 signaling in lung fibrosis. *Open Rheumatol* J 2012; 6:116-122

[123] Trambath RC, Thomson JR, Machado RD, Morgan NV, Atkinson C et al. Clinical and molecular genetic features of pulmonary hypertension in patients with hereditary hemorrhagic talengiectasia. *N. Eng. J. Med.* 2001, 345: 325-334

[124] Tuder RM, Groves B, Badesch DB, Voelkel NF. Exuberant endothelial cell growth and elements of inflammation are present in plexiform lesions of pulmonary hypertension. *Am J Path* 1994; 144:275-285

[125] Tuder RM, Chacon M, Alger L, Wang J, Taraseviciene-Stewart L et al. Expression of angiogenesis-related molecules in plexiform lesions in severe pulmonary hypertension: evidence for a process of disordered angiogenesis. *J Pathol* 2001; 195:367-374

[126] Urbich C, Kuehbacher A, Dimmeler S. Role of microRNAs in vascular diseases, inflammation and angiogenesis. *Cardiovasc Res* 2008; 79:581-588

[127] van Loon RL, Roofthooft MT, Hillege HL, ten Harkel AD, van Osch-Gevers M et al. Pediatric pulmonary hypertension in Netherlands: Epidemiology and characterization during period 1991 to 2005. *Circulation* 2011; 124:1755-1764

[128] Wagenvoort CA, Wagenvoort N. Primary pulmonary hypertension:a pathologic study of the lung vessels in 165 clinically diagnosed cases. *Circulation* 1970; 42:1163-1184

[129] Wang XM, Zhang Y, Kim HP, Zhou Z, Feghali-Bostwick CA et al. Caveolin-1 : a critical regulator of lung fibrosis in interstitial pulmonary fibrosis. *J Exp Med* 2006; 203:2895-2906

[130] Wang XM, Nadeau PE, Lin S, Abbott JR, Mergia A. Caveolin-1 inhibits HIV replication by transcriptional repression mediated through NF-κB. *J Virol* 2011; 85:5483-5493

[131] Weber M, Baker MB, Moore JP, Searles CD. Mir-21 is induced in endothelial cells by shear stress and modulates apoptosis and eNOS activity. *Biochem Biophys Res Comm* 2010; 393:643-648

[132] Yu PB, Deng DY, Beppu H, Hong CC, Lai C et al. Bone morphogenetic protein (BMP) type II receptor is required for BMP-mediated growth arrest and differentiation in pulmonary artery smooth muscle cells. *J Biol Chem.* 2008; 283:3877-3888

[133] Zhang B, Pan X, Cobb GP, Anderson TA. MicroRNAs as oncogenes and tumor suppressors. *Dev Biol* 2007; 302:1-12

Chapter 4

Nitric Oxide in Pathophysiology and Treatment of Pulmonary Hypertension

Junko Maruyama, Ayumu Yokochi, Erquan Zhang,
Hirofumi Sawada and Kazuo Maruyama

Additional information is available at the end of the chapter

http://dx.doi.org/10.5772/55680

1. Introduction

All conditions causing pulmonary hypertension (PH) are characterized by three major changes in the pulmonary vasculature: vasoconstriction, vascular remodeling, and thrombosis [1,2,3]. Vascular remodeling includes muscularization of normally non-muscular peripheral pulmonary arteries, increase in medial wall thickness of muscular arteries, and increase in vascular connective tissue such as collagen and elastin [1,2,3]. Imbalance of vasoconstrictive and vasodilatory mediators might explain the increased vascular tone [1,2,3]. Endothelial cells synthesize and release prostacylin and nitric oxide for vasodilation as well as endothelin and thromboxane for vasoconstriction. Approved treatments for pulmonary arterial hypertension (PAH) include prostacyclins, endothelin receptor blockers, and phosphodiesterase-5 inhibitors as well as inhaled NO for persistent pulmonary hypertension of the neonate (PPHN) [2].

Studies have demonstrated that short- and long-term NO inhalation improves arterial oxygenation and reduces pulmonary artery (PA) pressure in animal models of PH [4,5,6,7,8,9,10] and clinical disease such as post-operative congenital heart disease [11,12], chronic obstructive pulmonary disease (COPD) [13], pulmonary fibrosis [14], and acute respiratory distress syndrome (ARDS) [15]. In chronic hypoxia-induced PH in rats, we showed that low-dose NO (less than 5ppm) induces a submaximal reduction in pulmonary artery pressure, which does not correlate with the severity of pulmonary vascular changes [4]. Clinically, the effect of inhaled NO is based on pulmonary vasorelaxation. In experimental settings, NO inhibits vascular smooth muscle cell proliferation directly through regulating protein kinases modulating gene expression for cell growth and/or indirectly through reducing pressure on the vascular cells by cyclic guanosine-3′,5′-monophosphate (cGMP) dependent vascular relaxation. In this chapter we will discuss NO and its regulation and function with special references to the development of PH as well as pulmonary vascular reactivity in PH.

2. Biological effects of NO

2.1. NO acts through the sGC pathway and S-nitrosylation of target proteins

NO activates soluble guanylyl cyclase (sGC) stimulating cGMP production and subsequent activation of cGMP-dependent protein kinase (PKG). This sGC-cGMP-PKG pathway plays a major role in NO-mediated regulation. In addition to this pathway, NO directly binds to proteins and induces conformational changes with subsequent functional alterations, like phosphorylation. Thus, S-nitration is also called S-nitrosylation, the term which emphasizes a biological effect of the chemical reaction of S-nitration [16]. S-nitrosylation modifies the activity of some kinases and phosphatases, thus raising the possibility that NO modifies phosphorylation and dephosphorylation through S-nitrosylation.

NO reacts with oxygen, transitional metal ions, thiols, and superoxides, exerting its effects via cGMP-dependent and/or -independent pathways. cGMP effector molecules include cGMP-dependent protein kinases type-I and –II, cGMP-activated phosphodiesterases, and cGMP-gated ion channels. Similar to phosphorylation, S-nitrosylation regulates protein function allosterically or by direct modification of cysteine.

In the vascular system, NO reacts with sGC forming cGMP, which activates cGMP-dependent protein kinase decreasing vascular smooth muscle cell cytoplasmic Ca^{2+} concentration by 1) activation of proteins such as Ca^{2+}-sensitive potassium channels which decrease membrane potential thereby causing hyperpolarization and closing voltage dependent Ca^{2+} channels; 2) phosphorylation of voltage- and receptor-operated sarcolemmal Ca^{2+} channels, causing them to close; 3) inhibition of the inositol 1,3,5-trisphospate-sensitive Ca^{2+} release channel of the sarcoplasmic reticulum [17].

2.2. NO prevents the development of PH

NO mediates vasorelaxation, anticoagulation, and anti-proliferation, as well as neurotransmission. Several earlier studies demonstrated that NO inhibits smooth muscle cell growth by a cGMP-dependent mechanism [18] in addition to inhibiting growth regulating enzymes such as ribonucleotide reductase and thymidine kinase [19,20]. NO also suppresses the hypoxia-induced increase in ET-1 and platelet-derived growth factor-B, both of which have vasoconstriction and growth effects [21]. These effects of NO led investigators to determine whether administration of NO prevents the development of PH. Chronic NO inhalation ameliorates the development of hypertensive pulmonary vascular changes of chronic hypoxia-induced PH in rats [22], but not in monocrotaline (MCT)-induced PH [23]. In contrast, supplementation with the NO precursor, L-arginine, but not D-arginine prevented the development of PH in both models [24]. The reason for the different effects of NO inhalation is unclear, but may be a result of differing pathogenic mechanisms in the two models of PH: the increase in pulmonary pressures precedes the vascular structural changes in chronic hypoxia-induced PH, whereas the reverse sequence of events occurs in MCT-induced PH. Endogenous NO from L-arginine could prevent the development of new muscularization of peripheral pulmonary arteries in both models, whereas exogenous inhaled NO would be effective only in hypoxia-induced PH because of the reduction in pulmonary vascular pressures caused by NO mediated vasodilation.

Inhaled NO likely attenuates the hypertensive vascular structural changes through pulmonary vasodilation by a cGMP-mediated mechanism. Endogenous NO from L-arginine might also prevent the development of structural changes through a cGMP-mediated mechanism. This hypothesis is supported by another study that showed that pulmonary gene transfection of atrial natriuretic peptide (ANP), another inducer of cGMP, attenuates the development of chronic hypoxia-induced pulmonary vascular changes [25]. Treatment to increase NO production in the pulmonary vascular bed by eNOS gene transfection ameliorates the development of PH. Studies have demonstrated that eNOS transfected smooth muscle cell administration prevented the development of MCT-induced PH [26] and that eNOS transfected bone marrow-derived endothelial-like progenitor cell venous administration reversed established MCT-induced PH [27].

3. Endogenous NO production

3.1. Nitrate (NO_3^-) and nitrite (NO_2^-) as sources of NO (Figure 1)

NO is produced from L-arginine by nitric oxide synthase (NOS) in the presence of oxygen, tetrahydrobiopterin (BH4), and reduced NADPH[3]. Recent studies have indicated that inorganic anions, nitrate (NO_3^-) and nitrite (NO_2^-), can be recycled to NO in vivo as alternative sources of NO in addition to the classical NOS-NO pathway. The source of nitrate includes the endogenous NOS-NO synthase pathway and the diet. Green vegetables such as lettuce and spinach provide nitrate and preservatives in cured meat and bacon include nitrite. Basically reduction of nitrate and nitrite produce NO, thus nitrate and nitrite are considered an 'endocrine reservoir' of NO [28].

Nitrate in the plasma is excreted into the saliva, whereas nitrate is reduced by the oral anerobic bacteria producing nitrite. These bacteria use nitrate as an electron acceptor instead of oxygen during respiration. During its subsequent movement into the stomach, nitrite undergoes further reduction to NO, thus leading to gastric NO formation, which may play a role in gastric mucosa maintenance. This is a entro-salivary circulation of nitrate. In the systemic circulation intravascular nitrite is reduced to NO by deoxyHb, respiratory chain enzymes, xanthine oxidoreductase, deoxygenated myoglobin, and protons (29). They facilitate the transfer of protons to NO_2^-, causing NO production which is intensified under acidic and hypoxic states. Artery-to-vein gradients in nitrite are observed.

Nitrite has a vasodilatory effect. Inhaled nebulized sodium nitrite reduces pulmonary artery pressure (PAP) without changes in systemic artery pressure in hypoxia- or thromboxane-

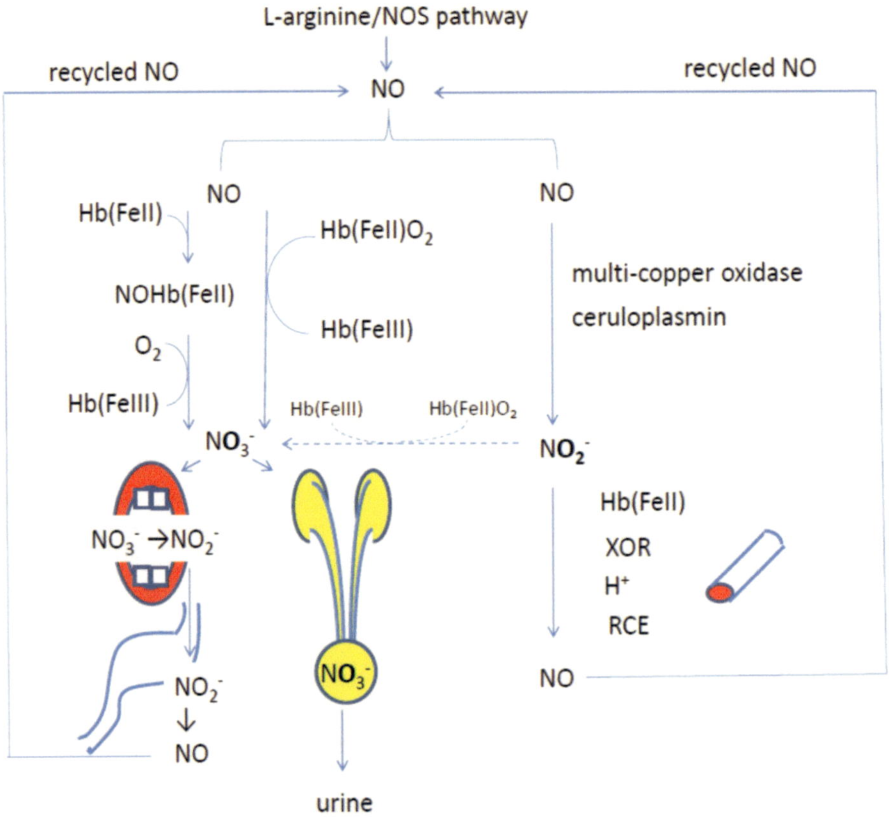

Figure 1. Recycling of NO from NO_2- Endogenous NO includes NO produced from L-arginine by NOS and recycled NO from NO_2^-. NO is converted to NO_3^- by the reaction with the Hb and /or to NO_2^- by the oxidation in the plasma with the aid of multicopper oxidase and NO oxidase ceruloplasmin. NO_3^- is excreted into urine by kidney and/or into oral cavity by salivary gland. In the oral cavity anaerobic bacteria reduces NO_3^- converting to NO_2^-, which goes down into stomach and is protonated under the gastric acidic state forming nitrous acid (HNO_2) with further decomposition to NO and/or other nitrogen oxides. NO_2^- in the plasma is reduced and converted to NO by the reductase activity of deoxygenated hemoglobin, xanthine oxidoreductase, respiratory chain enzymes, and hydrogen ion. Hb(FeII), deoxygenated hemoglobin;Hb(FeII)O_2, oxygenated hemoglobin; NO, nitric oxide; NOHb(FeII), nitrosylhemoglobin; NOS, nitric oxide synthase; NO_2^-, nitrite, NO_3^-, nitrate; XOR, xanthine oxidoreductase; Hb(FeIII), methemoglobin; REC, respiratory chain enzymes

induced PH [30]. Intravenous administration of sodium nitrite reverses PH induced by hypoxia or thromboxane analogs [31]. Furthermore, intermittent nebulization of sodium nitrite ameliorated the muscularization and hyperplasia of small pulmonary arteries, the development of right ventricular hypertrophy, and the rise in right ventricular pressure in chronic hypoxia- or MCT-induced PH in rats [32], which is similar to L-arginine administration[33].

The effects of inhaled NO are not restricted to the lung. Recent studies have shown that inhaled NO improves neurological and left ventricular dysfunction after successful cardiopulmonary resuscitation [34] as well as liver function after liver transplantation [35]. Inhaled NO is converted to nitrate and nitrite when it enters the blood [36, 37]. NO can be recycled from nitrite and be used to protect organs from ischemia reperfusion injury.

http://dx.doi.org/10.5772/55680

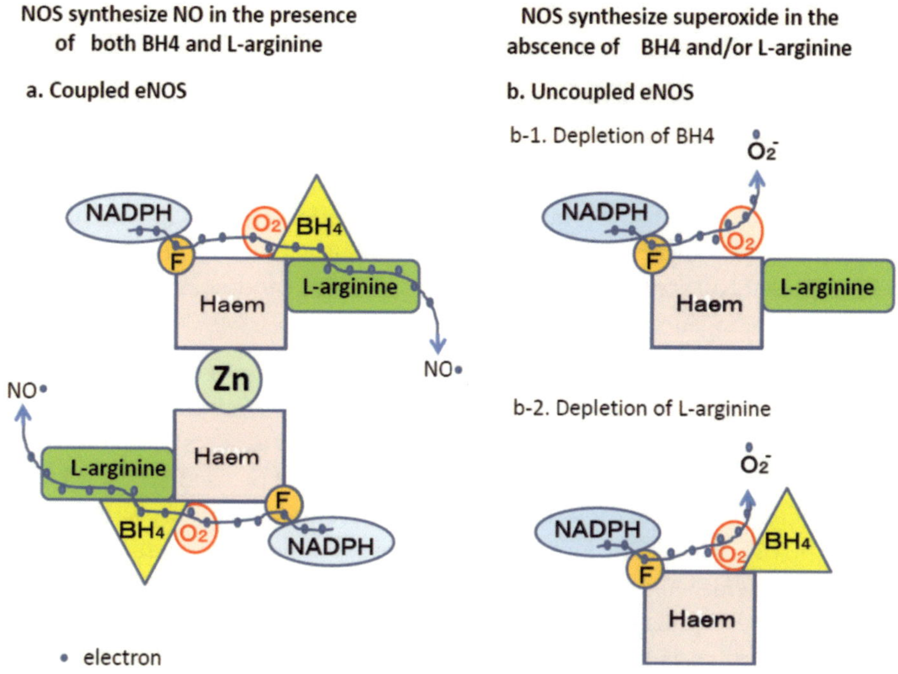

Figure 2. Coupled eNOS (eNOS homodimer) produces NO. (a) eNOS homodimer produces NO, whereas eNOS monomer produces superoxide. eNOS uncoupling occurs during the conversion of eNOS homodimer to eNOS monomer. Two eNOS monomers are connected with the aid of Zn^{2+}, making eNOS homodimer. BH4 strengthen the Zn^{2+} connection, maintaining the dimer form. In coupled NOS, an electron is transferred to L-arginine, producing NO and L-citrulline. (b) electron(•) from NADPH is transferred to O_2 in the uncoupled eNOS in absence of BH4(b-1) and/or L-arginine(b-2), thereby producing superoxide. BH4, tetrahydrobiopterin; eNOS, endothelial nitric oxide synthase; F, flavin; NADPH, nicotinamide adenine dinucleotide phosphate

3.2. NOS uncoupling: NOS produces NO and superoxide depending on whether it is a homodimer or monomer (Figure2)

In the process of NO formation from oxygen and L-arginine, oxygen molecules are incorporated in both NO and L-citrulline, showing that NOS is a dioxygenase [38]. NOS containes both a reductase domain and an oxygenase domain, where electron transfer occurs from the reductase domain to the oxygenase domain. NADPH and flavin bind to the reductase domain, while oxygen, BH4 and L-arginine bind to the oxgenase domain. Electrons are transferred from NADPH through the flavin containing reductase domain to the oxygenase domain [39]. Then two cascades of further electron transfer occur depending on the presence or absence of BH4 and L-arginine. When both BH4 and L-arginine are present, NO is synthesized by oxidative deamination of arginine by NOS, where the electron is transferred to L-arginine. The initial step of L-arginine oxidation is donation of electrons to the ferrous–dioxygen complex from BH4, where trihydrobiopterin is produced and the electron is supplied through flavin regaining BH4 [40]. In contrast, in the absence of L-arginine or BH4, NOS synthesizes the superoxide, where the electron is transferred to ferrous oxygen. Intracellular deficiency of BH4 induces superoxide generation from eNOS [40]. The term "eNOS uncoupling" means functionally that electron transfer to L-arginine is uncoupled, when the electron is transferred to ferrous-dioxygen instead of L-arginine, producing superoxide. NOS homodimer produces NO from L-arginine and oxygen, whereas NOS monomer produces superoxide [41]. Thus, the molecular basis of eNOS uncoupling is conversion of the NOS dimer to the NOS monomer. To maintain the NOS dimer, BH4 is essential and dihydrobiopterin (BH2) is the oxidized form of BH4. Peroxinitrite oxidizes BH4 to BH2, reducing the BH4 amount and/or the BH2/BH4 ratio, both of which induce eNOS uncoupling [42]. The effects of BH4 are mediated through the regulation of NO compared with superoxide synthesis by endothelial NOS. Since BH4 might both augment NO synthesis and decrease superoxide production, BH4 deficiency may play a role in the pathogenesis of PH.

eNOS uncoupling is evaluated by the eNOS dimer/monomer ratio in cold SDS-PAGE Western blot analysis. While oxidative stress reduces the eNOS dimer/monomer ratio in a cardiac hypertrophic model suggesting eNOS uncoupling, exogenous BH4 restored the eNOS dimer/monomer ratio [43]. Administration of exogenous BH4 might be used for eNOS uncoupling diseases. BH4 deficiency might cause PH in mice and BH4 augmentation might ameliorate the development of PH. Mice with low BH4 tissue levels develop PH which is reversed by increasing BH4 with targeted transgenic overexpression of the rate-limiting enzyme in BH4 synthesis, guanosine triphosphate(GTP) cyclohydrolase [44]. Lung BH4 availability is controlled by pulmonary vascular tone, right ventricular hypertrophy, and vascular structural remodeling. BH4 is a cofactor of NOS in the production of NO. BH4 deficiency causes decreased NO production with concomitant production of superoxide by NOS. Chronic administration of BH4 analogues improves NO-mediated pulmonary artery dilatation in rats with chronic hypoxic pulmonary hypertension [45]. Copresence of increased levels of NOS and reduced NO bioactivity might be explained by the deficiency of BH4 and/or L-arginine.

Long-term increases in NO might increase eNOS expression and eNOS uncoupling, thereby producing superoxide. Long-term administration of nitroglycerin (TNG) increased eNOS mRNA and protein expression and vascular superoxide ($O_2^{\bullet-}$) in intact vessels monitored using ESR spectroscopy [46]. An earlier study showed that endothelial denudation improves vascular relaxation induced by TNG in isolated vessels from nitrate-tolerant animals [47].

3.3. Caveolin and NOS (Figure 3)

Caveolae are flask-shaped invaginations on the cell surface, which contain structural proteins called caveolin and other signaling proteins. In endothelial cells, eNOS is inactivated when it is conjugated to caveolin-1, a structural protein of endothelial caveolae; eNOS is activated when it dissociates from caveolae. Stimulation of β2 adrenergic receptors cause this dissociation through phosphorylation of Tyr in caveolin-1. The mouse pulmonary endothelial β2 adrenergic receptor coupled to Gi/o proteins causes phosphorylation of caveolon-1 by Src kinase and eNOS phosphorylation at ser^{1177} by the Src kinase - phosphatidylinositol 3 kinase (PI3kinase) - Akt kinase pathway [48]. Thus, stimulation of the β2 adrenergic receptor causes endothelial NO synthase-dependent relaxation.

Loss of caveolin-1 induces chronic activation of eNOS and subsequent tyrosine nitration of PKG in lungs from patients with idiopathic pulmonary hypertension, where activated eNOS is uncoupled eNOS, producing superoxide [49]. Genetic deletion of caveolin in mice causes PH and treatment with a superoxide scavenger and/or a NOS inhibitor prevents PH associated vascular remodeling [49]. Although caveolin expression in total lung determined by Western blotting is not altered in severe PH, its immunohistological expression in plexiform lesions is absent or decreased [50].

A 90-kDa heat shock protein (HSP90) is a molecular chaperone of proteins that modulates protein functions. Along with many other proteins, eNOS and sGC are targets for HSP90. HSP90 interacts with eNOS and HSP90 facilitates the displacement of eNOS from caveolin 1, activating eNOS. HSP90 activity is dependent on adenosine triphosphate (ATP). Asymmetric dimethylarginine (ADMA) inhibits HSP90 activity in pulmonary endothelial cells through mitochondrial dysfunction, caused by ADMA induced eNOS uncoupling with subsequent superoxide production and nitration of mitochondrial protein, which reduce ATP production [51].

3.4. eNOS expression and activity in PH

To examine whether the change in eNOS expression and its activity is associated with vascular endothelial dysfunction in PH, many studies have been performed in several species of animals and humans, using isolated lung, isolated pulmonary artery, and in vivo. eNOS is expressed in not only vascular endothelial cells, but lung epithelial cells. In addition, eNOS expression and/or activity might be different between conduit PAs and resistance PAs.

Animal models

mRNA and protein expression of eNOS in rat lung and eNOS expression localized in pulmonary vascular endothelial cells and epithelial cells is upregulated in acute hypoxia [52]. In that study, nitrate/nitrite in rat lung homogenate also increased, suggesting augmented eNOS activity. The enhancement of eNOS activity in hypoxic pulmonary vasoconstriction (HPV) in normal rat lung also has been shown in other studies using NOS inhibitors [53, 54] (see sect. 3.1). eNOS protein expression was time-dependently increased in rats in chronic hypoxia-induced PH [55,56], while phosphorylated eNOS (peNOS), active form, was impaired [55]. MCT-induced PH rats showed decreased expression of both eNOS [57,58,59] and peNOS [59].

Human

Many studies of eNOS expression and its activity have been performed in adult human PAH. However, the results are not consistent: eNOS expression is reduced in pulmonary vessels from adults with primary and secondary PH, but is increased in plexiform lesions [60]. Western blot analysis showed that eNOS expression is not changed in the lung tissue of idiopathic PAH (IPAH) patients [61]. However, several studies reported lower exhaled nitrate/nitrite (NOx) in PAH patients [62,63]. Overall, these results suggest that eNOS activity might be depressed in adult human PAH.

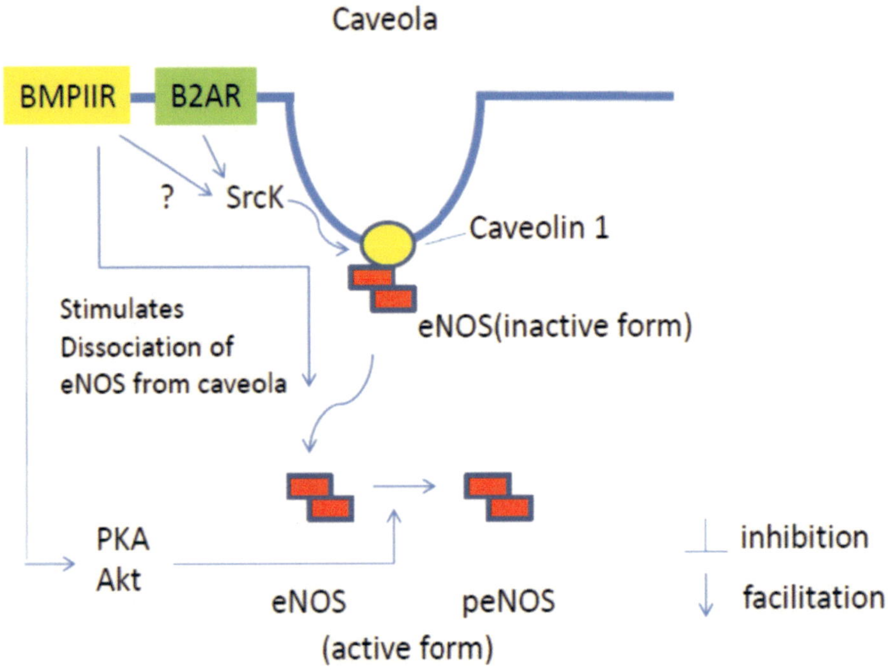

Figure 3. Inactive form of eNOS associated with caveola. eNOS is associated with caveola, which is the inactive form of eNOS. The active form of eNOS is dissociated from caveola. Stimulation of BMPIIR induces dissociation of eNOS from caveola as well as phosphorylation of eNOS through PKA and/or Akt activation. eNOS, endothelial nitric oxide synthase; B2-AR, beta 2-adrenergic receptor; SrcK, src kinase; peNOS, phosphorylated eNOS; BMPIIR, bone morphogenetic ptotein II receptor; PKA, cyclic AMP-dependent protein kinase

4. Endothelium-dependent and -independent NO-mediated relaxation in pulmonary circulation

4.1. Role of endothelium-derived NO in basal tone

L-NMMA (N omega-monomethyl–L-arginine), L-NNA (N omega-nitro-L-arginine), L-NAME (N omega-nitro-L-arginine methyl ester), L-NA(N omega-nitro-L-arginine) and other NOS inhibitors have been used to examine the physiological role of NO in pulmonary vascular tone. The increase in vascular tone in the presence of NOS inhibitors may indirectly represent NO production and/or release in the pulmonary circulation.

Animals

L-NMMA [53] and L-NNA [64,65] did not change pulmonary basal tone in normal rat PA rings. Normal isolated perfused lungs were not affected by NOS inhibitors such as L-NMMA [53], L-NNA [64], and L-NA [66] except for a few studies showing a moderate increase with L-NAME [67]. In chronic hypoxia, many studies showed markedly enhanced vascular tone by L-NNA [64] or L-NAME [67]. Although these NOS inhibitors caused different results, the findings suggested that 1) NO might not be involved in vascular basal tone in normal pulmonary circulation, and 2) basal NO production might be increased in hypoxia-induced chronic

PH. On exposure to acute hypoxia, NOS inhibitors augmented vascular contraction in normal [53,67,68] and hypoxia-induced PH rat models [67]. This finding suggests that NO production in HPV is increased in both normal and hypoxic PH rats.

Humans

Inhibition of NO production by L-NMMA caused the reduction of pulmonary flow in conscious healthy adults [69,70], suggesting the possible role of continuous production of NO in maintaining basal vascular tone. In PAH patients, several studies reported decreased expression of NOS. Although several studies reported decreased exhaled nitrogen oxide (NOx) levels in PAH patients, others have reported higher levels. The results therefore remain inconclusive.

4.2. Vasoreactivity to endothelium-dependent and independent NO-related relaxing substances in rat lung

Many studies have been performed using acetylcholine (Ach) and sodium nitroprusside (SNP), endothelium-dependent and -independent NO-related vasorelaxants, to examine functional changes in vascular endothelial and smooth muscle cells in PH. As Ach-induced relaxation was abolished by NOS inhibitors [64] and restored with L-arginine [71,72], reactivity may partly reflect changes in NOS expression and/or activity.

Rats with hypoxic PH

The relaxation response to Ach is impaired in rat isolated conduit pulmonary arteries (PAs) [65,73,74,75,76]. Many of these studies also described an impaired relaxation response to SNP in conduit PAs [65,74,76]. These results suggested 1) decreased production and release of NO in endothelial cells or 2) decreased responsiveness to NO in smooth muscle cells, or both. Impaired relaxation in Ach and SNP was partially restored after exposure to chronic hypoxia. As the recovery process was different between the responses of Ach and SNP [65], it was speculated that NO-related functional abnormalities in endothelial and smooth muscle cells occurred independently.

In contrast, in hypoxic vasoconstriction resistant rat PA rings, the relaxation response to Ach was not changed [74,75] or augmented [77] in chronic hypoxia. It is likely that Ach-reactive NO production and/or release varies in a vascular site-specific manner. Conduit arteries produce and release more eNOS than peripheral arteries. The vascular functional change in response to stimuli such as abnormal shear stress, circumferential wall stretch and hypoxia itself may occur in conduit PAs more than in peripheral resistant arteries. Although conduit arteries do not directly relate to pulmonary vascular resistance, the pathophysiological change in conduit arteries may play a key role in pulmonary vascular remodeling [78].

Impaired response to Ach was partly restored in the presence of a non-selective inhibitor of cyclooxygenase (COX) [65] or prostaglandin (PG) H_2 / thromboxane (TX) A_2 receptor antagonist [79], suggesting the possibility of 1) imbalance between the production of vasocontracting and vasorelaxing prostanoid in vascular endothelial cells, and 2) simultaneously release of vasocontracting prostanoids such as PGH_2 and/or TXA_2. Pidgeon et al. showed that the basal expression of COX2, otherwise known as PGH synthase, was increased in rat lungs in chronic hypoxia, and a PGH_2/TXA_2 receptor antagonist attenuated the rise in PAP induced by chronic hypoxia [80].

MCT-induced PH in rats

PA vascular functional changes in rats with MCT-induced PH have been compared with PAs from animals with chronic hypoxia-induced PH. Many vasodilation studies have reported a depressed relaxation response to Ach in MCT-induced rat conduit PA rings [76,81,82,83,84]. Many of these studies described impaired SNP relaxation, [76,82] with the exception of one study [84]. While Ach-induced relaxation was impaired in the pulmonary circulation in MCT-induced PH, the SNP relaxation response has been reported to be impaired [85] or not impaired [86]. Taken together, in MCT-induced PH, vascular endothelial dysfunction is observed from proximal to distal PAs; however, smooth muscle functional alteration is not apparent in peripheral PAs.

5. Superoxide scavenges NO producing peroxynitrite (Figure 4)

5.1. Oxidative stress

In pulmonary hypertension, endothelial NOS expression is increased, which may not necessarily indicate an increase in NO production [87]. NOS might produce superoxide, which is due to uncoupling of NOS [88]. Increased levels of NOS and reduced NO bioactivity might be explained by the deficiency of BH4 and/or L-arginine. Oxidative stress induces the changes of BH4 to BH2. Oxidative stress also induces S-glutathionylation and subsequent eNOS uncoupling [39], in which S-glutathionylation of eNOS reversibly decreases NOS activity with an increase in $O_2^{\bullet-}$ generation primarily from the reductase and endothelium-dependent relaxation is impaired. Oxidative stress upregulates nuclear factor (NF)-kappaB, a key transcription factor that is involved in vascular tissue remodeling. NF-kappaB nuclear localization and vascular cell adhesion molecule 1(VCAM-1) expression is temporally and spatially associated with the development of MCT-induced PH in rats, which is ameliorated by administering a NF-kappaB inhibitor, pyrrolidine dithiocarbamate(PDTC)[89].

5.2. Production of superoxide in PH: role of NADPH oxidase and SOD

NAD(P)H oxidase enzyme complex catalyzes one electron reduction of oxygen using NADPH or NADH as an electron donor, which produces superoxide : $NAD(P)H + 2O_2 \rightarrow NAD(P)^+ + H^+ + 2O_2^{-}$ NADPH oxidase expression is increased in pulmonary arteries from a lamb model of persistent pulmonary hypertension of the newborn (PPHN) [90]. The expression was determined by the Western blotting of the levels of $p67^{phox}$ a subunit of the NADPH oxidase complex and immunostaining of the pulmonary vessels in lung sections. Another study demonstrated that expression and activity of the NADPH oxidase complex are upregulated in PH with increased pulmonary blood flow [91].

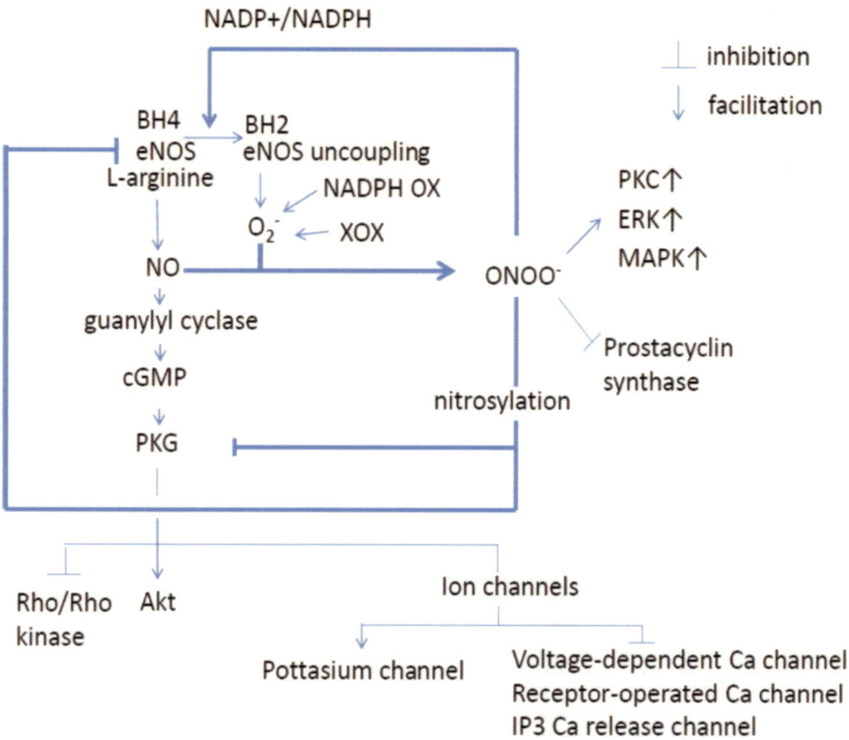

Figure 4. Peroxynitrite production from NO and superoxide. Superoxide ($O_2^{\cdot-}$) is produced by uncoupled eNOS, NADPH oxidase, and xanthine oxidase. NO reacts with $O_2^{\cdot-}$ producing peroxynitrite(ONOO$^-$) with subsequent nitrosylation of protein kinases, thereby activating or suppressing their activities. PKG phosphorylates Rho kinase, Akt, and ion channels. Phosphorylation of ion channels makes Ca^{2+} ion channels closed and potassium channel open. Peroxynitrite further oxidize BH4 to BH2, inducing eNOS uncoupling with subsequent superoxide production. BH4, tetrahydrobiopterin; BH2, dihydrobiopterin; eNOS, endothelial nitric oxide synthase; ERK, extracellular signal-regulated kinase; IP3, inositol triphosphate receptor; MAPK, mitogen-activated protein kinase; OX, oxidase; ONOO$^-$, peroxynitrite; PKC, protein kinase C; PKG, cyclic-GMP dependent protein kinase(protein kinase G); XOX, xanthine oxidase;

Deficiency of superoxide dismutase (SOD) may play a role in the development of PH. Expression and activity of mitochondrial SOD2 in patients and animal models of PH is decreased [92,93] in pulmonary arteries and plexiform lesions. SOD produces H_2O_2 from mitochondrial superoxide. H_2O_2 is less potent than superoxide and acts as a signaling molecule to inhibit transcriptional factors such as hypoxia-inducible factor-1α. Epigenetic suppression of SOD with selective hypermethylation of CpG islands in SOD2 gene induces excessive proliferation and decreases apoptosis in pulmonary artery smooth muscle cells [92], suggesting a causative role of SOD deficiency in PH.

NO reacts with superoxide more rapidly than SOD producing peroxinitrite. Peroxynitrite is a more potent and versatile oxidant than NO or superoxide, in which HO^{+} and NO_2 produced from peroxynitrous acid (HOONO) and/or its reactive activated isomer (HOONO*) attacks biological targets [94] including cyclic GMP-dependent protein kinase (PKG). In the setting of eNOS uncoupling, eNOS synthesizes superoxide which reacts with NO to create peroxynitrite. Nitrosylation of PKG by ONOO$^-$ depresses the function of PKG (42).

6. Prevention of hypertensive pulmonary vascular remodeling through NOS/NO pathway

6.1. NO precursor L-arginine ameliorates PH

Arginase, an enzyme in the urea cycle, converts arginine to ornithine and urea. NOx concentrations in exhaled gas and serum are decreased in PH patients compared with normal persons [95], suggesting decreased NO availability in PH. The deficiency of the NO precursor L-arginine, the substrate depletion of NOS, might partly explain the decrease in NO availability. Lower levels of arginine in the cell might be due to the increased activity of arginase. In PH patients, lower levels of arginine correlate with higher pulmonary artery pressures. Serum arginase activity is higher and the serum arginine-ornithine ratio is lower in PH patients than in healthy controls, indirectly suggesting increased intracellular arginase activity [33]. Animal studies showed that prolonged administration of L-arginine ameliorated the development of monocrotaine-induced PH [24,96] and chronic hypoxia-induced PH [96]. In patients with PH L-arginine treatment reduces PAP [97]. In addition to functioning as the substrate for NO formation, L-arginine prevents eNOS uncoupling, serves as a direct radical scavenger, and competes with the endogenous eNOS inhibitor ADMA, which decreases superoxide and increases NO formation [41].

6.2. ATRA increases NO production (Figure 5)

The level of asymmetrical dimethylarginine (ADMA) is increased in patients with PAH and MCT-induced PH in rats [98]. Since ADMA is an endogenous competitive inhibitor of NOS and suppresses NOS activity, increases in ADMA inhibit NO production. In atherosclerotic arteries from patients with high serum ADMA, endothelium-dependent relaxation by acetylcholine was impaired and $O_2^{\bullet-}$ production was increased [99]. Dysregulation of ADMA might cause PH through the decrease in NO in the lung as well. Dimethylarginine dimethyaminohydrolase (DDAH) is a metabolizing enzyme of ADMA. Thus the increase in DDAH activity reduces ADMA and induces subsequent increases in NOS activity. DDAH has two isoforms: DDAH 1 and DDAH 2. DDHA 1 and DDAH 2 are expressed predominantly in tissues containing neuronal NOS (nNOS) and eNOS, respectively [100]. Phosphodiesterase (PDE) 3/4 inhibitors reduce ADMA and raise NO/cGMP levels [2]; PDE3/4 inhibitors activate the cAMP/protein kinase A (PKA) pathway and induce subsequent activation of the promoter region of DDAH2. Western blot analysis of lung from PH rats 28 days after the injection of MCT showed decreases in eNOS, pNOS, AKT, and DDAH2 and increases in lung and serum ADMA levels [101]. In this PH model, 1) decreased Akt reduces eNOS phosphorylation and thereby decreases eNOS activity 2) decreased DDAH2 reduces ADMA breakdown and thereby the increase in ADMA inhibits eNOS activity. This study showed that rosuvastatin ameliorates MCT-induced PH through the normalization of Akt, eNOS and DDAH2 expression and ADMA levels [101].

Endothelial cells express retinoid receptors and all-trans-retinoic acid (ATRA) increased DDHA2 mRNA levels in endothelial cells. Although eNOS mRNA expression is not increased with ATRA treatment, ATRA increases NO production, suggesting that ATRA increases activity of expressed eNOS indirectly through the decrease in ADMA due to increased DDHA2 [102]. ATRA also upregulates NO production in vascular endothelial cells through the PI3 kinase/Akt pathway [103]. ATRA induces eNOS phosphorylation at ser^{1177} and Akt phosphorylation at ser^{473} without changes in protein expression such as occur during DDAH2 upregulation. In terms of inducible NOS(iNOS), interleukin(IL)-1β increases iNOS mRNA levels and ATRA reduces this increase in vascular smooth muscle cell culture [104]. Because iNOS inhibition by the iNOS inhibitor N6-(1-iminoethyl-L-lysine, dihydrochloride(L-NIL) prevented the development of PH [105], the inhibitory effect of ATRA on iNOS expression might reduce the development of PH. Peroxisome proliferator-activated receptors (PPARγs) are a nuclear hormone receptor superfamily of ligand-activated transcription factors of retinoid hormone receptors other than steroid and thyroid hormones. PPARγ or retinoid X receptor (RXR) agonists inhibit smooth muscle proliferation. The PPARγ agonist rosiglitazone attenuates the development of chronic hypoxia-induced vascular structural remodeling [106], although it has little effect on the vasoconstriction component of PH. Since PPARγ mediates effects through the RXR, retinoids might also ameliorate PH vascular changes. PPARγ ligands increase the release of NO from endothelial cells through a transcriptional mechanism probably through the increase in DDAH mRNA expression without changes in eNOS expression [107]. These results suggest that ATRA might prevent the development of experimental PH in rats. ATRA ameliorated the development of MCT-induced PH [108], but not chronic hypoxia-induced PH [109]. These differences in the effect of ATRA on the development of PH may be due to a more pronounced inflammatory response in MCT-induced PH and a more subtle inflammatory reaction in chronic hypoxia-induced PH; endothelial damage precedes the rise in PAP in MCT model whereas the rise in PAP precedes endothelial changes in the chronic hypoxic model [110,111].

6.3. BMPIIR activates eNOS

Mutation of the bone morphogenetic protein receptor type II (BMPIIR) gene is one of the causes of familial PAH. The link between BMPIIR and eNOS partly explains the mechanism for the development of PH caused by BMPIIR mutations. Stimulation of BMPIIR induces eNOS phosphorylation, primarily through the cyclic-AMP dependent protein kinase and partially through serine-threonine kinase Akt [112]. Stimulation of BMPIIR also causes dissociation of eNOS from caveolin-1 and increases the eNOS-HSP90 interaction, which facilitates electron transfer through eNOS[112]. Thus, impaired BMPIIR or loss of BMPIIR stimulation might disturb the pulmonary vascular homeostasis, thereby causing PH.

6.4. VEGF increases eNOS expression

Vascular endothelial growth factor (VEGF) stimulates NO production initially by increasing intracellular Ca^{++} levels and subsequent Ca^{++}-calmodulin dependent activation of eNOS, and later by increasing intracellular eNOS message and protein levels [113]. VEGF stimulates vasodilation, microvascular hyperpermeability, and angiogenesis. Plexiform lesions show striking expression of VEGF associated with endothelial proliferation. NOS inhibition prevents

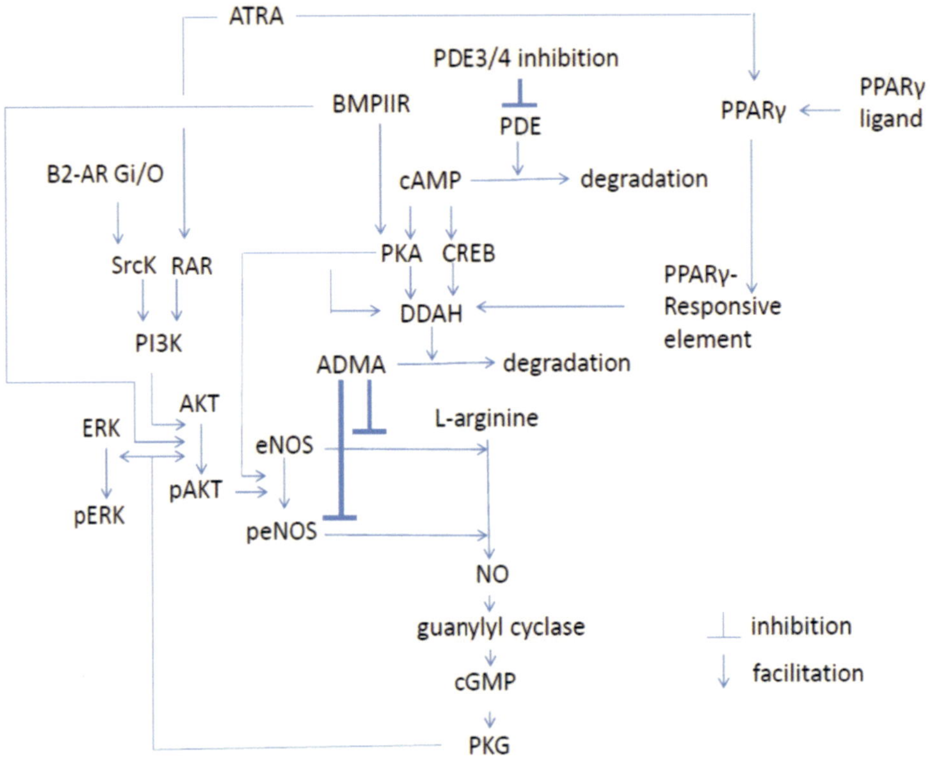

Figure 5. Possible pathway to enhance NO production by ATRA, DDAH, PDE3/4 inhibition, and BMPIIR. ADMA supresses NOS activity. DDAH is the enzyme that metabolizes ADMA. The cAMP/PKA pathway activates the promoter region of DDAH2, thereby increasing DDAH2 expression. ATRA increases DDAH2 mRNA, stimulates RAR with a subsequent increase in PI3K activity as well as PI3K protein and mRNA expression, and thereby enhances Akt and eNOS phosphorylation without increasing eNOS expression. Phosphorylated Akt(pAkt) phosphorylates eNOS making peNOS, the activated form of NOS. B2-AR stimulation activates SrcK via Gi/o protein. Activated SrcK phosphorylates PI3K and induces subsequent its downstream eNOS phosphorylation as well as phosphorylation of caveolin -1 to dissociate eNOS from caveola (Figure 3]. ADMA, asymmetric dimethylarginine; ATRA, all trans retinoic acid; B2-AR, beta 2-adrenergic receptor; BMPIIR, bone morphogenetic ptotein II receptor; CREB, cAMP responsive element binding protein; cAMP, cyclic adenosine monophosphate; DDAH, dimethylarginine dimethylaminohydrolase; eNOS, endothelial nitric oxide synthase; peNOS, phosphorylated eNOS; ERK, extracellular signal-regulated kinase; pERK, phosphorylated ERK; Gi/o, GTP binding protein subunit Gi/o; PDE, phosphodiesteras; PI3K, phosphoinositide 3-kinase; PKA, cAMP dependent protein kinase; PKG, cyclic GMP-dependent protein kinase ; PPARγ, peroxisome proliferator-activated receptor; Srck, src kinase; RAR, retinoic acid receptor;

VEGF-induced proliferation in cultured microvascular endothelial cells, associated with the decrease in cGMP levels [114], suggesting that VEGF-induced proliferation is in part mediated by the NOS-NO-cGMP pathway. VEGF induces translocation of eNOS and caveolin-1 from caveola to the nucleus, where NO production activates transcriptional factors thereby inducing the early growth response gene, c-fos [115] and possibly inducing angiogenesis, and endothelial cell growth. VEGF receptor 2 (VEGF2R) blockade combined with chronic hypoxic exposure causes PH with plexiform like lesions, where decreased expression of VEGF2R, Src, Akt, phosphorylated Akt protein in lung have been demonstrated [116]. Studies have demonstrated that reduced Src and Akt attenuate eNOS phosphorylation [101].

http://dx.doi.org/10.5772/55680

6.5. Elastase inhibition by NO

Earlier studies have shown that vascular elastase activity is increased in MCT-induced PH and chronic hypoxia-induced PH in rats [3,117], and that elastase inhibition prevents the development of pulmonary hypertension, right ventricular hypertrophy, muscularization of peripheral pulmonary arteries and medial hypertrophy of muscular arteries [3,117,118]. NO might reduce the elastase activity through its scavenging effect of superoxide. Reactive oxygen species inactivates endogenous elastase inhibitor, α1-protease inhibitor, and might increase elastase activity [119]. Furthermore NO might reduce elastase expression by inhibiting its transcriptional factor, acute myeloid leukemia factor 1 (AML-1), through extracellular signal-regulated kinase mitogen-activated protein kinase (ERK MAPK) inhibition which is mediated by cGMP dependent protein kinase activation [120].

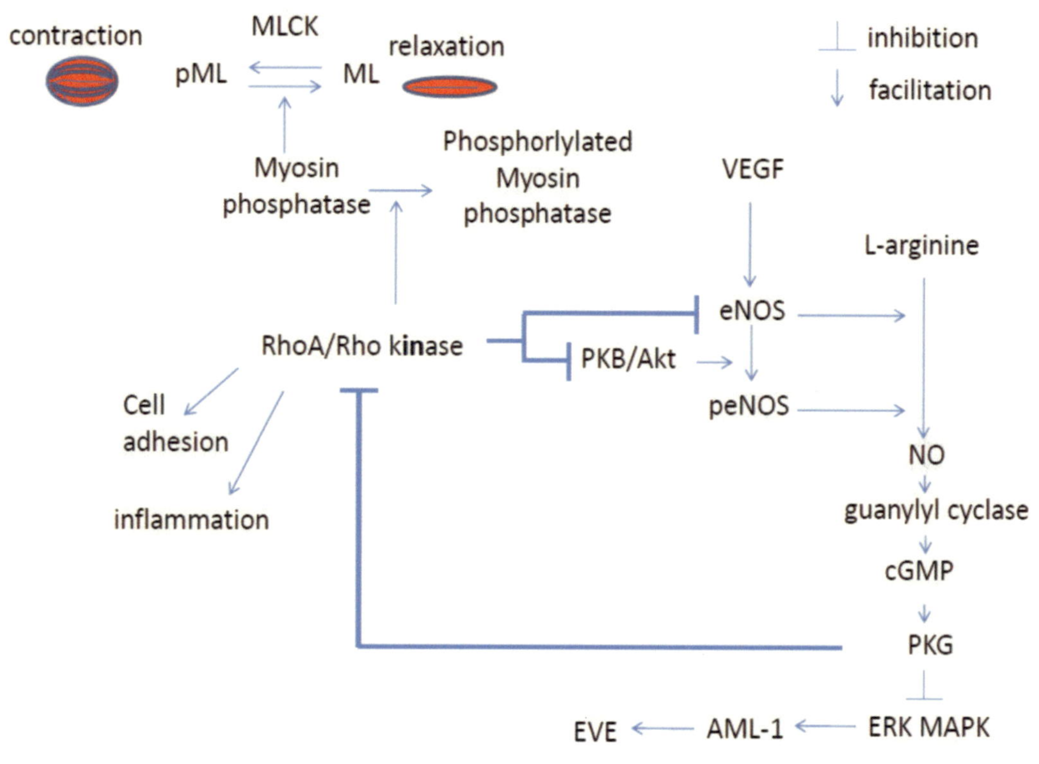

Figure 6. Rho/Rho kinase pathway inhibits eNOS/NO/cGMP pathway Rho kinase is activated by the guanosine triphosphate (GTP)-bound, active form of RhoA (GTP RhoA). Activated Rho kinase phosphorylates and subsequently inactivates myosin phosphatase, causing smooth muscle contraction, which is the RhoA/Rho kinase pathway. PKG phosphorylates Rho A at Ser[188] and inhibits Rho A function, thereby inactivating the RhoA/Rho kinase pathway. Activated RhoA/Rho kinase decreases eNOS mRNA and protein expression, inactivates Akt, and inhibits PKG activity, thereby supressing the eNOS/ NO/cGMP pathway. VEGF upregulates eNOS mRNA and protein expression. AML-1, acute myeloid leukemia factor 1(transcriptional factor); EVE, endogenous vascular elastase; PKG, cyclic GMP-dependent protein kinase(G kinase); PKB, protein kinase B(=Akt), AML-1, acute myeloid leukemia factor 1; ML, myosin light chain; pML, phosphorylated myosin light chain; MLCK, myosin light chain kinase; ERK MAPK, extracellular signal-regulated kinase mitogen activated protein kinase; VEGF, vascular endothelial growth factor.

6.6. Rho-kinase inhibitor upregulates NOS in PH (Figure 6)

Myosin light chain (MLC) phosphorylation by myosin light chain kinase (MLCK) causes vascular smooth muscle contraction. In contrast, myosin light chain dephosphorylation by myosin light chain phosphatase causes relaxation. The phosphorylation status of MLC phosphatase determines the contractility of smooth muscle at the same Ca^{++} concentration, thereby regulating the Ca^{++} sensitivity for contraction; the stronger the phosphatase activity, the weaker the vascular tone at the same Ca^{++} concentration. RhoA/Rho-kinase activation augments the phosphorylation of MLC phosphatase, which results in inhibition of MLC phosphatase. Studies have shown that Rho-kinase in circulating neutrophils is increased in patients with PH and that Rho-kinase expression is upregulated in isolated lung tissue on transplantation [121]. Rho-kinase activity in pulmonary arteries is enhanced in experimental PH [122,123]. NO-cGMP-cGMP dependent protein kinase pathway suppresses Rho/Rho kinase activity [124]. On the other hand Rho/Rho-kinase activation downregulates eNOS expression and eNOS phosphorylation through the inhibition of the protein kinase B/Akt pathway [125].

Author details

Junko Maruyama, Ayumu Yokochi, Erquan Zhang, Hirofumi Sawada and Kazuo Maruyama

Department of Anesthesiology and Critical Care Medicine, Mie University School of Medicine and Department of Clinical Engineering, Suzuka University of Medical Science, Mie, Japan

References

[1] Farber HW, Loscalzo J. Pulmonary arterial hypertension. N Engl J Med. 2004 Oct 14;351(16):1655-65.

[2] Archer SL, Weir EK, Wilkins MR. Basic science of pulmonary arterial hypertension for clinicians: new concepts and experimental therapies. Circulation. 2010 May 11;121(18):2045-66.

[3] Rabinovitch M. Molecular pathogenesis of pulmonary arterial hypertension. J Clin Invest. 2008 Jul;118(7):2372-9.

[4] Jiang BH, Maruyama J, Yokochi A, Amano H, Mitani Y, Maruyama K. Correlation of inhaled nitric-oxide induced reduction of pulmonary artery pressure and vascular changes. Eur Respir J. 2002 Jun;,20(1),52-8.

[5] Jiang BH, Maruyama J, Yokochi A, Iwasaki M, Amano H, Mitani Y, Maruyama K. Prolonged nitric oxide inhalation fails to regress hypoxic vascular remodeling in rat lung. Chest. 2004 Jun;125(6):2247-52.

[6] Kobayashi T, Gabazza EC, Shimizu S, Yasui H, Yuda H, Hataji O, Maruyama K, Yamauchi T, Suzuki K, Adachi Y, Taguchi O. Long-term inhalation of high-dose nitric oxide increases intraalveolar activation of coagulation system in mice. Am J Respir Crit Care Med. 2001 Jun;163(7):1676-82.

[7] Maruyama J, Jiang BH, Maruyama K, Takata M, Miyasaka K. Prolonged nitric oxide inhalation during recovery from chronic hypoxia does not decrease nitric oxide-dependent relaxation in pulmonary arteries. Chest. 2004 Dec;126(6):1919-25.

[8] Maruyama J, Maruyama K, Mitani Y, Kitabatake M, Yamauchi T, Miyasaka K. Continuous low-dose NO inhalation does not prevent monocrotaline-induced pulmonary hypertension in rats. Am J Physiol. 1997 Jan;272(1 Pt 2):H517-24.

[9] Katayama Y, Hatanaka K, Hayashi T, Onoda K, Namikawa S, Yuasa H, Yada I, Maruyama K, Kitabatake M, Kusagawa M. Effects of inhaled nitric oxide in single lung transplantation in rats with monocrotaline-induced pulmonary hypertension. J Heart Lung Transplant. 1995 May-Jun;14(3):486-92.

[10] Katayama Y, Hatanaka K, Hayashi T, Onoda K, Yada I, Namikawa S, Yuasa H, Kusagawa M, Maruyama K, Kitabatake M. Effects of inhaled nitric oxide in rats with chemically induced pulmonary hypertension. Respir Physiol. 1994 Aug;97(3):301-7.

[11] Shimpo H, Mitani Y, Tanaka J, Mizumoto T, Onoda K, Tani K, Yuasa H, Yada I, Maruyama K. Inhaled low-dose nitric oxide for postoperative care in patients with congenital heart defects. Artif Organs. 1997 Jan;21(1):10-3.

[12] Ashida Y, Miyahara H, Sawada H, Mitani Y, Maruyama K. Anesthetic management of a neonate with vein of Galen aneurysmal malformations and severe pulmonary hypertension. Paediatr Anaesth. 2005 Jun;15(6):525-8.

[13] Yoshida M, Taguchi O, Gabazza EC, Kobayashi T, Yamakami T, Kobayashi H, Maruyama K, Shima T. Combined inhalation of nitric oxide and oxygen in chronic obstructive pulmonary disease. Am J Respir Crit Care Med. 1997 Feb;155(2):526-9.

[14] Yoshida M, Taguchi O, Gabazza EC, Yasui H, Kobayashi T, Kobayashi H, Maruyama K, Adachi Y. The effect of low-dose inhalation of nitric oxide in patients with pulmonary fibrosis. Eur Respir J. 1997 Sep;10(9):2051-4.

[15] Maruyama K, Zhang E, Maruyama J. Clinical application of inhaled nitric oxide. In Yoshikawa/Naito (eds) Gas Biology Research in Clinical Practice. Basel Karger 2011, pp43-55

[16] Nakamura T, Lipton SA. Redox modulation by S-nitrosylation contributes to protein misfolding, mitochondrial dynamics, and neuronal synaptic damage in neurodegenerative diseases. Cell Death and Differentiation 18; 1478-1486, 2011

[17] Hampl V, Herget J. Role of nitric oxide in the pathogenesis of chronic pulmonary hypertension. Physiol Rev. 2000 Oct;80(4):1337-72.

[18] Garg UC, Hassid A. Nitric oxide-generating vasodilators and 8-bromo-cyclic guanosine monophosphate inhibit mitogenesis and proliferation of cultured rat vascular smooth muscle cells. J Clin Invest. 1989 May;83(5):1774-7.

[19] Garg UC, Hassid A Mechanisms of nitrosothiol-induced antimitogenesis in aortic smooth muscle cells. Eur J Pharmacol. 1993 Jun 24;237(2-3):243-9.

[20] Kwon NS, Stuehr DJ, Nathan CF. Inhibition of tumor cell ribonucleotide reductase by macrophage-derived nitric oxide. J Exp Med. 1991 Oct 1;174(4):761-7

[21] Kourembanas S, McQuillan LP, Leung GK, Faller DV. Nitric oxide regulates the expression of vasoconstrictors and growth factors by vascular endothelium under both normoxia and hypoxia. J Clin Invest. 1993 Jul;92(1):99-104

[22] Kouyoumdjian C, Adnot S, Levame M, Eddahibi S, Bousbaa H, Raffestin B. Continuous inhalation of nitric oxide protects against development of pulmonary hypertension in chronically hypoxic rats. J Clin Invest. 1994 Aug;94(2):578-84.

[23] Maruyama J, Maruyama K, Mitani Y, Kitabatake M, Yamauchi T, Miyasaka K. Continuous low-dose NO inhalation does not prevent monocrotaline-induced pulmonary hypertension in rats. Am J Physiol. 1997 Jan;272(1 Pt 2):H517-24.

[24] Mitani Y, Maruyama K, Sakurai M. Prolonged administration of L-arginine ameliorates chronic pulmonary hypertension and pulmonary vascular remodeling in rats. Circulation. 1997 Jul 15;96(2):689-97.

[25] Mitani Y, Maruyama J, Jiang BH, Sawada H, Shimpo H, Imanaka-Yoshida K, Kaneda Y, Komada Y, Maruyama K. Atrial natriuretic peptide gene transfection with a novel envelope vector system ameliorates pulmonary hypertension in rats. J Thorac Cardiovasc Surg. 2008 Jul;136(1):142-9. Epub 2008 May 12

[26] Campbell AI, Kuliszewski MA, Stewart DJ. Cell-based gene transfer to the pulmonary vasculature: Endothelial nitric oxide synthase overexpression inhibits monocrotaline-induced pulmonary hypertension. Am J Respir Cell Mol Biol. 1999 Nov;21(5): 567-75

[27] Zhao YD, Courtman DW, Deng Y, Kugathasan L, Zhang Q, Stewart DJ. Rescue of monocrotaline-induced pulmonary arterial hypertension using bone marrow-derived endothelial-like progenitor cells: efficacy of combined cell and eNOS gene therapy in established disease. Circ Res. 2005 Mar 4;96(4):442-50. Epub 2005 Feb 3

[28] Zuckerbraun BS, George P, Gladwin MT. Nitrite in pulmonary arterial hypertension: therapeutic avenues in the setting of dysregulated arginine/nitric oxide synthase signalling. Cardiovasc Res. 2011 Feb 15;89(3):542-52. Epub 2010 Dec 22. Review

[29] Lundberg JO, Weitzberg E, Gladwin MT. The nitrate-nitrite-nitric oxide pathway in physiology and therapeutics. Nat Rev Drug Discov. 2008 Feb;7(2):156-67. Review.

[30] Hunter CJ, Dejam A, Blood AB, Shields H, Kim-Shapiro DB, Machado RF, Tarekegn S, Mulla N, Hopper AO, Schechter AN, Power GG, Gladwin MT.Inhaled nebulized nitrite is a hypoxia-sensitive NO-dependent selective pulmonary vasodilator. Nat Med. 2004 Oct;10(10):1122-7. Epub 2004 Sep 12.

[31] Casey DB, Badejo AM Jr, Dhaliwal JS, Murthy SN, Hyman AL, Nossaman BD, Kadowitz PJ. Pulmonary vasodilator responses to sodium nitrite are mediated by an allopurinol-sensitive mechanism in the rat. Am J Physiol Heart Circ Physiol. 2009 Feb; 296(2):H524-33. Epub 2008 Dec 12

[32] Zuckerbraun BS, Shiva S, Ifedigbo E, Mathier MA, Mollen KP, Rao J, Bauer PM, Choi JJ, Curtis E, Choi AM, Gladwin MT. Nitrite potently inhibits hypoxic and inflammatory pulmonary arterial hypertension and smooth muscle proliferation via xanthine oxidoreductase-dependent nitric oxide generation. Circulation. 2010 Jan 5;121(1): 98-109. Epub 2009 Dec 21.

[33] Xu W, Kaneko FT, Zheng S, Comhair SA, Janocha AJ, Goggans T, Thunnissen FB, Farver C, Hazen SL, Jennings C, Dweik RA, Arroliga AC, Erzurum SC. Increased arginase II and decreased NO synthesis in endothelial cells of patients with pulmonary arterial hypertension. FASEB J. 2004 Nov;18(14):1746-8. Epub 2004 Sep 13.

[34] Minamishima S, Kida K, Tokuda K, Wang H, Sips PY, Kosugi S, Mandeville JB, Buys ES, Brouckaert P, Liu PK, Liu CH, Bloch KD, Ichinose F. Inhaled nitric oxide improves outcomes after successful cardiopulmonary resuscitation in mice. Circulation. 2011 Oct 11;124(15):1645-53. Epub 2011 Sep 19.

[35] Lang JD Jr, Teng X, Chumley P, Crawford JH, Isbell TS, Chacko BK, Liu Y, Jhala N, Crowe DR, Smith AB, Cross RC, Frenette L, Kelley EE, Wilhite DW, Hall CR, Page GP, Fallon MB, Bynon JS, Eckhoff DE, Patel RP. Inhaled NO accelerates restoration of liver function in adults following orthotopic liver transplantation. J Clin Invest. 2007 Sep;117(9):2583-91

[36] Yoshida K, Kasama K, Kitabatake M, Okuda M, Imai M. Metabolic fate of nitric oxide. Int Arch Occup Environ Health. 1980;46(1):71-7.

[37] Yoshida K, Kasama K, Kitabatake M, Imai M. Biotransformation of nitric oxide, nitrite and nitrate. Int Arch Occup Environ Health. 1983;52(2):103-15.

[38] Moncada S, Palmer RM, Higgs EA. Nitric oxide: physiology, pathophysiology, and pharmacology. Pharmacol Rev. 1991 Jun;43(2):109-42.

[39] Chen CA, Wang TY, Varadharaj S, Reyes LA, Hemann C, Talukder MA, Chen YR, Druhan LJ, Zweier JL. S-glutathionylation uncouples eNOS and regulates its cellular and vascular function. Nature. 2010 Dec 23;468(7327):1115-8.

[40] Crabtree MJ, Tatham AL, Al-Wakeel Y, Warrick N, Hale AB, Cai S, Channon KM, Alp NJ. Quantitative regulation of intracellular endothelial nitric-oxide synthase (eNOS) coupling by both tetrahydrobiopterin-eNOS stoichiometry and biopterin re-

dox status: insights from cells with tet-regulated GTP cyclohydrolase I expression. J Biol Chem. 2009 Jan 9;284(2):1136-44. Epub 2008 Nov 14

[41] Gielis JF, Lin JY, Wingler K, Van Schil PE, Schmidt HH, Moens AL. Pathogenetic role of eNOS uncoupling in cardiopulmonary disorders. Free Radic Biol Med. 2011 Apr 1;50(7):765-76. Epub 2010 Dec 21.

[42] Tabima DM, Frizzell S, Gladwin MT. Reactive oxygen and nitrogen species in pulmonary hypertension. Free Radic Biol Med. 2012 May 1;52(9):1970-86. Epub 2012 Mar 6.

[43] Moens AL, Takimoto E, Tocchetti CG, Chakir K, Bedja D, Cormaci G, Ketner EA, Majmudar M, Gabrielson K, Halushka MK, Mitchell JB, Biswal S, Channon KM, Wolin MS, Alp NJ, Paolocci N, Champion HC, Kass DA. Reversal of cardiac hypertrophy and fibrosis from pressure overload by tetrahydrobiopterin: efficacy of recoupling nitric oxide synthase as a therapeutic strategy. Circulation. 2008 May 20;117(20):2626-36. Epub 2008 May 12

[44] Khoo JP, Zhao L, Alp NJ, Bendall JK, Nicoli T, Rockett K, Wilkins MR, Channon KM. Pivotal role for endothelial tetrahydrobiopterin in pulmonary hypertension. Circulation. 2005 Apr 26;111(16):2126-33. Epub 2005 Apr 11.

[45] Kunuthur SP, Milliken PH, Gibson CL, Suckling CJ, Wadsworth RM. Tetrahydrobiopterin analogues with NO-dependent pulmonary vasodilator properties. Eur J Pharmacol. 2011 Jan 10;650(1):371-7. Epub 2010 Oct 13.

[46] Münzel T, Li H, Mollnau H, Hink U, Matheis E, Hartmann M, Oelze M, Skatchkov M, Warnholtz A, Duncker L, Meinertz T, Förstermann U. Effects of long-term nitroglycerin treatment on endothelial nitric oxide synthase (NOS III) gene expression, NOS III-mediated superoxide production, and vascular NO bioavailability. Circ Res. 2000 Jan 7;86(1):E7-E12.

[47] Münzel T, Sayegh H, Freeman BA, Tarpey MM, Harrison DG. Evidence for enhanced vascular superoxide anion production in nitrate tolerance. A novel mechanism underlying tolerance and cross-tolerance. J Clin Invest. 1995 Jan;95(1):187-94.

[48] Banquet S, Delannoy E, Agouni A, Dessy C, Lacomme S, Hubert F, Richard V, Muller B, Leblais V. Role of G(i/o)-Src kinase-PI3K/Akt pathway and caveolin-1 in β2-adrenoceptor coupling to endothelial NO synthase in mouse pulmonary artery. Cell Signal. 2011 Jul;23(7):1136-43. Epub 2011 Mar 6

[49] Zhao YY, Zhao YD, Mirza MK, Huang JH, Potula HH, Vogel SM, Brovkovych V, Yuan JX, Wharton J, Malik AB. Persistent eNOS activation secondary to caveolin-1 deficiency induces pulmonary hypertension in mice and humans through PKG nitration. J Clin Invest. 2009 Jul;119(7):2009-18.

[50] Achcar RO, Demura Y, Rai PR, Taraseviciene-Stewart L, Kasper M, Voelkel NF, Cool CD. Loss of caveolin and heme oxygenase expression in severe pulmonary hypertension. Chest. 2006 Mar;129(3):696-705.

[51] Sud N, Wells SM, Sharma S, Wiseman DA, Wilham J, Black SM. Asymmetric dimethylarginine inhibits HSP90 activity in pulmonary arterial endothelial cells: role of mitochondrial dysfunction. Am J Physiol Cell Physiol. 2008 Jun;294(6):C1407-18. Epub 2008 Apr 2

[52] Rus A, Peinado MA, Castro L, Del Moral ML. Lung eNOS and iNOS are reoxygenation time-dependent upregulated after acute hypoxia. Anat Rec (Hoboken). 2010 ; 293(6):1089-98.

[53] Archer SL, Tolins JP, Raij L, Weir EK. Hypoxic pulmonary vasoconstriction is enhanced by inhibition of the synthesis of an endothelium derived relaxing factor. Biochem Biophys Res Commun. 1989 15;164(3):1198-205.

[54] Fox GA, Paterson NA, McCormack DG. Effect of inhibition of NO synthase on vascular reactivity in a rat model of hyperdynamic sepsis. Am J Physiol. 1994 ;267(4 Pt 2):H1377-82.

[55] Murata T, Kinoshita K, Hori M, Kuwahara M, Tsubone H, Karaki H, Ozaki H. Statin protects endothelial nitric oxide synthase activity in hypoxia-induced pulmonary hypertension. Arterioscler Thromb Vasc Biol. 2005 ;25(11):2335-42.

[56] Blumberg FC, Wolf K, Arzt M, Lorenz C, Riegger GA, Pfeifer M. Effects of ET-A receptor blockade on eNOS gene expression in chronic hypoxic rat lungs. J Appl Physiol. 2003 ;94(2):446-52.

[57] Kanno S, Wu YJ, Lee PC, Billiar TR, Ho C. Angiotensin-converting enzyme inhibitor preserves p21 and endothelial nitric oxide synthase expression in monocrotaline-induced pulmonary arterial hypertension in rats. Circulation. 2001;104(8):945-50.

[58] Mawatari E, Hongo M, Sakai A, Terasawa F, Takahashi M, Yazaki Y, Kinoshita O, Ikeda U. Amlodipine prevents monocrotaline-induced pulmonary arterial hypertension and prolongs survival in rats independent of blood pressure lowering. Clin Exp Pharmacol Physiol. 2007 ;34(7):594-600.

[59] Pei Y, Ma P, Wang X, Zhang W, Zhang X, Zheng P, Yan L, Xu Q, Dai G. Rosuvastatin attenuates monocrotaline-induced pulmonary hypertension via regulation of Akt/eNOS signaling and asymmetric dimethylarginine metabolism. Eur J Pharmacol. 2011 ;666(1-3):165-72.

[60] Mason NA, Springall DR, Burke M, Pollock J, Mikhail G, Yacoub MH, Polak JM. High expression of endothelial nitric oxide synthase in plexiform lesions of pulmonary hypertension. J Pathol. 1998 ;185(3):313-8.

[61] Zhao YY, Zhao YD, Mirza MK, Huang JH, Potula HH, Vogel SM, Brovkovych V, Yuan JX, Wharton J, Malik AB. Persistent eNOS activation secondary to caveolin-1 deficiency induces pulmonary hypertension in mice and humans through PKG nitration. J Clin Invest. 2009 ;119(7):2009-18.

[62] Kaneko FT, Arroliga AC, Dweik RA, Comhair SA, Laskowski D, Oppedisano R, Thomassen MJ, Erzurum SC. Biochemical reaction products of nitric oxide as quantita-

tive markers of primary pulmonary hypertension. Am J Respir Crit Care Med. 1998 ; 158(3):917-23.

[63] Malinovschi A, Henrohn D, Eriksson A, Lundberg JO, Alving K, Wikström G. Increased plasma and salivary nitrite and decreased bronchial contribution to exhaled NO in pulmonary arterial hypertension. Eur J Clin Invest. 2011 ;41(8):889-97

[64] Oka M, Hasunuma K, Webb SA, Stelzner TJ, Rodman DM, McMurtry IF. EDRF suppresses an unidentified vasoconstrictor mechanism in hypertensive rat lungs. Am J Physiol. 1993 ;264:L587-97.

[65] Maruyama J, Maruyama K. Impaired nitric oxide-dependent responses and their recovery in hypertensive pulmonary arteries of rats. Am J Physiol. 1994 ;266(6 Pt 2):H2476-88.

[66] Ferrario L, Amin HM, Sugimori K, Camporesi EM, Hakim TS. Site of action of endogenous nitric oxide on pulmonary vasculature in rats. Pflugers Arch. 1996 ;432(3): 523-7.

[67] Igari H, Tatsumi K, Sugito K, Kasahara Y, Saito M, Tani T, Kimura H, Kuriyama T. Role of EDRF in pulmonary circulation during sustained hypoxia. J Cardiovasc Pharmacol. 1998 ;31(2):299-305.

[68] Bardou M, Goirand F, Marchand S, Rouget C, Devillier P, Dumas JP, Morcillo EJ, Rochette L, Dumas M. Hypoxic vasoconstriction of rat main pulmonary artery: role of endogenous nitric oxide, potassium channels, and phosphodiesterase inhibition. J Cardiovasc Pharmacol. 2001 Aug;38(2):325-34.

[69] Stamler JS, Loh E, Roddy MA, Currie KE, Creager MA. Nitric oxide regulates basal systemic and pulmonary vascular resistance in healthy humans. Circulation. 1994;89(5):2035-40.

[70] Cooper CJ, Landzberg MJ, Anderson TJ, Charbonneau F, Creager MA, Ganz P, Selwyn AP. Role of nitric oxide in the local regulation of pulmonary vascular resistance in humans. Circulation. 1996 15;93(2):266-71.

[71] Eddahibi S, Adnot S, Carville C, Blouquit Y, Raffestin B.L-arginine restores endothelium-dependent relaxation in pulmonary circulation of chronically hypoxic rats. Am J Physiol. 1992 ;263:L194-200.

[72] Goret L, Tanguy S, Guiraud I, Dauzat M, Obert P. Acute administration of l-arginine restores nitric oxide-mediated relaxation in isolated pulmonary arteries from pulmonary hypertensive exercise trained rats. Eur J Pharmacol. 2008 26;581(1-2):148-56.

[73] Shaul PW, Wells LB, Horning KM.Acute and prolonged hypoxia attenuate endothelial nitric oxide production in rat pulmonary arteries by different mechanisms. J Cardiovasc Pharmacol.1993;22(6):819-27.

[74] Oka M. Phosphodiesterase 5 inhibition restores impaired ACh relaxation in hypertensive conduit pulmonary arteries. Am J Physiol Lung Cell Mol Physiol. 2001;280(3):L432-5.

[75] Elmedal B, de Dam MY, Mulvany MJ, Simonsen U. The superoxide dismutase mimetic, tempol, blunts right ventricular hypertrophy in chronic hypoxic rats. Br J Pharmacol. 2004;141(1):105-13.

[76] Mam V, Tanbe AF, Vitali SH, Arons E, Christou HA, Khalil RA. Impaired vasoconstriction and nitric oxide-mediated relaxation in pulmonary arteries of hypoxia- and monocrotaline-induced pulmonary hypertensive rats. J Pharmacol Exp Ther. 2010;332(2):455-62.

[77] MacLean MR, McCulloch KM. Influence of applied tension and nitric oxide on responses to endothelins in rat pulmonary resistance arteries: effect of chronic hypoxia. Br J Pharmacol. 1998;123(5):991-9.

[78] Tian L, Lammers SR, Kao PH, Reusser M, Stenmark KR, Hunter KS, Qi HJ, Shandas R. Linked opening angle and histological and mechanical aspects of the proximal pulmonary arteries of healthy and pulmonary hypertensive rats and calves. Am J Physiol Heart Circ Physiol. 2011;301(5):H1810-8.

[79] Maruyama J, Yokochi A, Maruyama K, Nosaka S. Acetylcholine-induced endothelium-derived contracting factor in hypoxic pulmonary hypertensive rats. J Appl Physiol. 1999;86(5):1687-95.

[80] Pidgeon GP, Tamosiuniene R, Chen G, Leonard I, Belton O, Bradford A, Fitzgerald DJ. Intravascular thrombosis after hypoxia-induced pulmonary hypertension: regulation by cyclooxygenase-2. Circulation. 2004 26;110(17):2701-7.

[81] Mathew R, Zeballos GA, Tun H, Gewitz MH. Role of nitric oxide and endothelin-1 in monocrotaline-induced pulmonary hypertension in rats. Cardiovasc Res. 1995 ;30(5): 739-46.

[82] Fullerton DA, Hahn AR, McIntyre RC Jr. Mechanistic imbalance of pulmonary vasomotor control in progressive lung injury. Surgery. 1996;119(1):98-103.

[83] Gout B, Quiniou MJ, Khandoudi N, Le Dantec C, Saïag B. Impaired endothelium-dependent relaxation by adrenomedullin in monocrotaline-treated rat arteries. Eur J Pharmacol. 1999 3;380(1):23-30.

[84] Ozturk EI, Uma S. Effects of atorvastatin and L-arginine treatments on electrical field stimulation-mediated relaxations in pulmonary arterial rings of monocrotaline-induced pulmonary hypertensive rats. J Cardiovasc Pharmacol. 2010 ;56(5):498-505.

[85] Baber SR, Deng W, Master RG, Bunnell BA, Taylor BK, Murthy SN, Hyman AL, Kadowitz PJ. Intratracheal mesenchymal stem cell administration attenuates monocrotaline-induced pulmonary hypertension and endothelial dysfunction. Am J Physiol Heart Circ Physiol. 2007 ;292(2):H1120-8.

[86] Prié S, Stewart DJ, Dupuis J. EndothelinA receptor blockade improves nitric oxide-mediated vasodilation in monocrotaline-induced pulmonary hypertension. Circulation. 1998 2;97(21):2169-74.

[87] Demiryürek AT, Karamsetty MR, McPhaden AR, Wadsworth RM, Kane KA, MacLean MR. Accumulation of nitrotyrosine correlates with endothelial NO synthase in pulmonary resistance arteries during chronic hypoxia in the rat. Pulm Pharmacol Ther. 2000;13(4):157-65

[88] Weerackody RP, Welsh DJ, Wadsworth RM, Peacock AJ. Inhibition of p38 MAPK reverses hypoxia-induced pulmonary artery endothelial dysfunction. Am J Physiol Heart Circ Physiol. 2009 May;296(5):H1312-20. Epub 2009 Feb 6.

[89] Sawada H, Mitani Y, Maruyama J, Jiang BH, Ikeyama Y, Dida FA, Yamamoto H, Imanaka-Yoshida K, Shimpo H, Mizoguchi A, Maruyama K, Komada Y. A nuclear factor-kappaB inhibitor pyrrolidine dithiocarbamate ameliorates pulmonary hypertension in rats. Chest. 2007 Oct;132(4):1265-74

[90] Brennan LA, Steinhorn RH, Wedgwood S, Mata-Greenwood E, Roark EA, Russell JA, Black SM. Increased superoxide generation is associated with pulmonary hypertension in fetal lambs: a role for NADPH oxidase. Circ Res. 2003 Apr 4;92(6):683-91. Epub 2003 Feb 27.

[91] Grobe AC, Wells SM, Benavidez E, Oishi P, Azakie A, Fineman JR, Black SM Increased oxidative stress in lambs with increased pulmonary blood flow and pulmonary hypertension: role of NADPH oxidase and endothelial NO synthase. Am J Physiol Lung Cell Mol Physiol. 2006 Jun;290(6):L1069-77.

[92] Archer SL, Marsboom G, Kim GH, Zhang HJ, Toth PT, Svensson EC, Dyck JR, Gomberg-Maitland M, Thébaud B, Husain AN, Cipriani N, Rehman J. Epigenetic attenuation of mitochondrial superoxide dismutase 2 in pulmonary arterial hypertension: a basis for excessive cell proliferation and a new therapeutic target. Circulation. 2010 Jun 22;121(24):2661-71. Epub 2010 Jun 7.

[93] Bonnet S, Michelakis ED, Porter CJ, Andrade-Navarro MA, Thébaud B, Bonnet S, Haromy A, Harry G, Moudgil R, McMurtry MS, Weir EK, Archer SL. An abnormal mitochondrial-hypoxia inducible factor-1alpha-Kv channel pathway disrupts oxygen sensing and triggers pulmonary arterial hypertension in fawn hooded rats: similarities to human pulmonary arterial hypertension. Circulation. 2006 Jun 6;113(22): 2630-41. Epub 2006 May 30

[94] Pryor WA, Squadrito GL. The chemistry of peroxynitrite: a product from the reaction of nitric oxide with superoxide. Am J Physiol. 1995 May;268(5 Pt 1):L699-722.

[95] Kaneko FT, Arroliga AC, Dweik RA, Comhair SA, Laskowski D, Oppedisano R, Thomassen MJ, Erzurum SC Biochemical reaction products of nitric oxide as quantitative markers of primary pulmonary hypertension. Am J Respir Crit Care Med. 1998 Sep; 158(3):917-23.

[96] Sasaki S, Asano M, Ukai T, Nomura N, Maruyama K, Manabe T, Mishima A. Nitric oxide formation and plasma L-arginine levels in pulmonary hypertensive rats. Respir Med. 2004 Mar;98(3):205-12

[97] Morris CR, Morris SM Jr, Hagar W, Van Warmerdam J, Claster S, Kepka-Lenhart D, Machado L, Kuypers FA, Vichinsky EP. Arginine therapy: a new treatment for pulmonary hypertension in sickle cell disease? Am J Respir Crit Care Med. 2003 Jul 1;168(1):63-9. Epub 2003 Mar 5

[98] Pullamsetti S, Kiss L, Ghofrani HA, Voswinckel R, Haredza P, Klepetko W, Aigner C, Fink L, Muyal JP, Weissmann N, Grimminger F, Seeger W, Schermuly RT Increased levels and reduced catabolism of asymmetric and symmetric dimethylarginines in pulmonary hypertension. FASEB J. 2005 Jul;19(9):1175-7. Epub 2005 Apr 12

[99] Antoniades C, Shirodaria C, Leeson P, Antonopoulos A, Warrick N, Van-Assche T, Cunnington C, Tousoulis D, Pillai R, Ratnatunga C, Stefanadis C, Channon KM. Association of plasma asymmetrical dimethylarginine (ADMA) with elevated vascular superoxide production and endothelial nitric oxide synthase uncoupling: implications for endothelial function in human atherosclerosis. Eur Heart J. 2009 May;30(9): 1142-50. Epub 2009 Mar 18

[100] Zweier JL, Talukder MA. Targeting dimethylarginine dimethylaminohydrolases in pulmonary arterial hypertension: a new approach to improve vascular dysfunction? Circulation. 2011 Mar 22;123(11):1156-8. Epub 2011 Mar 7.

[101] Pei Y, Ma P, Wang X, Zhang W, Zhang X, Zheng P, Yan L, Xu Q, Dai G. Rosuvastatin attenuates monocrotaline-induced pulmonary hypertension via regulation of Akt/ eNOS signaling and asymmetric dimethylarginine metabolism. Eur J Pharmacol. 2011 Sep;666(1-3):165-72. Epub 2011 May 30

[102] Achan V, Tran CT, Arrigoni F, Whitley GS, Leiper JM, Vallance P. all-trans-Retinoic acid increases nitric oxide synthesis by endothelial cells:a role for the induction of dimethylarginine dimethylaminohydrolase. Circ Res. 2002 Apr 19;90(7):764-9.

[103] Uruno A, Sugawara A, Kanatsuka H, Kagechika H, Saito A, Sato K, Kudo M, Takeuchi K, Ito S. Upregulation of nitric oxide production in vascular endothelial cells by all-trans retinoic acid through the phosphoinositide 3-kinase/Akt pathway. Circulation. 2005 Aug 2;112(5):727-36. Epub 2005 Jul 25.

[104] Hirokawa K, O'Shaughnessy KM, Ramrakha P, Wilkins MR. Inhibition of nitric oxide synthesis in vascular smooth muscle by retinoids. Br J Pharmacol. 1994 Dec;113(4): 1448-54

[105] Hampl V, Bíbová J, Banasová A, Uhlík J, Miková D, Hnilicková O, Lachmanová V, Herget J. Pulmonary vascular iNOS induction participates in the onset of chronic hypoxic pulmonary hypertension. Am J Physiol Lung Cell Mol Physiol. 2006 Jan; 290(1):L11-20. Epub 2005 Aug 19

[106] Crossno JT Jr, Garat CV, Reusch JE, Morris KG, Dempsey EC, McMurtry IF, Stenmark KR, Klemm DJ. Rosiglitazone attenuates hypoxia-induced pulmonary arterial remodeling. Am J Physiol Lung Cell Mol Physiol. 2007 Apr;292(4):L885-97. Epub 2006 Dec 22

[107] Calnek DS, Mazzella L, Roser S, Roman J, Hart CM. Peroxisome proliferator-activated receptor gamma ligands increase release of nitric oxide from endothelial cells. Arterioscler Thromb Vasc Biol. 2003 Jan 1;23(1):52-7.

[108] Qin Y, Zhou A, Ben X, Shen J, Liang Y, Li F. All-trans retinoic acid in pulmonary vascular structural remodeling in rats with pulmonary hypertension induced by monocrotaline. Chin Med J (Engl). 2001 May;114(5):462-5.

[109] Zhang E, Jiang B, Yokochi A, Maruyama J, Mitani Y, Ma N, Maruyama K. Effect of all-trans-retinoic acid on the development of chronic hypoxia-induced pulmonary hypertension. Circ J. 2010 Aug;74(8):1696-703. Epub 2010 Jul 1.

[110] Rosenberg HC, Rabinovitch M. Endothelial injury and vascular reactivity in monocrotaline pulmonary hypertension. Am J Physiol. 1988 Dec;255(6 Pt 2):H1484-91

[111] Rabinovitch M, Gamble W, Nadas AS, Miettinen OS, Reid L. Rat pulmonary circulation after chronic hypoxia: hemodynamic and structural features. Am J Physiol. 1979 Jun;236(6):H818-27

[112] Gangopahyay A, Oran M, Bauer EM, Wertz JW, Comhair SA, Erzurum SC, Bauer PM. Bone morphogenetic protein receptor II is a novel mediator of endothelial nitric-oxide synthase activation. J Biol Chem. 2011 Sep 23;286(38):33134-40. Epub 2011 Aug 1

[113] Hood JD, Meininger CJ, Ziche M, Granger HJ. VEGF upregulates ecNOS message, protein, and NO production in human endothelial cells. Am J Physiol. 1998 Mar; 274(3 Pt 2):H1054-8

[114] Morbidelli L, Chang CH, Douglas JG, Granger HJ, Ledda F, Ziche M. Nitric oxide mediates mitogenic effect of VEGF on coronary venular endothelium. Am J Physiol. 1996 Jan;270(1 Pt 2):H411-5.

[115] Feng Y, Venema VJ, Venema RC, Tsai N, Caldwell RB. VEGF induces nuclear translocation of Flk-1/KDR, endothelial nitric oxide synthase, and caveolin-1 in vascular endothelial cells. Biochem Biophys Res Commun. 1999 Mar 5;256(1):192-7.

[116] Taraseviciene-Stewart L, Kasahara Y, Alger L, Hirth P, Mc Mahon G, Waltenberger J, Voelkel NF, Tuder RM Inhibition of the VEGF receptor 2 combined with chronic hypoxia causes cell death-dependent pulmonary endothelial cell proliferation and severe pulmonary hypertension. FASEB J. 2001 Feb;15(2):427-38.

[117] Maruyama K, Ye CL, Woo M, Venkatacharya H, Lines LD, Silver MM, Rabinovitch M. Chronic hypoxic pulmonary hypertension in rats and increased elastolytic activity. Am J Physiol. 1991 Dec;261(6 Pt 2):H1716-26

[118] Ilkiw R, Todorovich-Hunter L, Maruyama K, Shin J, Rabinovitch M. SC-39026, a serine elastase inhibitor, prevents muscularization of peripheral arteries, suggesting a mechanism of monocrotaline-induced pulmonary hypertension in rats. Circ Res. 1989 Apr;64(4):814-25.

[119] Carp H, Janoff A. In vitro suppression of serum elastase-inhibitory capacity by reactive oxygen species generated by phagocytosing polymorphonuclear leukocytes. J Clin Invest. 1979 Apr;63(4):793-7

[120] Mitani Y, Zaidi SH, Dufourcq P, Thompson K, Rabinovitch M. Nitric oxide reduces vascular smooth muscle cell elastase activity through cGMP-mediated suppression of ERK phosphorylation and AML1B nuclear partitioning. FASEB J. 2000 Apr;14(5): 805-14

[121] Do e Z, Fukumoto Y, Takaki A, Tawara S, Ohashi J, Nakano M, Tada T, Saji K, Sugimura K, Fujita H, Hoshikawa Y, Nawata J, Kondo T, Shimokawa H. Evidence for Rho-kinase activation in patients with pulmonary arterial hypertension. Circ J. 2009 Sep;73(9):1731-9. Epub 2009 Jul 9.

[122] Abe K, Shimokawa H, Morikawa K, Uwatoku T, Oi K, Matsumoto Y, Hattori T, Nakashima Y, Kaibuchi K, Sueishi K, Takeshit A. Long-term treatment with a Rho-kinase inhibitor improves monocrotaline-induced fatal pulmonary hypertension in rats. Circ Res. 2004 Feb 20;94(3):385-93. Epub 2003 Dec 11

[123] Nagaoka T, Morio Y, Casanova N, Bauer N, Gebb S, McMurtry I, Oka M. Rho/Rho kinase signaling mediates increased basal pulmonary vascular tone in chronically hypoxic rats. Am J Physiol Lung Cell Mol Physiol. 2004 Oct;287(4):L665-72. Epub 2003 Sep 5.

[124] Sauzeau V, Le Jeune H, Cario-Toumaniantz C, Smolenski A, Lohmann SM, Bertoglio J, Chardin P, Pacaud P, Loirand G. Cyclic GMP-dependent protein kinase signaling pathway inhibits RhoA-induced Ca2+ sensitization of contraction in vascular smooth muscle. J Biol Chem. 2000 Jul 14;275(28):21722-9.

[125] Ming XF, Viswambharan H, Barandier C, Ruffieux J, Kaibuchi K, Rusconi S, Yang Z. Rho GTPase/Rho kinase negatively regulates endothelial nitric oxide synthase phosphorylation through the inhibition of protein kinase B/Akt in human endothelial cells. Mol Cell Biol. 2002 Dec;22(24):8467-77.

Chapter 5

Angiogenesis and Pulmonary Hypertension

Aureliano Hernández and Rafael A. Areiza

Additional information is available at the end of the chapter

http://dx.doi.org/10.5772/56054

1. Introduction

The aim of this chapter is to present an overview of salient findings in human beings and animal models (particularly in the chicken), as related to known participating molecules in angiogenesis within the lung as a response to induced and natural environmental hypoxia, in the framework of the pathobiology of pulmonary hypertension (PH).

Hypoxic PH is now recognized as an important disease within the PH types. More than 140 million human beings are settled in geographical zones located 2500 m above sea level (Peñaloza and Arias, 2007). Animals which provide proteins for human consumption, have different degrees of susceptibility to develop PH, especially the commercial chicken, which is particularly prone to develop PH, either from hypoxia (Gómez et al., 2007, 2008; Vásquez and Hernández, 2011; Areiza et al, 2011 and others) or low temperatures (Pakdel et al., 2005; Pan et al., 2005). The chicken has been proposed as a model to study PH in humans (Al-Ruyabe et al., 2010; Wideman and Hamal, 2011).

Exposure to hypoxia has been reported to cause different effects on the pulmonary vasculature. These include increasing the extent of pulmonary vascular network, increased vascular tone, vascular remodeling and in some cases quantitative reduction of microvessels. Neo-formation of blood vessels in the lung, takes place through a mechanism not fully understood and often controversial. Remodeling of pulmonary arterioles has been thoroughly studied. It includes thickening of the medial muscle and adventitia layers. Many tasks have been directed to discover the role of the endothelium in maintaining pulmonary vascular tone and in the PH remodeling process. Endothelial dysfunction leads to chronically impaired production of vasodilators such as nitric oxide (NO) and prostacyclin along with prolonged over expression of vasoconstrictors such as endothelin-1 (ET-1). These changes affect vascular tone and promote vascular remodeling. Given that most of these mediators affect the growth of smooth muscle cells, an alteration in their production may facilitate the development of pulmonary vascular hypertrophy and structural remodeling, which are characteristic of PH (Budhiraja et al., 2004; Humbert et al., 2004; reviewed by Hernández and Sandino de, 2011).

Both processes, angiogenesis and remodeling of pulmonary arterioles, appear to share the participation of similar molecules. In fact, some of them, known to increase pulmonary blood vessels tone during hypoxic exposure, are also involved in generating pulmonary blood vessels. In this framework, three main research cellular targets can be identified: the endothelium, the smooth muscle cells of the wall of pulmonary arterioles and, adventitial connective tissue cells.

PH has been related with malfunction of potassium channels and over-regulation of calcium channels on the cell membrane of vascular muscle cells as well as endothelial dysfunction. The latter, as it pertains with decreasing NO and prostacyclin (vasodilators) delivering and increment of vasocontrictors, such as endothelin-1 (ET-1) Inagami *et al.*, 1995; Voelkel and Tuder, 2000)

In adult subjects, angiogenesis could be taken as a compensatory process during hypoxic exposure. This process would be in addition to the well-known mechanisms of augmenting blood perfusion in less vascularized areas in the lung, hyperventilation and erythropoiesis. Those areas might be a potentially available area for *de novo* vascular formation. Human beings living in highlands, have developed a greater lung capacity through evolution, as an adaptive mechanism to hypobaric hypoxia (Frisancho, 1970). Also, high landers show increased lung capillary density than lowlanders, which was interpreted as an effect of hypoxia on angiogenesis (Bisschop et al, 2010).

Ooi et al (2000) and Howell et al (2002, 2003) determined that hypoxic hypoxia (10% oxygen) provoked augmentation in volume and total length in pulmonary blood vessels in rats, together with an increment in endothelial superficial area and cells numbers. In another work, chronically hypoxic rats, which exhibited a greater degree of vascular development through angiogenesis, had higher cardiac mass index values than the correspondent ones in animals subjected to hypoxia and hypercapnia or normoxia (Howell et al., 2004). In mice subjected to hypoxia, Pascaud et al (2003) gave evidence that inhibition of hypoxia-induced angiogenesis, enhanced the degree of PH.

Angiogenesis is regulated by angiogenic and anti-angiogenic molecules (Pascaud et al., 2003; Maharaj and D`Amore, 2007). Genetic and epigenetic factors permit blood vessels formation (Pauling and Vu, 2004). Taraseviciene-stewart et al (2001) found that plexiform lesions in idiopathic pulmonary hypertension (iPAH) were associated with disordered angiogenesis due to exaggerated mitosis of endothelial cells. Tuder and Voelkel (2002) reported endothelial cell proliferation in cases of primary PH, and, since these cells exhibited markers of angiogenesis, the authors named this process a "disordered or misguided angiogenesis". In this context, endothelium progenitor cells are now claimed to be therapeutic targets in PH due to their possible involvement in PH pathobiology. Nitric oxide synthases (eNOs), vascular endothelial growth factor (VEGF), angiopoietins and their receptor tie-2, which are associated with vascular remodeling, were all expressed in a monocrotaline induced model of PH (Cho et al.,

2009). Furthermore, induced ischemia results in pronounced cell proliferation and consequent lung vascularization in mice, within a period of 20 days (Wagner et al, 2006).

If vascular growth in the lung is an adapting mechanism to hypoxia, genetically predisposed individuals will develop hypoxic PH, and have a diminished pulmonary vascular growth capacity. Hence, angiogenesis might be the expression of genetic adaptation or predisposition to PH inducers.

2. Angiogenic promoting factors

The hypoxia inducible factor (HIF) system is oxygen sensitive. It includes HIF-1 and HIF-2. They bind and activate many of the same genes, but differ in their participation during hypobaric hypoxia. For instance, HIF-2 alone is responsible for the liberation of erythropoietin through stimulation of connective tissue cells in the kidney (Paliege et al., 2010) and other hematological reactions to hypoxia (reviewed by Tissot van Patot and Gassmann, 2011). HIF-1 is a key molecule in regulating the expression of several angiogenic molecules. Among the hypoxia-inducible genes which have important HIF-1 binding sites and are believed to participate in the pathogenesis of PH and angiogenesis as well, are those encoding VEGF (Liu et al., 1995), the VEGF receptor 1 (Gerber et al, 1997), and ET-1 (Hu et al., 1998). Expression of VEGF and its receptor Fetal Liver Kinase 1 receptor (FLK-1) was enhanced in hypoxic pulmonary hypertensive rats (Christou et al., 1998). Rats maintained under hypoxic hypoxia (exposure to 10% oxygen) showed augmented volume and total length of pulmonary blood vessels (Howell et al. 2002, 2003; Ooi et al., 2000). In another study, rats exposed to hypobaric hypoxia, exhibited reduced Angiopoietin-1/Tie2 and VEGF expression, together with a diminished number of arterial blood vessels in the lung (Yamamoto et al., 2008).

Sands et al (2012) gave insight on the interaction of members of the VEGF family in hypoxic PH. They found that VEGFB and the placental growth factor (PGF) inhibit or potentiate the actions of VEGFA, according to their relative concentrations, which change in the lungs of rats subjected to hypoxic hypoxia. The same authors stated that the abovementioned effects *in vivo* depend on specific concentrations of VEGF and PGF within the alveolar wall during adaptation to hypoxia. In this context, human subjects developing acute mountain sickness had higher levels of plasma VEGF on ascend to altitude as compared to their own values obtained under normoxic conditions. This variation did not occur in healthy subjects (Tissot van Patot et al., 2005).

VEGF exerts its angiogenic effect through four different pathways, which include NO participation (proposed by Gramatikoff, 1999). In a previous study, adrenomedullin mRNA expression was greater in the lungs of chickens with pulmonary hypertension compared with those without pulmonary hypertension (Gómez et al., 2008) and Vadivel et al (2010) demonstrated that adrenomedullin promotes angiogenesis in the lung. Hence, two vasodilators of pulmonary blood vessels, NO and adrenomedullin, may also have angiogenic properties.

Fahra et al (2011) found that CD34(+) and CD133(+) progenitor cell numbers are higher in the bone marrow, blood, and pulmonary arteries of pulmonary hypertensive subjects as compared to healthy controls. The blood levels of (hypoxia inducible myeloid-activating factors such as erythropoietin, the stem cell factor (SCF), and hepatocyte growth factor (HGF) were higher than normal levels in diseased individuals, and related to PH severity. Similarly, Davie et al (2004) found that progenitor cells from bone marrow origin contribute to neo-vascularization in pulmonary arteries of hypoxic calves, based on quantitative morphometric analyses of lung tissue from normoxic and hypoxic individuals. Their results showed adventitial growth in *vasa vasorum* of pulmonary arteries. This change was attributed to the transformation of cells from the bone marrow, which would be mobilized into the circulation, and differentiate into endothelial and smooth muscle cells. This model was supposed to entail an increase in the expression of c-kit(+), VEGF, fibronectin, and thrombin, as responses to hypoxia.

PH is linked to myeloid abnormalities, some of which may be related to increased production of HIF-inducible factors by a diseased pulmonary vasculature, but findings in non-affected subjects, suggest that myeloid abnormalities may be intrinsic to the disease process. Pro-angiogenic cell progenitors, and endothelial cells that have pathologic expression of hypoxia-inducible factor 1 alpha (HIF-1 alpha), were shown to be quantitatively higher in PH bone marrow, blood, and pulmonary arteries than in healthy controls. Also, the HIF-inducible myeloid-activating factors erythropoietin, stem cell factor (SCF), and hepatocyte growth factor (HGF) showed higher than normal levels in blood of pulmonary hypertensive subjects, and related to disease severity (Samar et al., 2011). In addition, endothelial progenitor cells with angiogenic capacity were found in the pulmonary circulation (Yoder, 2011). Epidermal growth factor promotes both angiogenesis and vascular remodeling (Janakidevi et al., 1995; Toby et al., 2010).

Bone morphogenetic protein (BMP) is compromised in endothelial repair within the pulmonary microvessels, and its expression is reduced in hypoxic PH, due to an increment in endothelial cell-derived Gremlin 1 and Gremlin 2, which antagonize BMP 2 type receptor expression (Cahill et al., 2012).

3. Inhibitors of angiogenesis

Angiogenesis is inhibited by thrombospondin-1 (TSP-1), a molecule produced by endothelial cells. Its secretion is induced by hypoxia and, experimentally, by NO inhibitors. In mesangial and smooth muscle cells, the cyclic guanosine monophosphate (GMPc) and kinase GMPc dependent protein, negatively regulate TSP-1 expression. CD36, a TSP-1 receptor, inhibits endothelial cell quimiotaxis (Isenberg el al., 2005). Low doses of NO stimulate endothelial cell proliferation, their motility and adhesion to collagen I matrixes, but the opposite is true for correspondent high doses. Exogenous TSP-1 treatment inhibits endothelial cell motility (Isenberg et al., 2005) and suppresses the angiogenic response provoked by low dose NO treatment (Ridnour et al., 2005).

Endogenous endostatin inhibits angiogenesis (Wickstrom et al., 2002; Paddenberg et al., 2006); it blocks the G1 phase of the cell cycle in endothelial cells, the attachment of $VEGF_{165}$ and $VEGF_{121}$ to the receptor VEGFR2 (Ribatti, 2009), and triggers endothelial cell apoptosis

(Dhanabal et al., 1999). Endostatin interferes with the assembly of the actin cytoskeleton of endothelial cells and inhibits their proliferation and participation in angiogenesis (Abdollahi et al., 2004; Skovseth et al., 2005). Endostatin expression on the surface of the smooth muscle cells of pulmonary arterioles in the mouse, is provoked by hypoxic exposure (Paddenberg et al., 2006). NO, in culture, induces endostatin production. Hence, endothelial apoptosis is also induced (Deininger et al., 2003). In human endothelial cell cultures, addition of endostatin reduces angiogenic activity by reducing HIF-1α, VEGF, VEGFR2, HGH and EGFR gene expression. Furthermore, expression of some anti-angiogenic genes, such HIF1An (a HIF antagonist), Kininogen, TSP-1 and a Vasostatin precursor is increased (Abdollahi et al., 2004). However, it appears that the mode of action of endostatin, in this context, needs to be fully elucidated (Deininger et al., 2003; Skovseth et al., 2005).

Adiponectin (ADPN) reinforces the vasodilatory action of NO in pulmonary blood vessels (Summer et al, 2009), and as stated, if NO contributes to the control of angiogenesis, ADPN will be a potential inhibitor of vascularization. Also, Le Cras et al (2003) found that alpha transforming growth factor (TGF-α) overexpression induced a diminution in pulmonary vascular development, which was accompanied by severe PH and vascular remodeling.

Oxidative stress is higher in the lungs of pulmonary hypertensive chickens (Iqbal y col., 2001a, b), which has been associated, in another species, with decreasing numbers of blood vessels (Murfee and Schmid-Schonbein, 2008). Oxidative stress, occurring in chronically hypoxic mice, can enhance endostatin production (Deininger et al., 2003) (Paddenberg et al., 2006).

4. Highlights on vascular development under hypoxia or normoxia in the chicken model

Angiogenesis in the mature pulmonary circulation could be a structural adaptation that may have important beneficial consequences for gas exchange (Howell et al., 2003). In contrast, Yamamoto et al (2008) reported a chronic hypoxia-induced pulmonary blood vessels loss, an event sometimes called "rarefaction" or "pruning".

Although there is no definitive evidence of less vascularized areas in the avian lung, it is feasible that during hypoxia, vasculogenesis and angiogenesis occur to augment the gas exchange area. Hypoxia exposure for 3 to 4 weeks, does not affect pulmonary growth in current commercial chicken strains (Vásquez and Hernández, 2011; Areiza et al., 2011). These findings appear to be controversial, since alveolar and vascular neo-formation should both increase in the pulmonary response to hypoxia (reviewed by Bhattacharya, 2008). If this is not the case, less vascularized areas within the lung could gain new blood vessels, which might not significantly affect the whole organ's weight. It should be noticed that arteriogenesis might also play a role in neo-vascularization (Deindi and Schaper, 2008)

The final goal of angiogenesis in the lung, should be to construct a complete functional arterio-venous tree. Therefore, vascular density would be represented by different types of blood vessels, such as arterioles or pre-capillaries. In this framework, using the chicken as a model, quantitative and molecular studies were undertaken to test the potentiality of hypobaric hypoxia to induce angiogenesis, to detect possible differences in vascular density in pulmonary hypertensive chickens and to correlate these findings with mRNA expression of some key genes for angiogenesis. Under hypobaric hypoxic conditions (altitude 2638 m above sea level, (oxygen tension: approximately 111 mmHg), both, healthy and pulmonary hypertensive birds, had more blood vessels with diameter ranges between >100-200, >200-300 and >300-500 μm, as compared to healthy chickens maintained under relative, normobaric, normoxic conditions (460 meters above sea level (oxygen tension: approximately 152 mmHg). However, the opposite was encountered when comparing values obtained for blood vessels within the ≥50-100 μm range. Coincident with this result, decreased expression of hepatocyte growth factor (HGF), HIF-2α, VEGF, Flk-1, and HGFR genes was encountered in the lung of chickens exposed to hypoxia. The same mRNA expression pattern did not show coincidence with observations for blood vessels within the range of 100-500 μm (Areiza et al., 2011, 2012).

It is interesting that the mRNA expression of various genes compromised in both, angiogenesis and vascular remodeling, varies in pulmonary hypertensive (susceptible chickens) versus non-pulmonary hypertensive chickens, which indicates different degrees of resistance or susceptibility to hypobaric hypoxia (Gómez et al, 2007, 2008; Areiza et al., 2012). This coincidence reinforces the idea that among all the known compensatory mechanisms for low pO2 in the airways and hypoxemia, angiogenesis is one of them, but it might be a long term one.

5. Final remarks

Promoting angiogenesis, vasculogenesis, or arteriogenesis could represent a possible palliative treatment in individuals chronically exposed to hypobaric hypoxia. It is clear that it would be useful to establish some characteristics of vascular development in the lung of susceptible individuals subjected to chronic hypoxia, in order to design long term treatments, such as vascular neo-formation enhancement. In this context, it is desirable to further investigate the chronology of angiogenesis in the hypoxic lung.

Again, mesodermal derivatives particularly bone marrow cells, the endothelium, and fibroblasts, act in two different but possibly complementary ways, as a response to hypoxia: the remodeling process and pulmonary vascular neo-formation. However, as has been presently highlighted, some results are controversial, which could not be currently explained, since there is not enough information on the vascular development in the lung, as a result of hypoxic exposure of susceptible and non-susceptible individuals, which would allow for the understanding of the molecular framework of angiogenesis at different stages of development and possibly, the correspondent genes involved.

Angiogenesis is a distinct mechanism to compensate for the hypoxic conditions within the alveoli (or respiratory capillaries in birds). However, addition of new blood vessels to the lung as a compensatory mechanism, might be a time-dependent process, as it occurs in the placenta, where distinct factors intervene at different times during gestation (Hamilton et al., 1995; Athanassiades and Lala, 1998; Matsumoto et al., 2002; Wulff et al., 2002), and further studies are needed in this matter. Evidence in this direction was given by Sands et al (2011), as related to the adapting process to hypoxia. They found that the *in vivo* actions of VEGFB and PGF can either inhibit or potentiate the actions of VEGFA. Those effects depend on their relative concentrations within the lung, which change in the hypoxic lung.

At this point, it is noted that ET-1, one the most studied molecules, has been chosen as a target molecule, in works aimed to design PH alleviation, by blocking its A receptor with bosentan (Weber et al., 1996; Lim et al., 2009). Also, vasoactive intestinal peptide was found to be a more potent ET-1 A receptor blocking agent than bosentan (Hamidi et al., 2011). Stromal derived factor 1 (SDF1), angiopoietin 2 (ANGPT2), placental growth factor (PGF), platelet-derived growth factor B (PDGFB), and stem cell factor (SCF) are also included as target molecules (reviewed by Rey and Semenza, 2010).

It is clear that both, angiogenesis and vascular remodeling as seen in PH, share common biological pathways and the endothelium appears to be the main participating structure in this regard. This coincidence might be an advantage in the design of therapeutic measures.

Some apparent differences in quantitative findings related to vascular neo-formation appear to depend on genetic differences and/or time of exposure to hypoxic conditions.

Author details

Aureliano Hernández* and Rafael A. Areiza

*Address all correspondence to: ahernandezv@unal.edu.co

Facultad de Medicina Veterinaria y de Zootecnia, Universidad Nacional de Colombia, Bogotá, Colombia

References

[1] Abdollahi, A, Hahnfeldt, P, Maercker, C, et al. (2004). Endostatin`s Antiangiogenic Signaling Network. Molecular Cell , 13, 649-663.

[2] Al-ruyabe, A. A. K, Kirshnamoorthy, S, Anthony, N. B, et al. (2010). Genetic Analysis Of Pulmonary Hypertension And Ascites In The Chicken. Plant & Animal Genomes XVIII Conference. XVIII-W492.

[3] Alvarez, D. F, Huang, L, King, J. A, et al. (2007). Lung microvascular endothelium is enriched with progenitor cells that exhibit vasculogenic capacity. American Journal of Physiology and Lung Cell and Molecular Physiology L, 419-430.

[4] Areiza, R. A, Rivas, P. C, & Hernández, A. (2011). A Quantitative Study of the Pulmonary Vascular Bed and Pulmonary Weight : Body Weight Ratio in Chickens Ex-

posed to Relative Normoxia and Chronic Hypobaric Hypoxia. The journal of poultry science , 48(4), 267-274.

[5] Areiza, R, Caminos, J. E, & Hernández, A. (2012). Diminished pulmonary expression of hypoxia-inducible factor 2-alpha, vascular endothelial growth factor and hepatocyte growth factor in chickens exposed to chronic hypobaric hypoxia. The journal of poultry science. , 49, 205-211.

[6] Athanassiades, A, & Lala, P. (1998). Role of placenta growth factor (PlGF) in human extravillous trophoblast proliferation, migration and invasiveness. Placenta , 17, 545-555.

[7] Bhattacharya, J. (2008). Lung neovascularization: a tale of two circulations Am J Physiol Lung Cell Mol Physiol March 2008 294:LL418, 417.

[8] Bisschop, D. E. C, Kiger, L, & Marden, M. C. (2010). Pulmonary capillary blood volume and membrane conductance in Andeans and lowlanders at high altitude: A cross-sectional study. Nitric Oxide , 23, 187-193.

[9] Budhiraja, R, Tuder, R. M, & Hassoun, P. M. (2004). Endothelial dysfunction in pulmonary hypertension. Circulation, , 109, 159-165.

[10] Cahill, E, Costello, C. M, Rowan, S. C, et al. (2012). Gremlin Plays a Key Role in the Pathogenesis of Pulmonary Hypertension. Circulation: U241., 125(7), 920.

[11] Cho, Y. J, Han, J. Y, Lee, S. J, et al. (2009). Temporal changes in angiopoietins and tie expression in rat lungs after monocrotaline-induced pulmonary hypertension. Comparative medicine. , 59, 350-356.

[12] Christou, H, Yoshida, A, Arthur, V, Morita, T, & Kourembanas, S. (1998). Increased vascular endothelial growth factor production in the lungs of rats with hypoxia-induced pulmonary hypertension. American Journal of Respiratory and Cell Molecular Biology , 18, 768-776.

[13] Dhanabal, M, Ramchandran, R, Waterman, M. J, et al. (1999). Endostatin induces endothelial cell apoptosis. Journal of Biological Chemistry , 274, 11721-11726.

[14] Davie, N. J, Crossno, J. T, Frid, M. G, et al. (2004). Hypoxia-induced pulmonary artery adventitial remodeling and neovascularization: contribution of progenitor cells. American Journal of Physiology-Lung Cellular and Molecular Physiology 286: L, 668-678.

[15] Deininger, M. H, Wybranietz, W. A, Graepler, F. T. C, et al. (2003). Endothelial endostatin release is induced by nitric oxide/cGMP pathway. The FASEB Journal, l, 17, 1267-1276.

[16] Deindi, E, & Schaper, W. (2005). The art of arteriogenesis. Cell biochemistry and biophysics , 43, 1-15.

[17] Farha, S, Asosingh, K, & Hypoxia-inducible, X. U, W. L. factors in human pulmonary arterial hypertension: a link to the intrinsic myeloid abnormalities. Blood , 117, 3485-3493.

[18] Frisancho, A. R. (1970). Developmental responses to high altitude hypoxia. American Journal of Physical Anthropology 32., 401-407.

[19] Gerber, H, Condorelli, P, Park, F, & Ferrara, J. N. (1997). Differential transcriptional regulation of the two vascular endothelial growth Factor receptor genes: Flt-1, but not Flk-1, is upregulated by hypoxia. Journal of Biological Chemistry , 272, 23659-23667.

[20] Gómez, A. P, Moreno, M. J, Iglesias, A, et al. (2007). Endothelin 1, its endothelin type a receptor, connective tissue growth factor, platelet-derived growth factor, and adrenomedullin expression in lungs of pulmonary hypertensive and nonhypertensive chickens. Poultry Science , 86, 909-916.

[21] Gómez, A. P, Moreno, M. J, Baldrich, R. M, & Hernández, A. (2008). Endothelin-1 Molecular Ribonucleic Acid Expression in Pulmonary Hypertensive and non-hypertensive Chickens. Poultry Science , 87, 1395-1401.

[22] Hamidi, S. A, Lin, R. Z, et al. (2011). VIP and endothelin receptor antagonist: An effective combination against experimental pulmonary arterial hypertension. Respiratory Research , 12, 141-147.

[23] Hamilton, G, Lysiak, J, Watson, A, & Lala, P. (1995). Autocrine growth stimulatory role of CSF-1 for the first trimester human trophoblast. American Journal of Reproductive Immunology , 33, 316-322.

[24] Hernández, A. Sandino de M., (2011). Hypoxic pulmonary hypertension in the chicken model. In: Pulmonary hypertension. From bench research to clinical challenges. Edited by: Sulica, R., Preston, I. IntechRijeka, Croatia, , 111-150.

[25] Howell, K, Hopkins, N, & Mcloughlin, P. (2002). Combined Confocal Microscopy and Stereology: a Highly Efficient and Unbiased Approach to Quantitative Structural Measurement in Tissues. Exp Physiol. , 87(6), 747-756.

[26] Howell, K, Preston, R. J, & Mcloughlin, P. (2003). Chronic hypoxia causes angiogenesis in addition to remodelling in the adult rat pulmonary circulation. Jornal of Physiology (Lond). , 547, 133-145.

[27] Hu, J, Discher, D. J, Bishopric, N. H, & Webster, K. A. (1998). Hypoxia regulates expression of endothelin-1 gene through a proximal hypoxia-inducible factor-1 binding site on the antisense strand. Biochemical and biophysical research communications , 245, 894-899.

[28] Humbert, M, Silbon, O, & Simonneau, G. (2004). Treatment of pulmonary arterial hypertension. New England Journal of Medicine , 351, 1425-1436.

[29] Inagami, T, Mitsuhide, N, & Hoover, R. (1995). Endothelium as an endocrine organ. Annual Reviews of Physiology , 57, 171-189.

[30] Iqbal, M, Cawthon, D, Wideman, R. F J. R, & Bottje, W. G. (2001a). Lung mitochondrial dysfunction in pulmonary hypertension syndrome. I. Site-specific defects in the electron transport chain. Poultry Science , 80, 485-495.

[31] Iqbal, M, Cawthon, D, Wideman, R. F J. R, & Bottje, W. G. (2001b). Lung mitochondrial dysfunction in pulmonary hypertension syndrome. II. Oxidative stress and inability to improve function with repeated additions of adenosine diphosphate. Poultry Science, , 80, 656-665.

[32] Inagami, T, Mitsuhide, N, & Hoover, R. (1995). Endothelium as an endocrine organ. Annual Reviews of Physiology , 57, 171-189.

[33] Isenberg, J. S, Ridnour, L. A, Perruccio, E. M, et al. (2005). Thrombospondin-1 Inhibits Endothelial Cell Responses to Nitric Oxide in cGMP-Dependent Manner. Proceedings of the Natural Academy of Science. USA., 102, 13141-13146.

[34] Janakidevi, K, & Tiruppathi, C. del Vecchio, P.J., et al. (1995). Growth characteristics of pulmonary artery smooth muscle cells from fawn-hooded rats Am J Physiol Lung Cell Mol Physiol March 1, 1995 268:LL470, 465.

[35] Le crasT. D., hardie, W. D., fagan, K., et al. (2003). Disrupted Pulmonary Vascular Development and Pulmonary Hypertension in Transgenic Mice Overespressing Transforming Growth Factor-α. American Journal of Physiology Lung and Cellular Molecular Physiology 285: ll1054., 1046.

[36] Le CrasT. D., Hardie, W. D., Fagan, K., et aL. (2003). Disrupted Pulmonary Vascular Development and Pulmonary Hypertension in Transgenic Mice Overespressing Transforming Growth Factor-α. American Journal of Physiology Lung and Cellular Molecular Physiology l1054., 285, 1046.

[37] Lim, K. A, Shim, J. Y, Cho, S. H, & Kim, K. Ch., Han, J.J., Hong, Y.M. (2009). Effect of endothelin receptor blockade on monocrotaline-induced pulmonary hypertension in rats. Korean J Pediatr. , 52, 689-695.

[38] Liu, Y, Cox, S. R, Morita, T, & Kourembanas, S. (1995). Hypoxia regulates vascular endothelial growth factor gene expression in endothelial cells. Circulation Research , 77, 638-643.

[39] Maharaj, A. S. R, & Amore, D. P.A. (2007). Roles for VEGF in the Adult. Microvascular Research , 74, 100-113.

[40] Matsumoto, H, & Daikoku, M. A, W. T, et al. (2002). Cyclooxygenase-2 differentially directs uterine angiogenesis during implantation in mice. Journal of Biological Chemistry , 277, 29260-29267.

[41] Melillo, G, Musso, T, Sica, A, et al. (1995). A hypoxia-responsive element mediates a novel pathway of activation of the inducible nitric oxide synthase promoter. Journal of Experimental Medicine , 182, 1683-1693.

[42] Murfee, W. L, & Schmid-schonbein, G. W. (2008). Structure of microvascular networks in genetic hypertension. Methods in Enzymology, , 444, 271-284.

[43] Ooi, H, Cadogan, E, Sweeney, M, et al. (2000). Chronic hypercapnia inhibits hypoxic pulmonary vascular remodeling. Am. J. Physiol. Heart Circ. Physiol. 278: HH338., 331.

[44] Paddenberg, R, Faulhammer, P, Goldenberg, A, & Kummer, W. (2006). Hypoxia-induced increase of endostatin in murine aorta and lung. Histochemistry and Cell Biology, , 125, 497-508.

[45] Pakdel, A, Van Arendonk, J. A, Vereijken, A. L, & Bovenhuis, H. (2005). Genetic parameters of ascites-related traits in broilers: effect of cold and normal temperature conditions. British Poultry Science , 46(1), 35-42.

[46] Paliege, A, Rosenberger, C, Bondke, A, et al. (2010). Hypoxia-inducible factor-2alpha-expressing interstitial fibroblasts are the only renal cells that express erythropoietin under hypoxia-inducible factor stabilization. Kidney International , 77(4), 312-318.

[47] Pan, J. Q, Tan, X, et al. (2005). Effects of early feed restriction and cold temperature on lipid peroxidation, pulmonary vascular remodelling and ascites morbidity in broilers under normal and cold temperature. British Poultry Science , 46(3), 374-381.

[48] Pascaud, M. A, Griscelli, F, Raoul, W, et al. (2003). Lung Overexpression of Angiostatin Aggravates Pulmonary Hypertension in Chronically Hypoxic Mice. American Journal of Respiratory and Cell Molecular Biology , 29, 449-457.

[49] Pauling, M, & Vu, T. H. (2004). Mechanisms and Regulation of Lung Vascular Development. Current Topics in Developmental Biology , 64, 73-99.

[50] Peñaloza, D, & Arias, S. J. (2007). The heart and pulmonary circulation at high altitudes: healthy highlanders and chronic mountain sickness. Circulation , 115(9), 1132-46.

[51] Rey, S, & Semenza, G. L. (2010). Hypoxia-inducible factor-1-dependent mechanisms of vascularization and vascular remodelling. Cardiovascular research , 86, 236-242.

[52] Ridnour, L. A, Isenberg, J. S, Espey, M. G, et al. (2005). Nitric Oxide Regulates Angiogenesis Through a Functional Switch Involving Thrombospondin-1. Proceedings of the Natural Academy of Science. USA. , 102, 13147-13152.

[53] Samar, F, Kewall, A, Weiling, X, et al. (2011). Hypoxia-inducible factors in human pulmonary arterial hypertension: a link to the intrinsic myeloid abnormalities. Blood , 117, 3485-3493.

[54] Sands, M, Howell, K, Costello, C. M, & Mcloughlin, P. (2011). Placental growth factor and vascular endothelial growth factor B expression in the hypoxic lung. Respiratory Research , 12, 17-29.

[55] Skovseth, D. K, Veuger, M. J. T, Sorensen, D. R, et al. (2005). Endostatin Dramatically Inhibits Endothelial Cell Migration, Vascular Morphogenesis, and Perivascular Cell Recruitment in vivo. Blood. , 105, 1044-1051.

[56] Summer, R, Fiack, C. A, Ikeda, Y, et al. (2009). Adiponectin deficiency: a model of pulmonary hypertension associated with pulmonary vascular disease. American Journal of Physiology and Lung Cell Molecular Physiology 297:L, 432-438.

[57] Taraseviciene-stewart, L, Kasahara, Y, Alger, L, et al. (2001). Inhibition of the vegf receptor 2 combined with chronic hypoxia causes cell death-dependent pulmonary endothelial cell proliferation and severe pulmonary hypertension. FASEB Journal, 15, 427-438.

[58] Tissot van Patot MC., Leadbetter G., Keyes, L.E., et al. (2005). Greater free plasma VEGF and lower VEGF receptor-1 in acute mountain sickness. Journal of applied physiology , 98, 1626-1629.

[59] Tissot van PatotM.C., Gassman, M. (2011). Hypoxia: Adapting to High Altitude by Mutating EPAS-1, the Gene Encoding HIF-2. High altitude medicine and biology , 12, 157-167.

[60] Toby, I. T, Chicoine, L. G, Cui, H, et al. (2010). Hypoxia-induced proliferation of human pulmonary microvascular endothelial cells depends on epidermal growth factor receptor tyrosine kinase activation. American journal of physiology and lung cell molecular physiology 298:L-L606., 600.

[61] Tuder, R. M, & Voelkel, N. F. (2002). Angiogenesis and pulmonary hypertension: A unique process in a unique disease. Antioxidants & Redox Signaling , 4, 833-843.

[62] Vadivel, A, Abozaid, S, Van Haaften, T, et al. (2010). Adrenomedullin Promotes Lung Angiogenesis, Alveolar Development, and Repair. American Journal of Respiratory Cell and Molecular Biology., 43, 152-160.

[63] Vásquez, I. C, & Hernández, A. (2012). Hipertensión pulmonar en pollos, lapso de exposición a la hipoxia hipobárica y relación peso pulmonar: peso corporal, bajo condiciones de temperatura controlada. Revista Colombiana de Ciencias Pecuarias , 25, 81-89.

[64] Voelkel, N. F, & Tuder, R. M. (2000). Hypoxia-induced pulmonary vascular remodelling: a model for what human disease?. Journal of Clinical Investigation , 106, 733-738.

[65] Wagner, E:M, Petrache, I, Schofield, B, & Mitzner, W. (2006). Pulmonary ischemia induces lung remodeling and angiogenesis. Journal of Applied Physiology , 100, 587-593.

[66] Weber, C, Schmitt, R, Birnboeck, H, Hoptgartner, G, Van Marle, S. P, Peeters, P. A, Jonkman, J. H, & Jones, C. R. (1996). Pharmacokinetics and pharmacodynamics of the endothelin antagonist bosentan in healthy human subjects. Clin Pharmacol Ther , 60, 124-137.

[67] Wideman, R. F, & Hamal, K. R. (2011). Idiopathic Pulmonary Arterial Hypertension: An Avian Model for Plexogenic Arteriopathy and Serotonergic Vasoconstriction. Journal of Pharmacological and toxicological methods , 63, 283-295.

[68] Wickstrom, S. A, Alitalo, K, & Keski-oja, J. (2003). Endostatin Associates with Lipid Rafts and Induces Reorganization of the Actin Cytoskeleton via Down-Regulation of RhoA Activity. Journal of Biological Chemistry , 278, 37895-37901.

[69] Wulff, C, Wilson, H, Dickson, S. E, et al. (2002). Hemochorial placentation in the primate: expression of endothelial growth factor, angiopoietins, and their receptors throughout pregnancy. Biology of Reproduction , 66, 802-8012.

[70] Yoder, M. C. (2011). Progenitor Cells in the Pulmonary Circulation. Proceedings of the American Thoracic Society , 2011, 8-466.

[71] Yamamoto, A, Takahashi, H, Kojima, Y, et al. (2008). Downregulation of Angiopoietin-1 and Tie2 in Chronic Hypoxic Pulmonary Hipertension. Respiration. , 75, 328-338.

Chapter 6

Acute Thromboembolic Pulmonary Hypertension

Jean M. Elwing and Ralph J. Panos

Additional information is available at the end of the chapter

http://dx.doi.org/10.5772/56719

1. Introduction

Acute pulmonary thromboembolism is a common and life-threatening condition that requires prompt evaluation and management to improve outcomes. In severe cases, acute pulmonary thromboembolism causes a rapid rise in pulmonary pressures precipitating compromised right ventricular (RV) function. Acute elevation in pulmonary pressures with RV failure is associated with poor outcome. When pulmonary thromboembolic disease is detected, further assessment of its impact on cardiac function is required for risk stratification and to determine appropriate therapy. This evaluation requires appropriate diagnosis of pulmonary thromboembolic disease as well as assessment of hemodynamics and RV function with electrocardiograms (ECG), echocardiography and commonly available biomarkers (Tapson 2012).

2. Epidemiology and prevalence

Venous thromboembolism is the third most common acute cardiovascular disease after myocardial infarction and stroke (Giuntini 1995). The incidence of venous thromboembolism is estimated to be 100-300 per 100,000 individuals but is age dependent increasing from 5 per 100,000 in childhood to 500-600 per 100,000 in those over 75 years of age (Douma 2010). Based upon the International Cooperative Pulmonary Embolism Registry (ICOPER), 4.2% of PE are classified as massive and are associated with systemic hypotension and cardiogenic shock (Stein 2003). In the Emergency Medicine Pulmonary Embolism in the Real World Registry (EMPEROR), 58 of 1875 patients (3.1%) presented with massive PE and their 30-day mortality was 14% (Lin 2012). The mortality rate for individuals with hemodynamically stable acute PE is 2-8% (Goldhaber 1999, Nijkeuter 2007) and the main cause of death is RV failure (Schoefp 2004, Kasper 1997, Wood 2002). However, in the first 3 months after acute PE, the case fatality rate increases to 15-18% (Goldhaber 1999).

2.1. Clinical presentation

Risk factors for PE are summarized in table 1 (Stein and Matta Curr Probl Cardiol 2010). Conditions predisposing to the development of deep venous thrombosis (DVT) include malignancy (especially pancreatic and brain cancers), chronic obstructive pulmonary disease, stroke, pregnancy, obesity, and immobilization, especially after lower extremity trauma or after surgery (hip and knee replacement). Hypercoagulable states may be acquired or inherited. Deficiencies in antithrombin, protein C, or protein S, factor V Leiden mutation, prothrombin gene 20210 mutation, and antiphospholipid antibodies predispose individuals to the development of venous thrombosis and subsequent PE.

Condition	Prevalence (%)
Immobilization	44
Surgery ≤ 3 month	35
Malignancy	18
Thrombophlebitis	16
Myocardial infarction	13
Trauma ≤ 3 months Lower extremity	11
Heart failure	9
Asthma	9
COPD	8
Stroke, paresis, or paralysis	8
Prior PE	5
Travel >4 hr in past month	4
Collagen vascular disease	4
Pneumonia (current)	1

Table 1. Predisposing conditions in patients with PE (based upon data from PIOPED I and II; (adapted from Stein and Matta 2010)

2.2. Clinical manifestations

The clinical manifestations and presentation of acute PE are not specific and range from mild breathlessness to hemodynamic collapse. Dyspnea either at rest or with exertion occurs in approximately three quarters of patients diagnosed with PE (Stein 2010). Pleuritic or non-pleuritic chest discomfort occurs less frequently. Hemoptysis occurs in 5-15% of patients with PE. Approximately one third of patients with DVT have clinically asymptomatic PE (Stein 2010). The clinical presentation of PE has been classified recently into three categories: 1)

http://dx.doi.org/10.5772/56719

syndrome of pulmonary hemorrhage or infarction with pleuritic chest pain or hemoptysis; 2) syndrome of isolated dyspnea, breathlessness with no accompanying chest discomfort, hemoptysis, or hemodynamic alteration; and 3) syndrome of circulatory collapse with loss of consciousness, hypotension, or cardiogenic shock (Ouellette 2012).

Alterations in vital signs occur frequently in patients with PE. Respiratory and heart rates are often increased; elevated temperatures occur less frequently. Blood pressure is reduced in hemodynamically significant PE. Physical examination findings are often not specific and are usually detected in only a minority of patients. Cardiac examination may reveal tachycardia, elevated jugular venous pressure, right ventricular lift, and increased sound of pulmonic valve closure. Pulmonary auscultation may identify crackles, rales, wheezes, diminished breath sounds, or rarely a pleural friction rub. Lower extremity swelling, edema, or tenderness is detected infrequently.

3. Diagnostic studies

Because the clinical presentation and manifestations of PE are not specific, further diagnostic testing is required to establish the diagnosis definitively. Patients are usually categorized by the clinical probability, either high or intermediate/low, based upon the clinician's suspicion for the presence of PE. Several evaluation systems have been developed to assess the clinical probability for the presence of PE and the most widely used algorithms are the Wells score and the revised Geneva score (Wells 2000, LeGal 2006). If the suspicion for PE is intermediate or low, a D-dimer assay is performed. D-dimer is formed during the degradation of cross-linked fibrin and its presence is very sensitive for intravascular thrombosis due to either venous thrombosis or PE. The threshold value for D-dimer testing depends upon the assay but a value below the threshold indicates a very low risk for the presence of thrombosis. However, a value above the threshold is not specific for thrombosis and further evaluation is required. Compression ultrasonography is the currently preferred evaluation for suspected DVT and chest computed tomographic pulmonary angiography (CTPA) is used to diagnose PE.

3.1. Laboratory abnormalities

Troponin I and T and brain natriuretic peptide (BNP) are cardiac biomarkers that are released into the circulation when cardiac myocytes are stretched or injured as may occur during right ventricular dysfunction after an acute pulmonary embolism (Samama 2006). Elevation of these biomarkers identifies patients who are normotensive but have an increased risk of mortality (Pruszcyk 2003). Neither biomarker is a sensitive assay for the diagnosis of pulmonary embolism (Meyer 2003).

Measurement of P_aO_2 and P_aCO_2 are routinely performed in patients presenting with breathlessness or pleurisy. In patients suspected to have PE, the sensitivity and specificity of a P_aCO_2<36 mmHg are 45% and 60%, respectively, and a P_aO_2<80 mmHg are 57% and 53%, respectively (Rodger 2000).

3.2. Electrocardiogram

The electrocardiographic manifestations of pulmonary embolism vary greatly from sinus tachycardia to conduction delays to patterns of RV strain (Panos 1988). Up to one quarter of patients with acute PE have normal electrocardiograms. Rhythm disturbances include tachycardia which is most common, atrial fibrillation, and atrial flutter. Conduction abnormalities include first degree AV block, and left and right bundle branch block. The S1Q3T3 pattern may occur in 25-50% of patients.

4. Imaging studies

Multi-detector computed tomography pulmonary angiography (CTPA) is the current best imaging study for the diagnosis of acute PE (Mos 2012, Klok 2011). Image acquisition is timed to occur during opacification of the pulmonary arterial bed after an intravenous injection of contrast. This technique has both high sensitivity, 96-100%, and specificity, 97-98% (Remy-Jardin 2007). The use of intravenous contrast may be contraindicated in patients with allergies to iodinated contrast and those with renal insufficiency or who are at risk for contrast-induced nephropathy. A prospective study showed that 14 of 174 patients (8%) developed contrast-induced nephropathy after CTPA which significantly contributed to the adverse outcomes of patients suspected of having an acute PE (Mitchell 2012). The radiation exposure during a CTPA has been estimated to cause 150 excess cancer deaths per million scans (Remy-Jardin 2007). RV function can also be assessed during multi-detector CTPA and abnormal position of the interventricular septum, inferior vena cava contrast reflux, RV diameter to left ventricle (LV) diameter ratio > 1.0 and RV volume to LV volume ratio > 1.0 are predictive of poor outcomes and RV diameter to LV diameter ratio > 1.0 and RV volume to LV volume ratio > 1.0 are also predictive of 30 day mortality after acute PE (Kang 2011).

In patients who are unable to undergo CTPA, ventilation perfusion scintigraphy (V/Q scan) is the next best imaging procedure for acute PE (Mos 2012). A normal V/Q scan effectively identifies patients who do not need anticoagulation treatment whereas a high probability V/Q scan has a positive predictive value >90% (PIOPED 1990). However, up to half of patients with suspected PE may have intermediate scans and require further testing to exclude or establish a diagnosis of PE (Anderson 2007). Intermediate scans occur less often in patients with a normal chest x-ray and no prior cardiopulmonary disease (Calvo-Romero 2005).

4.1. Echocardiography

Transthoracic and transesophageal echocardiography (ECHO) can be used to image cardiac structure and function in patients with suspected PE. Rarely, intravascular thrombus can be visualized if the clot is large and located within the proximal pulmonary artery (Goldhaber 2002). Studies correlating perfusion lung scans with ECHO findings suggest that approximately 92% of patients with PE and occlusion of greater than one third of the pulmonary vasculature demonstrate right ventricular hypokinesis (Wolfe 1994, McConnell 1996). Other echocardiographic findings in acute PE include right ventricular dilation, septal flattening and paradoxical septal motion, pulmonary arterial hypertension, and patent foramen ovale (Goldhaber 2002).

ECHO may be used to risk stratify hemodynamically stable patients with acute PE. In a meta-analysis, Sanchez and colleagues found the unadjusted relative risk of RV dysfunction for predicting death in patients with acute PE and normal hemodynamics was 2.4 (95% CI 1.3-4.4) (Sanchez 2008). In a prospective study of patients with acute PE, RV dysfunction determined by ECHO had an odds ratio of 1.2 (95% CI 1.1-1.4) for adverse events including death, cardiogenic shock, and recurrent venous thromboembolism (Sanchez 2010).

5. Hemodynamic consequences of acute pulmonary embolism

5.1. RV response to Acute PE

The response of the RV to acute PE depends upon its pre-existing level of function and hemodynamic relationship with the LV, the extent of pulmonary artery bed occlusion, and the degree of pulmonary arterial vasoconstriction caused by hypoxemia, release of vasoactive and bronchoactive mediators from platelets and vascular endothelial cells, and neural responses.

5.2. Baseline cardiopulmonary status

Approximately half of patients with acute PE have RV dysfunction at presentation and 14-17% have persistently reduced RV function six months later (Klok 2011, Stevinson 2007). Serial echocardiograms show that the PA pressure declines and RV dysfunction improves rapidly over the 30 days after presentation in approximately 90% of patients with acute PE and that age greater than 70 years and PAP greater than 50 mmHg are associated with persistent PH and RV dysfunction (Ribeiro 1999).

5.3. Extent of pulmonary vascular occlusion

In a series of 690 patients diagnosed with PE, the number of occluded pulmonary artery segments ranged from 1 to 17 and was normally distributed with a mean of 9.2 segments representing 51.2% of the pulmonary arterial bed (Guintini 1995). Because the pulmonary vasculature is a high capacitance system, earlier studies suggested that occlusion of 70% or more of the pulmonary vasculature is required for the elevation of pulmonary pressures (Sabiston 1965, Wagenvort 1995). Subsequent studies using measures of pulmonary vascular bed occlusion such as the Miller index, the Walsh score, or the Qanadli index suggested that obstruction of at least 30-40% identifies greater than 90% of patients with RV dilation (Qanadli 2001). However, further studies have shown that the RV ejection fraction determined with or without electrocardiographic synchronization and the RV/LV ratio are better predictors of clinical outcome than the pulmonary artery obstruction index (van der Bijl 2011)

5.4. Effects of vasoactive and broncho-active mediators

5.4.1. Vasoactive mediators

In experimental animal models of occlusive pulmonary embolism, blockage of vasoconstricting mediators such as thromboxane A_2 (TxA_2), serotonin, endothelin-1, and prostaglandin F_2alpha decreases pulmonary vascular resistance (Smulders 2000, Jones 2003, Reeves 1976 Reeves 1983, Todd 1981, Todd 1983, Breuer 1985, Battistini 2003, Kapsch 1981) suggesting that these factors play a significant role in increased pulmonary vascular resistance and elevated pulmonary pressures after acute PE.

Platelets produce TxA_2 after activation; other less significant sources of TxA_2 are endothelial cells and monocytes (Smulders 2000). TxA_2 production occurs quickly after PE and the level of production correlates with mortality in animal models (Reeves 1983). Reduction of TxA_2 production by COX inhibitors diminishes the increase in pulmonary artery pressure by 40-60% in various models of PE (Weidner 1979Konstam 1987).

Within the lung, serotonin is produced by activated platelets and is a potent vasoconstrictor. Serotonin levels increase in the pulmonary circulation after PE and infusion of serotonin can produce hemodynamic changes similar to PE (Thompson 1986, Breuer 1985). Inhibition of monoamine oxidase which degrades serotonin accentuates the vascular response to PE and reduction of platelet serotonin by reserpine diminishes the hemodynamic effect of PE (Rosoff 1971, Miczoch 1978, Gurewich 1968). Serotonin inhibitors markedly reduce pulmonary vascular resistance in various animal models of PE and a combination of TxA_2 and serotonin inhibitors completely prevents mortality due to massive PE in rabbits (Todd 1981, Todd 1983).

Prostacyclin (PGI_2) is a vasodilator produced by endothelial cells that antagonizes many of the effects of TxA_2 and serotonin. Blocking PGI_2 production or its effects augments the deleterious hemodynamic effects of PE (Smulders 2000).

Endothelins are potent vasoconstrictors produced by various pulmonary cells including endothelial cells, epithelial cells, monocytes, and macrophages. These mediators are potent vascular and bronchial constrictors and induce increases in pulmonary vascular resistance, decreases in pulmonary compliance and hypoxemia due to deranged ventilation-perfusion relationships. The effect of endothelin receptor antagonists on the hemodynamic consequences of PE are complex and vary depending upon the PE model and animal species (Battistini 2003).

Intravascular hemolysis may also occur during acute PE releasing free hemoglobin that may decrease pulmonary nitric oxide which may promote pulmonary vasoconstriction (Kline 2009).

5.4.2. Neural factors

In the resting state, the pulmonary arterial tree is nearly maximally dilated with little or no resting tone (Stratmann 2003). Vasodilating innervation is variable throughout most of the pulmonary arterial system but is consistently present in arteries >700 micrometers in diameter. In contrast, noradrenergic vasoconstrictive innervation is present throughout the entire

http://dx.doi.org/10.5772/56719

pulmonary bed. The effect of acetylcholine and sympathomimetics on pulmonary artery pressure is dependent upon the resting pressure and the same mediator may have constricting or dilating effects depending upon whether the baseline pressure is normal or increased (Stratmann 2003). Acute PE may also trigger the short lived von Bezold-Jarisch reflex which is manifest by apnea, bradycardia, and hypotension and may contribute to sudden death associated with PE (Stratmann 2003). This reflex may be mediated by J receptors, pulmonary irritant receptors, and pulmonary C-fibers.

5.4.3. RV response to changes in the pulmonary vasculature

The obstructive and vasoconstricting effects of acute PE on the pulmonary vasculature cause a sudden increase in the RV afterload that elevates RV wall tension dilating the RV, reducing its contractility, and impairing systolic and diastolic function. Right ventricular dilation distorts the anatomic configuration of the heart. Acute tricuspid valve insufficiency may be precipitated by elevated pulmonary arterial pressures coupled with physical dilation of the valvular annulus that causes misalignment of the leaflets. In addition, as the RV dilates, the interventricular septum flattens or bows toward the LV impairing its filling. LV preload is thus reduced by decreased RV output, tricuspid insufficiency, and diminished left ventricular filling. As preload falls, left ventricular output decreases and systemic hypotension ensues. Right ventricular ischemia or infarction may be caused by reduced myocardial perfusion, increased right ventricular wall tension, and compression of the right coronary artery reducing blood flow. (Piazza 2005, 2013) Figure 1.

5.4.4. Myocardial inflammation

After acute PE, neutrophilic infiltration of the right ventricular outflow tract occurs within 6 hours and subsequently resolves over the ensuing week (Watts 2008). Histopathologically, there is evidence of myocyte lysis and necrosis (Begieneman 2008) Monocytes are also present during the acute period and persist for at least 6 weeks; however, their phenotype transforms from inflammatory to healing over this period (Watts 2008).

5.5. Diagnosis of acute pulmonary embolism

The diagnostic evaluation of PE often is a multistep process which includes clinical evaluation, examination, laboratory assessment, and both noninvasive as well as invasive testing. Pulmonary angiography remains the gold standard to prove the presence of PE. However, this invasive test is not always readily available and does carry procedural risk. Other diagnostic modalities such as CTPA and V/Q scanning are used routinely in the assessment of possible PE (Tapson 2012).

6. Clinical prediction rules

PE is suspected in many patients presenting with acute worsening of dyspnea or chest pain. When evaluating patients for the possibility of PE, the use of a validated tool to predict pretest

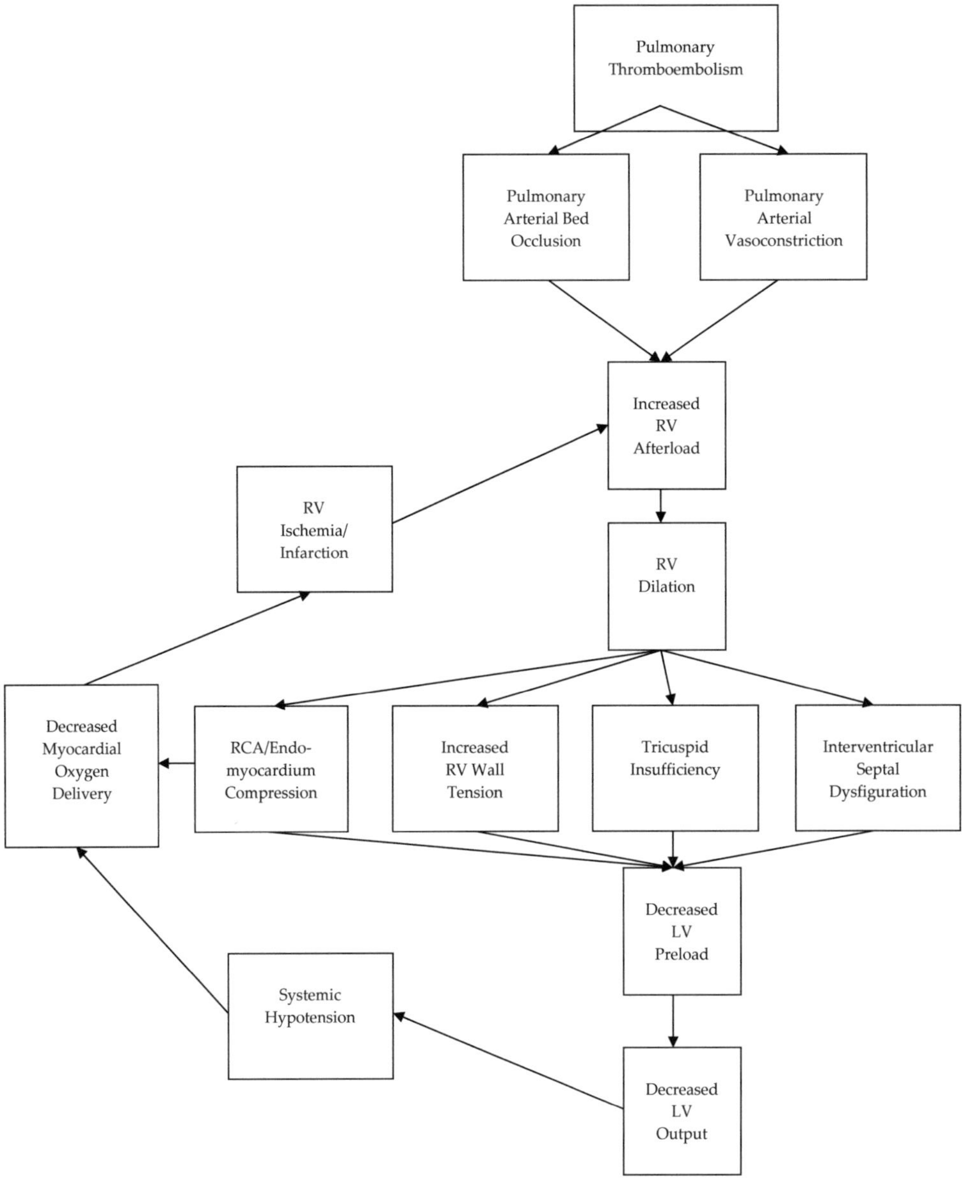

Figure 1. Acute pathophysiologic responses of the right ventricle to pulmonary thromboembolism (Adapted from Piazza and Goldhaber 2005)

probability of this diagnosis may be utilized. Several clinical prediction rules (CPRs) are available for the assessment of the clinical pretest probability for PE including but not limited to the Wells (Wells 1998), modified Wells (Bahia 2011), Geneva, and modified Geneva scores. In a meta-analysis performed by Ceriani et al (Ceriani 2010) in 2010, nine different clinical prediction tools for PE were reviewed. This meta-analysis suggests that all rules have comparable accuracy; however, there were differences in the extent of validation testing. The most extensively validated rules were the three-level Wells, two-level Wells, Geneva score, revised Geneva score, and the Charlotte rule (Ceriani 2010). The available CPRs incorporate patient's symptoms and the likelihood of alternative etiologies to determine the probability of PE as the cause of symptoms. These tools serve as valuable guides to assess the likelihood of PE as the cause of symptoms and often are used to determine the extent of testing performed during evaluation of suspected pulmonary thromboembolism. (Table 2)

Pulmonary Embolism Wells Score	
Symptoms of DVT	3 points
No alternative diagnosis better explains the illness	3 points
Tachycardia with pulse >100	1.5 points
Immobilization (≥3 days) or surgery in the previous four weeks	1.5 points
Prior history of DVT or pulmonary embolism	1.5 points
Presence of hemoptysis	1 point
Presence of malignancy	1 point
Total Criteria Point Count:	
	Pulmonary Embolism Score Interpretation
	Score > 6:High probability
	Score > 2 and < 6:Moderate probability
	Score < 2:Low Probability

Table 2. Wells Score to predict pulmonary embolism (adapted from Wells 2000)

7. D-dimer

The D-dimer antigen is a marker of fibrin degradation. It is formed by the sequential action of thrombin, Factor XIIIa and plasmin. D-dimer antigen can exist on fibrin degradation products derived from soluble fibrin before its incorporation into a fibrin gel or after the fibrin clot has been degraded by plasmin (Adam 2009). D-dimer has been found to be useful in evaluating outpatients for the presence of venous thromboembolism (VTE) (Wells 2001). D-dimer levels >500 ng/mL are considered elevated (Stein 2004). 95% of patients with proven PE will have an elevated D-dimer by ELISA assay (Stein 2004). Unfortunately, only 40-68% of patients without VTE have a negative D-dimer (Stein 2004). D-dimer elevation occurs in multiple other conditions besides PE including renal failure, surgery, cancer, sepsis, and pregnancy (Rathbun 2004). Thus, the use of d-dimer to evaluate VTE in hospitalized or otherwise chronically ill patients is limited. D-dimer is best used to exclude VTE in outpatients with low or moderate clinical suspicion for a thromboembolic event (Rathbun 2004, Wells 2000, Wells 2001, Stein 2006, Stein 2007).

8. Computed tomography pulmonary angiography (CTPA)

Over the last several decades, CTPA has become the first-line imaging modality for the assessment of PE. When compared with V/Q scanning in a randomized, single-blinded noninferiority clinical trial involving 1417 patients, CTPA was found to be non-inferior to V/Q scanning (Anderson 2007). CTPA is readily available and offers a high level of sensitivity and specificity for acute PE (Huisman 2013). PIOPED II found CTPA to be 83% sensitive and 96% specific for PE (Stein 2006). The newer generation multi-detector CTPA sensitivity is over 95% for segmental, lobar and centrally located PE (Huisman 2013) and is an extremely useful test to exclude PE (van Beek 2001). As with all other imaging modalities for pulmonary thromboembolism, CTPA should be used as part of an integrated approach in the evaluation of PE (Rathbun 2000, Van Strijen 2005) utilizing risk assessment tools to determine the appropriateness of proceeding to CTPA as this test does expose patients to radiation (Remy-Jardin 2007) and IV contrast.

9. Ventilation/perfusion scanning (V/Q scan)

An alternative diagnostic study to CTPA is V/Q scanning. V/Q scanning involves imaging of pulmonary perfusion and ventilation to evaluate for areas of mismatch that suggest the presence of PE. The average radiation exposure for a V/Q scan is 1.2 mSv. PIOPED evaluated the accuracy of V/Q scanning in the assessment of pulmonary embolism compared with the gold standard pulmonary angiogram (PIOPED 1990). Patients with a high clinical probability of PE and a high probability V/Q had a 95% likelihood of truly having a PE. Patients with a low clinical probability of PE and a low probability VQ scan had a 4% likelihood of having a PE (Gottschalk 2007). A normal V/Q scan virtually excluded PE (PIOPED 1990). Unfortunately, in patients with other combinations of clinical risk and V/Q results, the diagnostic accuracy of V/Q ranged from 15-86%. Therefore, additional diagnostic testing is required to determine the presence of PE in this group (Calvo-Romero 2005). (Table 3)

V/Q Scan Probability	**Clinical Probability of Pulmonary Embolism**		
	High	**Intermediate**	**Low**
High	96	88	56
Intermediate	66	28	16
Low	40	16	4
Normal or near normal	0	6	2

Table 3. Likelihood of pulmonary embolism according to scan category and clinical probability (based on PIOPED study 1990)

10. Pulmonary angiography

Pulmonary angiography is an invasive test that requires catheter placement in the pulmonary artery and directed IV contrast infusion to detect intraluminal vascular filling defects that might be caused by PE. This test requires performance and interpretation expertise and carries a risk of intracardiac catheter placement, radiation, and contrast exposure. In 1992, Stein et al (Stein 1992) reported 0.5% mortality, 1% nonfatal complications and 5% minor complications associated with this test in the 1,111 patients who underwent angiography in PIOPED. In most centers, pulmonary angiography has been replaced by CTPA as the standard for the diagnosis of PE (Hogg 2006). Currently, pulmonary angiography is only employed when other less invasive attempts at diagnosis are inconclusive.

11. Cardiac magnetic resonance imaging

Cardiac magnetic resonant imaging (MRI) is not a widely utilized tool in the evaluation of patients with PE. Magnetic resonance angiography (MRA) is often limited by motion artifact with resultant suboptimal resolution (Tapson 1997). When MRA was evaluated prospectively in 118 patients with dyspnea, MRA was positive in only 77% of patients with confirmed pulmonary embolism by conventional pulmonary angiography. Furthermore, in that study, MRA was positive in 100% of lobar PE, 84% of segmental PE and 40% of subsegmental PE (Oudkerk 2002). MRA may have promise in the future but requires further optimization of this imaging strategy prior to its routine use.

12. Assessment of right ventricle and pulmonary vasculature derangements

12.1. Electrocardiography

Electrocardiography (ECG) is an easily obtainable initial study in the evaluation of dyspnea and chest pain. It is often helpful in evaluating for acute coronary syndrome. Unfortunately, ECG has limited diagnostic value for acute PE (Rodger 2000). However, in the setting of known pulmonary thromboembolism, ECG is oftentimes abnormal and may be of some benefit in risk stratification. In 1997, Ferrari et al (Ferrari 1997) reported the results of 80 consecutive ECGs in hospitalized patients with documented pulmonary embolism. T-wave inversion in the precordial leads was shown to be the most common abnormality (68%) and correlated with PE severity. Anterior T wave inversions had a sensitivity of 90% and specificity of 81% for massive PE. The classic finding of acute RV failure with S1Q3 T3 was seen in 50% of ECGs in the setting of confirmed acute PE (Ferrari 1997) which is more frequent than previously reported, 12% (Stein 1975) to 28% (Cutforth 1958).

12.2. Cardiac echocardiography

Cardiac echocardiography (ECHO) is a useful tool in evaluation of a patient presenting with dyspnea and/or chest pain. Cardiac ECHO should not be used in the evaluation to confirm the diagnosis of acute PE as only 30-40% of all acute pulmonary thromboembolic events are associated with echocardiographic abnormalities (Gibson 2005). However, cardiac ECHO may be used in a supportive role in the diagnostic evaluation and for risk stratification. Several echocardiographic parameters should be assessed in the setting of presumed or confirmed PE including RV size, RV function, presence of RV thrombus, presence of McConnell's sign (mid-free wall akinesis but normal apical motion), and estimation of pulmonary artery pressures measured from tricuspid regurgitant jet velocity. RV dilation and dysfunction are associated with poor outcomes in PE accompanied by either normotension or hypotension. In 2005, Gibson et al (Gibson 2005) reported that RV dysfunction occurs in 30-40% of all normotensive patients with acute PE and is a positive predictor for short-term mortality (5%). This finding was also supported by Kucher et al (Kucher 2005) in 2005 who found decreased 30 day survival in patients with RV dysfunction in the setting of normotension (univariate hazard ratio of RV hypokinesis for predicting 30-day mortality of 2.11 (95% CI, 1.41-3.16; $P<.001$). In the setting of hypotension, RV dysfunction is a strong marker of poor outcome. In a retrospective assessment of 180 patients with acute PE, 70 were found to be hemodynamically stable without RV dysfunction, 74 hemodynamically stable with RV dysfunction and 36 hemodynamically unstable with RV dysfunction. The patients with hemodynamic instability and RV dysfunction had the highest mortality (27.8%, $p < 0.05$) and PE related deaths (16.7%, $p <0.05$) (Yoo 2012). McConnell's sign is a distinct pattern of regional RV dysfunction that may be seen in the setting of acute PE. McConnell's sign is characterized by akinesis of the mid-free wall but normal motion at the apex and is 77% sensitive and 94% specific for the diagnosis of acute PE with a positive predictive value of 71% and a negative predictive value of 96% (McConnell 1996).

12.3. Computed tomography pulmonary angiography (CTPA)

CTPA is a sensitive and specific diagnostic tool for PE (Huisman 2013). More recently, it has also been deemed an important study to assess thrombus burden and functions as a valuable indicator of RV decompensation. Thrombus burden can be assessed utilizing a modified Miller score (MMS) in which thrombus load is evaluated by the number of occluded segmental pulmonary arteries (9 on the right, 7 on the left) (Bankier 1997). In a retrospective analysis of 504 consecutive CTPA proven PE, higher MMS correlated with greater right ventricular (RV) to left ventricular (LV) ratio (RV:LV) indicating RV strain (Wong 2012). Furthermore, CTPA findings of high thrombus burden and RV strain are associated with increased PE mortality. In 81 consecutive patients with CTPA proven PE, RV:LV ratio, the shape of the interventricular septum, and the obstruction index were shown to be significant predictors of mortality ($p < 0.001$, $p = 0.04$, $p < 0.001$ respectively). The negative predictive value for mortality with an RV:LV ratio < or = 1.0 and the obstruction index of < 40% were 100% (Chaosuwannakit 2012).

http://dx.doi.org/10.5772/56719

13. Biomarkers

D-dimer, troponin I, troponin T, brain natruretic peptide (BNP) are commonly available biomarkers that are used to evaluate patients with PE. A recent meta-analysis evaluating D-dimer elevation and PE revealed that elevations greater than a defined threshold were associated with significantly increased short-term (3 months) mortality and the degree of pulmonary artery obstruction (Becattini 2012). Elevation in the cardiac biomarker, troponin I, when used in combination with CTPA predicts echocardiographically proven RV dysfunction associated with PE (Meyer 2012). Elevated high-sensitivity troponin T (hsTnT) has also been shown to be associated with poor outcomes in acute PE. hsTnT > 14 pg/ml is a predictor of early death and complications of venous thromboembolic disease. Furthermore, hsTnT, < 14 pg/ml is associated with a low risk of mortality in individuals with PE (Lankeit 2011). Various brain natruretic peptide assays are available for routine use to assess dyspnea. In a multicenter study including 570 patients with acute PE, ProBNP, BNP, and NT-proBNP values were significantly increased in patients with adverse outcomes after acute pulmonary embolism. However, the prognostic performance of proBNP for predicting adverse outcomes was lower than that of the other natriuretic peptides (Verschuren 2013).

14. Management of acute pulmonary embolism

Optimal management of the dyspneic patient includes rapid assessment for etiologies including PE. Complete history, physical examination and use of clinical prediction rules (CPRs) are essential to the initial evaluation. If the index of suspicion for PE is significant, radiologic imaging with CTPA or V/Q is often employed. If these noninvasive tests are inconclusive, pulmonary angiography is occasionally necessary to obtain a definitive diagnosis. Once PE is confirmed, additional risk assessment with hemodynamic assessment, echocardiography, CT determination of RV configuration, ECG, and biomarkers should be performed (Tapson 2008, Tapson 2012). Individual patient characteristics, level of hemodynamic compromise, and risk assessment should be used to determine optimal management. The 2011 Scientific Statement from the American Heart Association defined acute pulmonary thromboembolism as massive, sub-massive or low risk PE using these criteria: 1. Massive PE: Acute PE with sustained hypotension defined as a systolic blood pressure < 90 mmHg for at least 15 minutes or requiring inotropic support without other etiology; 2. Sub-massive PE: Acute PE without systemic hypotension but at risk of poor outcome based on evidence of either RV dysfunction or myocardial necrosis; 3. Low risk PE: Acute PE without the clinical markers defined in massive or submassive PE that portend a poor prognosis (Jaff 2011). (Table 4)

Massive	Sub-massive	Low-Risk
Acute PE with sustained hypotension	Acute PE without systemic hypotension	Low-risk PE
Systolic blood pressure < 90 mm Hg for at least 15 minutes or requiring inotropic support Hypotension not due to a cause other than PE •Including but not limited to arrhythmia, hypovolemia, sepsis, or LV dysfunction, pulselessness, or persistent profound bradycardia ◦Heart rate 40 bpm with signs or symptoms of shock.	Systolic blood pressure > 90 mm Hg but with either RV dysfunction or myocardial necrosis RV dysfunction defined as the presence of at least 1 of the following: •RV dilation (apical 4-chamber RV diameter divided by LV diameter 0.9) or RV systolic dysfunction on echocardiography •RV dilation (4-chamber RV diameter divided by LV diameter 0.9) on CT •Elevation of BNP (90 pg/mL) •Elevation of N-terminal pro-BNP (500 pg/mL); or •Electrocardiographic changes (new complete or incomplete right bundle-branch block, anteroseptal ST elevation or depression, or anteroseptal T-wave inversion) Myocardial necrosis is defined as either of the following: •Elevation of troponin I (0.4 ng/mL) •Elevation of troponin T (0.1 ng/mL)	Acute PE and the absence of the clinical markers of adverse prognosis that define massive or submassive PE

Table 4. Definitions of massive, submassive and low risk of pulmonary embolism (based on 2011 American Heart Association Scientific Statement)

15. Low risk pulmonary embolism

The mainstay of treatment for low risk PE is prompt initiation of anticoagulation. Importantly, if there is a high clinical suspicion for PE, anticoagulation should be initiated prior to confirmation of the diagnosis (Tapson 2012). The 2012 American College of Chest Physicians Evidence-Based Clinical Practice Guidelines (Kearon 2012) for Venous Thromboembolism

http://dx.doi.org/10.5772/56719

(VTE) recommend parenteral anticoagulants or oral factor Xa inhibition with rivaroxaban as the initial therapy for PE. Low-molecular-weight heparin (LMWH) or fondaparinux is endorsed over IV unfractionated heparin or subcutaneous unfractionated heparin. If there are no contraindications to anticoagulation, treatment is recommended for at least 3 months after acute PE with a more prolonged course when indicated (Kearon 2012).

16. Submassive pulmonary embolism

The treatment of submassive PE remains controversial. Patients with submassive PE carry an increased risk of adverse outcomes and early mortality (Piazza 2013); however, there is no clear evidence that thrombolysis in addition to heparin in this subset of patients improves mortality. In 2002, Konstantinides et al (Konstantinides 2002) evaluated 256 patients with submassive PE who were randomly assigned to receive heparin plus alteplase versus heparin plus placebo. Treatment with heparin plus placebo was associated with more frequent clinical deterioration requiring an escalation of treatment (11% versus 25%); however, no change in mortality was detected (Konstantinides 2002). Further study is required to determine appropriate management of this patient population. Currently, comprehensive evaluation weighing risks and benefits of anticoagulation with heparin versus thrombolysis is the usual approach.

17. Massive pulmonary embolism

The management of massive PE requires a multifaceted approach to resolve pulmonary vascular obstruction, reverse hemodynamic instability, and support respiratory insufficiency (Tapson 2008). Supportive measures often require volume resuscitation, vasopressors, supplemental oxygen, and occasionally mechanical ventilation (Tapson 2012). Current American College of Chest Physicians (ACCP) (Kearon 2012) and American Heart Association (AHA) (Jaff 2011) guidelines support the use of thrombolytic therapy in patients with acute massive PE and no contraindications. A 2004 meta-analysis revealed that thrombolysis significantly reduced recurrent PE and mortality (9.4% versus 19.0%; OR 0.45, 95% CI 0.22 to 0.92; number needed to treat=10) in patients with hemodynamically unstable PE (Wan 2004). There are limited clinical trial data to provide guidance on the best management of massive PE. A small prospective randomized clinical trial evaluating 8 patients with massive PE showed that streptokinase plus heparin improved hemodynamics within the first hour after treatment and survival at 2 years compared with heparin alone (Jerjes-Sanchez 1995). The heparin treated group had 100% mortality 1-3 hours after initial presentation. Autopsy studies in the heparin treated group revealed massive pulmonary emboli with RV infarction and no coronary artery obstruction (Jerjes-Sanchez 1995). Additional studies are required to determine the optimal management of patients with massive PE.

18. Embolectomy

Several interventional techniques including mechanical fragmentation, thrombus aspiration, and direct thrombolytic therapy are currently available for the treatment of acute PE. No clear guidelines can be provided regarding the use of interventional techniques for PE as there are no randomized controlled trials to assess these treatments. ACCP guidelines advise consideration of these interventions in the setting of massive PE with contraindications to systemic thrombolysis, failed thrombolysis, or likelihood of death before thrombolysis (Kearon 2012). Surgical embolectomy is infrequently required for management of acute PE. There are limited data guiding surgical interventions in this setting. Leacche et al (Leacche 2005) reported surgical outcomes in 47 consecutive patients with acute massive PE treated surgically. Indications for surgery included contraindications to thrombolysis (45%), failed medical treatment (10%) and right ventricular dysfunction (32%). Operative mortality and late mortality were 6% and 12% with the majority (83%) of the late mortality related to metastatic cancer. 86% and 83% of patients were alive 1 and 3 years after surgery, respectively (Leacche 2005). Specific instances when surgical intervention may be indicated are the presence of right atrial thrombus, paradoxical arterial embolism, or closure of a patent foramen ovale (Kearon 2012).

19. Late consequences of pulmonary embolism

Unresolved pulmonary thromboembolic disease can result in significant morbidity and mortality after acute PE and may lead to chronic thromboembolic pulmonary hypertension (CTEPH). The incidence of this condition is not well-documented. In 2012 Korkmaz et al (Korkmaz 2012) evaluated 325 consecutive patients after acute PE for residual thrombus and CTEPH. Residual chronic thrombus was detected in 48%, 27% and 18% of patients at 3, 6 and 12 months respectively. CTEPH (defined echocardiographically as estimated PAP ≥ 50 mmHg) was detected in 4.6% of follow-up echocardiograms. It is unclear if specific interventions at the time of PE could improve the rapidity or extent of thrombus resolution or decrease the likelihood of CTEPH development.

Recently, Kline et al (Kline 2009) reported baseline and 6 month follow-up echocardiography at a single center after acute PE. Elevated pulmonary pressures were defined as an RV systolic pressure (RVSP) ≥ 40 mmHg on echocardiogram. 200 normotensive patients with CTPA proven PE were enrolled. 21 received thrombolytic therapy with alteplase because of subsequent hemodynamic destabilization or respiratory failure. 180 (90%) survived to 6 months. 162 returned for a 6 month reevaluation after PE. In the heparin treated group, 35% had elevated pulmonary pressures initially and 7% were elevated at 6 months. 27% had increased estimated RVSP on subsequent echocardiograms. In the alteplase plus heparin group, 61% had elevated pulmonary pressures initially and 11% on follow-up echocardiogram without any increase in RVSP at follow-up (Kline 2009). These data suggest that thrombolytic therapy is associated with better reduction of RVSP than heparin alone; however, more detailed evaluation is necessary.

http://dx.doi.org/10.5772/56719

20. Summary

Acute pulmonary thromboembolism is the third most common acute cardiovascular disease (Giuntini 1995) and is associated with significant morbidity and mortality. Thromboembolic obstruction of the pulmonary vasculature frequently causes dyspnea, hypoxia, and chest pain. In severe cases, PE can cause an acute rise in pulmonary pressures precipitating RV dysfunction and hemodynamic instability. The increase in hemodynamic pressures is due to both mechanical obstruction of the pulmonary vascular bed as well as the release of vasoconstricting mediators and derangement of neural regulation of vasomotor tone. Hypotension, RV dysfunction, elevated biomarkers (BNP, troponin I, troponin T) and ECG abnormalities with T-wave inversions are markers of poor prognosis. Rapid evaluation and risk stratification are necessary for effective treatment. Hemodynamically stable PE, i.e. low risk PE, is routinely managed with heparin therapy and clinical monitoring. Hemodynamically unstable PE, i.e. massive PE, is frequently managed with thrombolysis. Optimal management of hemodynamically stable PE with high risk features, i.e. submassive PE, is unclear at this time. Further study to determine best practice in this group is ongoing. Unfortunately, acute PE has both short-term and long-term consequences. Additional evaluation and characterization of patients at risk to develop long term complications of pulmonary emboli are needed.

Author details

Jean M. Elwing[1,2*] and Ralph J. Panos[1,2]

*Address all correspondence to: jean.elwing@uc.edu

1 Pulmonary, Critical Care, and Sleep Medicine Division, Cincinnati Veterans Affairs Medical Center, Cincinnati, USA

2 Pulmonary, Critical Care, and Sleep Medicine Division, University of Cincinnati College of Medicine, Cincinnati, USA

References

[1] Adam SS, Key NS, Greenberg CS. D-dimer antigen: current concepts and future prospects. Blood. 2009 Mar 26;113(13):2878-87.

[2] Anderson DR, Kahn SR, Rodger MA, Kovacs MJ, Morris T, Hirsch A, Lang E, Stiell I, Kovacs G, Dreyer J, Dennie C, Cartier Y, Barnes D, Burton E, Pleasance S, Skedgel C, O'Rouke K, Wells PS.Computed tomographic pulmonary angiography vs ventilation-perfusion lung scanning in patients with suspected pulmonary embolism: a randomized controlled trial. JAMA. 2007 Dec 19;298(23):2743-53.

[3] Bahia A, Albert RK. The modified Wells score accurately excludes pulmonary embolus in hospitalized patients receiving heparin prophylaxis. J Hosp Med. 2011 Apr; 6(4):190-4.

[4] Bankier AA, Janata K, Fleischmann D, Kreuzer S, Mallek R, Frossard M, Domanovits H, Herold CJ. Severity assessment of acute pulmonary embolism with spiral CT: evaluation of two modified angiographic scores and comparison with clinical data. J Thorac Imaging. 1997 Apr; 12(2):150-8.

[5] Battistini B. Modulation and roles of the endothelins in the pathophysiology of pulmonary embolism. Can J Physiol Pharmacol. 2003 Jun; 81(6):555-569.

[6] Becattini C, Lignani A, Masotti L, Forte MB, Agnelli G. D-dimer for risk stratification in patients with acute pulmonary embolism. J Thromb Thrombolysis. 2012 Jan; 33(1): 48-57.

[7] Begieneman MP, van de Goot FR, van dB I, Noordegraaf AV, Spreeuwenberg MD, Paulus WJ, et al. Pulmonary embolism causes endomyocarditis in the human heart. Heart 2008; 94:450-456.

[8] Breuer J, Meshcig R, Breuer HWM, Arnold G. Effects of serotonin on the cardiopulmonary circulatory system with and without 5- HT2-receptor blockade by ketanserin. J Cardiovasc Pharmacol 1985; 7(suppl.7):S64–S66.

[9] Calvo-Romero JM, Lima-RodrÃguez EM, Bureo-Dacal P, PÃ©rez-Miranda M. Predictors of an intermediate ventilation/perfusion lung scan in patients with suspected acute pulmonary embolism.Eur J Emerg Med. 2005 Jun;12(3): 129-31.

[10] Ceriani E, Combescure C, Le Gal G, Nendaz M, Perneger T, Bounameaux H, Perrier A, Righini M. Clinical prediction rules for pulmonary embolism: a systematic review and meta-analysis. J Thromb Haemost. 2010 May; 8(5):957-70.

[11] Chaosuwannakit N, Makarawate P. Prognostic value of right ventricular dysfunction and pulmonary obstruction index by computed tomographic pulmonary angiography in patients with acute pulmonary embolism. J Med Assoc Thai. 2012 Nov; 95(11): 1457-65.

[12] Cutforth RH, Oram S. The electrocardiogram in pulmonary embolism.Br Heart J. 1958 Jan;20(1):41-60.

[13] Douma RA, Kamphuisen PW, Büller HR. Acute pulmonary embolism. Part 1: epidemiology and diagnosis. Nat Rev Cardiol. 2010 Oct;7(10):585-596.

[14] Ferrari E, Imbert A, Chevalier T, Mihoubi A, Morand P, Baudouy M. The ECG in pulmonary embolism. Predictive value of negative T waves in precordial leads--80 case reports. Chest. 1997 Mar;111(3):537-43.

[15] Gibson NS, Sohne M, Buller HR.Prognostic value of echocardiography and spiral computed tomography in patients with pulmonary embolism. Curr Opin Pulm Med. 2005 Sep;11(5):380-4.

[16] Giuntini C, Di Ricco G, Marini C, Melillo E, Palla A. Pulmonary embolism: epidemiology. Chest. 1995 Jan; 107(1 Suppl):3S-9S.

[17] Goldhaber SZ, Visani L, De Rosa M. Acute pulmonary embolism: clinical outcomes in the International Cooperative Pulmonary Embolism Registry (ICOPER). Lancet 1999; 353:1386–9.

[18] Goldhaber SZ. Echocardiography in the management of pulmonary embolism. Ann Intern Med. 2002; 136(9):691-700.

[19] Gottschalk A, Stein PD, Sostman HD, Matta F, Beemath A.Very low probability interpretation of V/Q lung scans in combination with low probability objective clinical assessment reliably excludes pulmonary embolism: data from PIOPED II.J Nucl Med. 2007 Sep; 48(9):1411-5.

[20] Gurewich V, Cohen ML, Thomas DP. Humoral factors in massive pulmonary embolism: an experimental study. Am Heart J 1968; 76:784–794.

[21] Hogg K, Brown G, Dunning J, Wright J, Carley S, Foex B, Mackway-Jones K. Diagnosis of pulmonary embolism with CT pulmonary angiography: a systematic review. Emerg Med J. 2006 Mar;23(3):172-8.

[22] Huisman MV, Klok FA. How I diagnose acute pulmonary embolism. Blood. 2013; 121(22):4443-4448.

[23] Jaff MR, McMurtry MS, Archer SL, Cushman M, Goldenberg N, Goldhaber SZ, Jenkins JS, Kline JA, Michaels AD, Thistlethwaite P, Vedantham S, White RJ, Zierler BK, American Heart Association Council on Cardiopulmonary, Critical Care, Perioperative and Resuscitation, American Heart Association Council on Peripheral Vascular Disease, American Heart Association Council on Arteriosclerosis, Thrombosis and Vascular Biology. Management of massive and submassive pulmonary embolism, iliofemoral deep vein thrombosis, and chronic thromboembolic pulmonary hypertension: a scientific statement from the American Heart Association. Circulation. 2011 Apr 26; 123(16):1788-830.

[24] Jerjes-Sanchez C, Ramírez-Rivera A, de Lourdes García M, Arriaga-Nava R, Valencia S, Rosado-Buzzo A, Pierzo JA, Rosas E. Streptokinase and Heparin versus Heparin Alone in Massive Pulmonary Embolism: A Randomized Controlled Trial. J Thromb Thrombolysis. 1995; 2(3):227-229.

[25] Jones AE, Watts JA, Debelak JP, Thornton LR, Younger JG, Kline JA. Inhibition of prostaglandin synthesis during polystyrene microsphere-induced pulmonary embolism in the rat. Am J Physiol Lung Cell Molec Physiol 2003; 284:L1072-1081.

[26] Kang DK, Thilo C, Schoepf UJ, Barraza JM Jr, Nance JW Jr, Bastarrika G, Abro JA, Ravenel JG, Costello P, Goldhaber SZ. CT signs of right ventricular dysfunction:

prognostic role in acute pulmonary embolism. JACC Cardiovasc Imaging. 2011; 4(8): 841-9.

[27] Kapsch DN, Metzler M, Silver D. Contributions of prostaglandin F2alpha and thromboxane A2 to the acute cardiopulmonary changes of pulmonary embolism. J Surg Res 1981; 30:522-529.

[28] Kasper W , Konstantinides S , Geibel A , Tiede N , Krause T , Just H . Prognostic significance of right ventricular afterload stress detected by echocardiography in patients with clinically suspected pulmonary embolism. Heart. 1997; 77(4):346-349 .

[29] Kearon C, Akl EA, Comerota AJ, Prandoni P, Bounameaux H, Goldhaber SZ, Nelson ME, Wells PS, Gould MK, Dentali F, Crowther M, Kahn SR, American College of Chest Physicians. Antithrombotic therapy for VTE disease: Antithrombotic Therapy and Prevention of Thrombosis, 9th ed: American College of Chest Physicians Evidence-Based Clinical Practice Guidelines. Chest. 2012 Feb; 141(2 Suppl):e419S-94S.

[30] Kline JA, Marchick MR, Hogg MM. Reduction in plasma haptoglobin in humans with acute pulmonary embolism causing tricuspid regurgitation. J Thromb Haemostasis 2009; 7:1597-9.

[31] Kline JA, Steuerwald MT, Marchick MR, Hernandez-Nino J, Rose GA. Prospective evaluation of right ventricular function and functional status 6 months after acute submassive pulmonary embolism: frequency of persistent or subsequent elevation in estimated pulmonary artery pressure. Chest. 2009 Nov; 136(5):1202-10.

[32] Klok FA, Mos IC, Kroft LJ, de Roos A, Huisman MV. Computed tomography pulmonary angiography as a single imaging test to rule out pulmonary embolism. Curr Opin Pulm Med. 2011; 17(5):380-6.

[33] Klok FA, S Romeih, LJM. Kroft, JJMWestenberg, MV Huisman, A de Roos Recovery of right and left ventricular function after acute pulmonary embolism Clinical Radiology 2011; 66: 1203-1207.

[34] Konstam MA, Hill NS, Bonin JD, Isner JM. Prostaglandin mediation of hemodynamic responses to pulmonary microembolism in rabbits: effects of ibuprofen and meclofenamate. Exp Lung Res 1987; 12:331–345.

[35] Konstantinides S, Geibel A, Heusel G, Heinrich F, Kasper W, Management Strategies and Prognosis of Pulmonary Embolism-3 Trial Investigators. Heparin plus alteplase compared with heparin alone in patients with submassive pulmonary embolism. N Engl J Med. 2002 Oct 10; 347(15):1143-50.

[36] Korkmaz A, Ozlu T, Ozsu S, Kazaz Z, Bulbul Y. Long-term outcomes in acute pulmonary thromboembolism: the incidence of chronic thromboembolic pulmonary hypertension and associated risk factors. Clin Appl Thromb Hemost. 2012 Jun; 18(3):281-8

[37] Kucher N, Rossi E, De Rosa M, Goldhaber SZ. Prognostic role of echocardiography among patients with acute pulmonary embolism and a systolic arterial pressure of 90 mm Hg or higher. Arch Intern Med. 2005; Aug 8-22; 165(15)1777-1781.

[38] Lankeit M, Jiménez D, Kostrubiec M, Dellas C, Hasenfuss G, Pruszczyk P, Konstantinides S. Predictive value of the high-sensitivity troponin T assay and the simplified Pulmonary Embolism Severity Index in hemodynamically stable patients with acute pulmonary embolism: a prospective validation study. Circulation. 2011 Dec 13; 124(24):2716-24.

[39] LeGal G, Righini M, Roy PM, et al. Prediction of pulmonary embolism in the emergency department: the revised Geneva score. Ann Intern Med 2006; 144: 165–71.

[40] Leacche M, Unic D, Goldhaber SZ, Rawn JD, Aranki SF, Couper GS, Mihaljevic T, Rizzo RJ, Cohn LH, Aklog L, Byrne JG. Modern surgical treatment of massive pulmonary embolism: results in 47 consecutive patients after rapid diagnosis and aggressive surgical approach. J Thorac Cardiovasc Surg. 2005 May; 129(5):1018-23.

[41] Lin BW, Schreiber DH, Liu G, Briese B, Hiestand B, Slattery D, Kline JA, Goldhaber SZ, Pollack CV Jr. Therapy and outcomes in massive pulmonary embolism from the Emergency Medicine Pulmonary Embolism in the Real World Registry. Am J Emerg Med. 2012; 30(9):1774-1781.

[42] McConnell MV, Solomon SD, Rayan ME, Come PC, Goldhaber SZ, Lee RT. Regional right ventricular dysfunction detected by echocardiography in acute pulmonary embolism. Am J Cardiol. 1996 Aug 15; 78(4):469-73.

[43] Meyer G, Roy PM, Sors H, Sanchez O. Laboratory tests in the diagnosis of pulmonary embolism. Respiration. 2003; 70(2):125-32.

[44] Meyer M, Fink C, Roeger S, Apfaltrer P, Haghi D, Kaminski WE, Neumaier M, Schoenberg SO, Henzler T. Benefit of combining quantitative cardiac CT parameters with troponin I for predicting right ventricular dysfunction and adverse clinical events in patients with acute pulmonary embolism. Eur J Radiol. 2012 Nov; 81(11): 3294-9.

[45] Miczoch J, Tucker A, Weir EK, Reeves JT, Grover RF. Platelet mediated pulmonary hypertension and hypoxia during pulmonary microembolism. Reduction by platelet inhibition. Chest 1978; 74:648–653.

[46] Mitchell AM, Jones AE, Tumlin JA, Kline JA. Prospective study of the incidence of contrast induced nephropathy among patients evaluated for pulmonary embolism by contrast-enhanced computed tomography. Acad Emerg Med. 2012; 19(6):618-25.

[47] Mos IC, Klok FA, Kroft LJ, de Roos A, Huisman MV. Imaging tests in the diagnosis of pulmonary embolism. Semin Respir Crit Care Med. 2012; 33(2):138-43

[48] Nijkeuter M , Söhne M , Tick LW , et al ; Christopher Study Investigators . The natural course of hemodynamically stable pulmonary embolism: clinical outcome and risk factors in a large prospective cohort study. Chest. 2007; 131(2):517-523.

[49] Oudkerk M, van Beek EJ, Wielopolski P, van Ooijen PM, Brouwers-Kuyper EM, Bongaerts AH, Berghout A.Comparison of contrast-enhanced magnetic resonance angiography and conventional pulmonary angiography for the diagnosis of pulmonary embolism: a prospective study.Lancet. 2002 May 11; 359(9318):1643-7.

[50] Ouellette DW, Patocka C. Pulmonary embolism. Emerg Med Clin North Am. 2012 May; 30(2):329-75

[51] Panos RJ, Barish RA, Whye DW Jr, Groleau G. The electrocardiographic manifestations of pulmonary embolism. J Emerg Med. 1988 Jul-Aug; 6(4):301-7.

[52] Piazza G, Goldhaber SZ.The acutely decompensated right ventricle: pathways for diagnosis and management. Chest. 2005 Sep; 128(3):1836-1852.

[53] Piazza G. Submassive pulmonary embolism. JAMA. 2013 Jan 9; 309(2):171-80.

[54] PIOPED. Value of the ventilation/perfusion scan in acute pulmonary embolism. Results of the prospective investigation of pulmonary embolism diagnosis (PIOPED). The PIOPED Investigators.JAMA. 1990 May 23-30; 263(20):2753-9.

[55] Pruszcyk P, Bochowicz A, Torbicki A, Szulc M, Kurzyna M, Fijalkowska A, Kuch-Wocial A. Cardiac troponin T monitoring identifies high-risk group of normotensive patients with acute pulmonary embolism. Chest 2003; 123(6):1947-1952.

[56] Qanadli SD, El Hajjam M, Vieillard-Baron A, Joseph T, Mesurolle B, Oliva VL, Barré O, Bruckert F, Dubourg O, Lacombe P. New CT index to quantify arterial obstruction in pulmonary embolism: comparison with angiographic index and echocardiography. AJR Am J Roentgenol. 2001 Jun; 176(6):1415-1420.

[57] Rathbun SW, Raskob GE, Whitsett TL.Sensitivity and specificity of helical computed tomography in the diagnosis of pulmonary embolism: a systematic review. Ann Intern Med. 2000 Feb 1; 132(3):227-32.

[58] Rathbun SW, Whitsett TL, Raskob GE. Negative D-dimer result to exclude recurrent deep venous thrombosis: a management trial. Ann Intern Med. 2004 Dec 7;141(11): 839-45.

[59] Rathbun SW, Whitsett TL, Vesely SK, Raskob GE. Clinical utility of D-dimer in patients with suspected pulmonary embolism and nondiagnostic lung scans or negative CT findings. Chest. 2004 Mar; 125(3):851-5.

[60] Reeves WC, Demers LM, Wood MA et al. The release of 168. thromboxane A and prostacyclin following experimental acute Pulmonary microembolism: attenuated pulmonary vasoconstriction with prostaglandin inhibitors and antihistamines. Prostaglandins 1976; 11:31– 41.

[61] Reeves WC, Demers LM, Wood MA, Skarlatos S, Copenhaver G, Whitesell L, et al. The release of thromboxane A2 and prostacyclin following experimental acute pulmonary embolism. Prostagland Leukotrienes Med 1983; 11:1-10.

[62] Remy-Jardin M, Pistolesi M, Goodman LR, et al. Management of suspected acute pulmonary embolism in the era of CT angiography: a statement from the Fleischner Society. Radiology 2007; 245(2):315–329

[63] Remy-Jardin M, Pistolesi M, Goodman LR, Gefter WB, Gottschalk A, Mayo JR, Sostman HD. Management of suspected acute pulmonary embolism in the era of CT angiography: a statement from the Fleischner Society.Radiology. 2007 Nov; 245(2): 315-29.

[64] Ribeiro A, Lindmarker P, Johnsson H, et al. Pulmonary embolism: oneyear follow-up with echocardiography Doppler and five-year survival analysis. Circulation 1999; 99:1325-1330.

[65] Rodger M, Makropoulos D, Turek M, Quevillon J, Raymond F, Rasuli P, Wells PS.Diagnostic value of the electrocardiogram in suspected pulmonary embolism. Am J Cardiol. 2000 Oct 1; 86(7):807-9.

[66] Rodger MA, Carrier M, Jones GN, Rasuli P, Raymond F, Djunaedi H, Wells PS: Diagnostic value of arterial blood gas measurement in suspected pulmonary embolism. Am J Respir Crit Care Med 2000; 162:2105–2108.

[67] Rosoff CB, Salzman EW, Gurewich V. Reduction of platelet serotonin and the response to pulmonary emboli. Surgery 1971; 70:12–19.

[68] Sabiston DC Wagner HN. The pathophysiology of pulmonary embolism: relationshpes to accurate diagnosis and choice of therapy. J Thorac Cardiovasc Surg. 1965 Sep; 50:339-56.

[69] Samama MM. Pulmonary embolism: controversies in laboratory studies. Pathophysiol Haemost Thromb. 2006; 35(1-2):157-161.

[70] Sanchez, O., Trinquart, L., Caille, V., Couturaud, F., Pacouret, G., Meneveau, N., Verschuren, F., Roy, P.M., Parent, F., Righini, M., Perrier, A., Lorut, C., Tardy, B., Benoit, M.O., Chatellier, G., Meyer, G. Prognostic factors for pulmonary embolism: the PREP study, a prospective multicenter cohort study. American Journal of Respiratory and Critical Care Medicine, 2010; 181:168–173.

[71] Sanchez, O., Trinquart, L., Colombet, I., Durieux, P., Huisman, M.V., Chatellier, G. & Meyer, G. Prognostic value of right ventricular dysfunction in patients with haemodynamically stable pulmonary embolism: a systematic review. European Heart Journal, 2008; 29:1569–1577.

[72] Schoepf UJ , Kucher N , Kipfmueller F , Quiroz R , Costello P , Goldhaber SZ . Right ventricular enlargement on chest computed tomography: a predictor of early death in acute pulmonary embolism . Circulation. 2004; 110 (20): 3276-3280 .

[73] Smulders YM. Pathophysiology and treatment of haemodynamic instability in acute pulmonary, embolism: the pivotal role of pulmonary vasoconstriction. Cardiovasc Res. 2000 Oct; 48(1):23-33.

[74] Stein PD, Athanasoulis C, Alavi A, Greenspan RH, Hales CA, Saltzman HA, Vreim CE, Terrin ML, Weg JG.Complications and validity of pulmonary angiography in acute pulmonary embolism.Circulation. 1992 Feb; 85(2):462-8.

[75] Stein PD, Dalen JE, McIntyre KM, Sasahara AA, Wenger NK, Willis PW 3rd.The electrocardiogram in acute pulmonary embolism. Prog Cardiovasc Dis. 1975 Jan-Feb; 17(4):247-57.

[76] Stein PD, Fowler SE, Goodman LR, Gottschalk A, Hales CA, Hull RD, Leeper KV Jr, Popovich J Jr, Quinn DA, Sos TA, Sostman HD, Tapson VF, Wakefield TW, Weg JG, Woodard PK; PIOPED II Investigators. Multidetector computed tomography for acute pulmonary embolism.N Engl J Med. 2006 Jun 1; 354(22):2317-27.

[77] Stein PD, Hull RD, Ghali WA, Patel KC, Olson RE, Meyers FA, Kalra NK. Tracking the uptake of evidence: two decades of hospital practice trends for diagnosing deep vein thrombosis and pulmonary embolism. Arch Intern Med. 2003; 163: 1213–1219.

[78] Stein PD, Hull RD, Patel KC, Olson RE, Ghali WA, Brant R, Biel RK, Bharadia V, Kalra NK. D-dimer for the exclusion of acute venous thrombosis and pulmonary embolism: a systematic review. Ann Intern Med. 2004 Apr 20; 140(8):589-602.

[79] Stein PD, Matta F, Musani M, et al. Silent pulmonary embolism in patients with deep venous thrombosis: a systematic review. Am J Med 2010; 123:426-431.

[80] Stein PD, Matta F. Acute pulmonary embolism. Curr Probl Cardiol. 2010 Jul;35(7): 314-76. Giuntini C, DiRicco G, Marini C, Melillo E, Palla A. Pulmonary embolism: epidemiology. Chest 1995; 107(suppl):3S-9S.

[81] Stein PD, Woodard PK, Weg JG, Wakefield TW, Tapson VF, Sostman HD, Sos TA, Quinn DA, Leeper KV Jr, Hull RD, Hales CA, Gottschalk A, Goodman LR, Fowler SE, Buckley JD; PIOPED II investigators.Diagnostic pathways in acute pulmonary embolism: recommendations of the PIOPED II investigators.Am J Med. 2006 Dec; 119(12):1048-55.

[82] Stein PD, Woodard PK, Weg JG, Wakefield TW, Tapson VF, Sostman HD, Sos TA, Quinn DA, Leeper KV Jr, Hull RD, Hales CA, Gottschalk A, Goodman LR, Fowler SE, Buckley JD; PIOPED II Investigators.Diagnostic pathways in acute pulmonary embolism: recommendations of the PIOPED II Investigators. Radiology. 2007 Jan; 242(1):15-21.

[83] Stevinson BG, Hernandez-Nino J, Rose G, et al. Echocardiographic and functional cardiopulmonary problems 6 months after first-timepulmonary embolism in previously healthy patients. Eur Heart J 2007; 28:2517-24.

[84] Stratmann G, Gregory GA. Neurogenic and humoral vasoconstriction in acute pulmonary thromboembolism. Anesth Analg. 2003 Aug; 97(2):341-54.

[85] Tapson VF. Acute pulmonary embolism. N Engl J Med. 2008 Mar 6; 358(10):1037-52.

[86] Tapson VF. Advances in the diagnosis and treatment of acute pulmonary embolism. F1000 Med Rep. 2012; 4:9.

[87] Tapson VF.Pulmonary embolism--new diagnostic approaches.N Engl J Med. 1997 May 15; 336(20):1449-51.

[88] Thompson JA, Millen JE, Glauser FL, Hess ML. Role of 5-HT2 receptor inhibition in pulmonary embolization. Circ Shock 1986; 20:299–309.

[89] Todd MH, Forrest JB, Cragg DB. The effects of aspirin and methysergide, singly and in combination, on systemic haemodynamic responses to pulmonary embolism. Can Anaesth Soc J 1981; 28:373-380.

[90] Todd MH, Forrest JB, Cragg DBJ. The effects of aspirin and methysergide on responses to clot induced pulmonary embolism. Am Heart J 1983; 105:769–776.

[91] van Beek EJ, Brouwerst EM, Song B, Stein PD, Oudkerk M.Clinical validity of a normal pulmonary angiogram in patients with suspected pulmonary embolism—a critical review.Clin Radiol. 2001 Oct; 56(10):838-42.

[92] van der Bijl N, Klok FA, Huisman MV, van Rooden JK, Mertens BJ, de Roos A, Kroft LJ. Measurement of right and left ventricular function by ECG-synchronized CT scanning in patients with acute pulmonary embolism: usefulness for predicting short-term outcome. Chest. 2011 Oct; 140(4):1008-15.

[93] Van Strijen MJ, De Monye W, Kieft GJ, Pattynama PM, Prins MH, Huisman MV.Accuracy of single-detector spiral CT in the diagnosis of pulmonary embolism: a prospective multicenter cohort study of consecutive patients with abnormal perfusion scintigraphy.J Thromb Haemost. 2005 Jan; 3(1):17-25. Erratum in: J Thromb Haemost. 2005 Mar;3(3):622.

[94] Verschuren F, Bonnet M, Benoit MO, Gruson D, Zech F, Couturaud F, Meneveau N, Roy PM, Righini M, Meyer G, et al. The prognostic value of pro-B-Type natriuretic peptide in acute pulmonary embolism. Thromb Res. 2013 Apr 4. [Epub ahead of print]

[95] Wagenvort CA. Pathology of pulmonary thromboembolism. Chst 1995; 107(1 Suppl): 10S-17S.

[96] Wan S, Quinlan DJ, Agnelli G, Eikelboom JW. Thrombolysis compared with heparin for the initial treatment of pulmonary embolism: a meta-analysis of the randomized controlled trials. Circulation. 2004 Aug 10; 110(6):744-9.

[97] Watts JA, Gellar MA, Obraztsova M, Kline JA, Zagorski J. Role of inflammation in right ventricular damage and repair following experimental pulmonary embolism in rats. Int J Exp Pathol 2008; 89:389-399.

[98] WeidnerWJ. Effects of indomethacin on pulmonary hemodynamics and extravascular lung water in sheep after pulmonary microembolism. Prostagl Med 1979; 3:71–80.

[99] Wells PS, Anderson DR, Rodger M, et al. Derivation of a simple clinical model to categorize patients probability of pulmonary embolism: increasing the models utility with the SimpliRED D dimer. Thromb Haemost 2000; 83: 416–20.

[100] Wells PS, Anderson DR, Rodger M, Ginsberg JS, Kearon C, Gent M, Turpie AG, Bormanis J, Weitz J, Chamberlain M, Bowie D, Barnes D, Hirsh J. Derivation of a simple clinical model to categorize patients probability of pulmonary embolism: increasing the models utility with the SimpliRED D-dimer.Thromb Haemost. 2000 Mar; 83(3): 416-20.

[101] Wells PS, Anderson DR, Rodger M, Stiell I, Dreyer JF, Barnes D, Forgie M, Kovacs G, Ward J, Kovacs MJ. Excluding pulmonary embolism at the bedside without diagnostic imaging: management of patients with suspected pulmonary embolism presenting to the emergency department by using a simple clinical model and d-dimer. Ann Intern Med. 2001 Jul 17; 135(2):98-107.

[102] Wells PS, Ginsberg JS, Anderson DR, Kearon C, Gent M, Turpie AG, Bormanis J, Weitz J, Chamberlain M, Bowie D, Barnes D, Hirsh J. Use of a clinical model for safe management of patients with suspected pulmonary embolism. Ann Intern Med. 1998 Dec 15; 129(12):997-1005.

[103] Wolfe MW, Lee RT, Feldstein ML, Parker JA, Come PC, Goldhaber SZ. Prognostic significance of right ventricular hypokinesis and perfusion lung scan defects in pulmonary embolism. Am Heart J. 1994; 127:1371-5.

[104] Wong LF, Akram AR, McGurk S, Van Beek EJ, Reid JH, Murchison JT. Thrombus load and acute right ventricular failure in pulmonary embolism: correlation and demonstration of a "tipping point" on CT pulmonary angiography. Br J Radiol. 2012 Nov; 85(1019):1471-6.

[105] Wood KE. Major pulmonary embolism: review of a pathophysiologic approach to the golden hour of hemodynamically significant pulmonary embolism. Chest. 2002; 121(3):87-905.

[106] Yoo JW, Hong SB, Lim CM, Koh Y. Clinical implications of right ventricular dysfunction in patients with acute symptomatic pulmonary embolism: short- and long-term clinical outcomes. J Crit Care. 2012 Jun; 27(3):325.e1-6.

Chapter 7

Chronic Thromboembolic Pulmonary Hypertension

Mehdi Badidi and M'Barek Nazi

Additional information is available at the end of the chapter

http://dx.doi.org/10.5772/54749

1. Introduction

Chronic thromboembolic pulmonary hypertension (CTEPH) is a form of pulmonary hypertension caused by obstruction and vascular remodeling of the pulmonary arteries after a pulmonary embolism [1]. Once considered rare, CTEPH is likely under-diagnosed and its true prevalence is still uncertain [2,3]. CTEPH is a consequence of the persistence and fibrous organization of clots in the pulmonary arteries after one or more acute pulmonary emboli. Recent research has provided evidence, suggesting that the old view of CTEPH as a disease caused solely by obliteration of pulmonary arteries by organized thrombus constitutes a very superficial understanding of the consequences of pulmonary thromboemboli [3]. In fact, pulmonary embolism, either as a single episode or as recurrent episodes, is probably the trigger followed by progressive pulmonary vascular remodeling leading to elevated pulmonary vascular resistance, progressing to right ventricular (RV) failure [4]. Thanks to enhanced vascular and cardiac imaging, less-invasive diagnostic work-up of CTEPH have become widely available. Doppler ultrasound echocardiography and pulmonary ventilation/perfusion (V/Q) scintigraphy are two excellent and complementary examinations for CTEPH [5]. Computed tomography (CT) and pulmonary angiography are the two best tools to decide on the operability of the endovascular lesions. [6]. Equally important, CTEPH is a type of pulmonary hypertension (PH) that is unique because it is potentially curable by PEA [7, 8]. Indeed, the prognosis of CTEPH was transformed by this technique [8]. The first surgery for CTEPH was performed in 1958 [9]. The mortality in the early surgical series was 22% but with advances in surgery and improved and perioperative care, it has decreased to about 4% [10, 11].

2. Epidemiology of CTEPH

Pulmonary embolism (PE) is a common condition with an annual incidence estimated at 50 per 100,000 persons [12]. This is an acute disease and usually reversible after anticoagulation and / or after thrombolysis. Patients are frequently deemed to be "cured" after treatment. However, studies based on V/Q lung or computed tomography pulmonary angiogram (CTPA) reported the presence of residual perfusion disorders after acute pulmonary embolism [13]. Other echocardiographic studies have also shown that 30% of patients with PAH have residual or impaired right ventricular wall motion abnormalities and functional impairment after acute pulmonary embolism [14]. These data suggest that a significant proportion of patients with acute symptomatic PE develop persistent pulmonary vascular sequelae with serious long-term consequences [14.15]. Initial estimates of the frequency of CTEPH are of the order of 0.1% to 0.5% of patients surviving an episode of acute pulmonary embolism [16, 17]. More recent data suggest that 1% to 4% of patients may develop CTEPH after a first episode of pulmonary embolism [18, 19]. This frequency is even higher after recurrent thromboembolic events [20].

In a series of 866 patients with acute pulmonary embolism, all patients who had not previously been diagnosed with pulmonary hypertension (PH) and had survived until inclusion in the study were asked to undergo echocardiography. Patients suspected of having PH by echocardiogram underwent complete assessment to test chronic thromboembolic pulmonary hypertension. This procedure includes V/Q scintigraphy and right heart catheterization. The results showed the incidence of CTEPH to be about 0.5% [21, 22].

In a prospective study, after a first episode of symptomatic pulmonary embolism for patients with unexplained persistent dyspnea, echocardiographic abnormality, a V/Q scan, pulmonary angiography, and right heart catheterization, the cumulative incidence of symptomatic CTEPH was 1.0% at six months, 3.1% at one year and 3.8% at two years [23]. In another study of 320 patients who presented with a symptomatic pulmonary embolism, V/Q scintigraphy results showed persistent perfusion defects 6 and 12 months after pulmonary embolism. The cumulative incidence of CTEPH was 0.9% to 1.3% [24]. The true incidence of CTEPH may have been underestimated due to exclusion of patients with a history of venous thromboembolism, thrombophilia or other potential causes of pulmonary hypertension. In addition, a significant proportion of patients with CTEPH have not shown any previous episode of symptomatic pulmonary embolism [25, 26]. The discrepancy between theoretical estimates and the number of patients diagnosed with CTEPH emphasizes that CTEPH is likely to be underdiagnosed. The time between an acute pulmonary embolism episode and the development of CTEPH is also a matter of debate. Most cases of CTEPH are diagnosed during the first two years after the acute symptomatic pulmonary embolism [23]. However, some patients may experience symptoms of CTEPH many years later [27, 28]. This variability was attributed to progressive vasculopathy which affected the distal small pulmonary arteries [29].

3. Risk factors for CTEPH

To better identify patients with pulmonary embolism who are more likely to develop CTEPH, many studies have assessed the potential risk factors for CTEPH including demographic factors, the specific details of pulmonary embolism, the presence of co-morbidities and underlying thrombophilia (table 1) [23, 30]. An increased risk of CTEPH is associated with splenectomy, cancer, chronic inflammatory diseases (Crohn's disease and ulcerative colitis), hypothyroidism, an atrioventricular shunt and infected cardiac pacemaker [30, 31]. Complications associated with pulmonary embolism such as acute perfusion defects, idiopathic, recurrent thromboemboli, massive pulmonary emboli, and delayed diagnosis may also predispose patients to CTEPH. Patients older than 70 years whose systolic pulmonary artery pressure is above 50 mmHg have a higher risk of persistent pulmonary hypertension one year after an acute pulmonary embolism [30, 32].

Independent clinical risk factors for CTEPH
• Splenectomy
• Ventriculo-atrial (VA) shunts
• Pacemaker leads
• Indwelling central venous catheters (e.g. Port, Hickman catheter)
• Chronic inflammatory diseases (osteomyelitis, inflammatory bowel diseases)
• Malignant diseases
• Thyroid hormone replacement therapy
Risk factors associated with CTEPH after symptomatic PE
• Previous pulmonary embolism
• Young age
• Large perfusion defect
• Idiopathic PE at presentation
Plasmatic risk factors associated with CTEPH
• Elevated factor VIII levels "/>250%
• APA/LAC
• Combined coagulation defects
• Fibrinogen mutations
APA, antiphospholipid antibodies; LAC, lupus anticoagulans.

Table 1. Risk factors for CTEPH [23].

Thrombolytics are frequently used to treat acute pulmonary emboli. The rapid and complete recanalization of the pulmonary arteries may decrease the subsequent development of CTEPH [33]. 23 of 40 patients who had angiographically proven pulmonary embolism and who had initially been randomized to an IV infusion of heparin (n = 11) or a thrombolytic agent (urokinase or streptokinase, n = 12) were restudied after a mean follow-up of 7.4 years to

Recommendation	Class of recommendation	Level of evidence
The diagnosis of CTEPH is based on the presence of pre-capillary PH (mean PAP ≥25 mmHg, PCWP ≤15 mmHg, PVR "/>2 Wood units) in patients with multiple chronic/organized occlusive thrombi/emboli in the elastic pulmonary arteries (main, lobar, segmental, subsegmental), persisting after effective anticoagulation over a minimum period of three months.	I	C
In patients with CTEPH, lifelong anticoagulation is indicated	I	C
Surgical pulmonary endarterectomy (PEA) is the recommended treatment for patients with CTEPH.	I	C
Once perfusion scanning and/or CT angiography shows signs compatible with CTEPH, the patient should be referred to a center with expertise in surgical pulmonary endarterectomy.	IIa	C
The selection of patients for surgery should be based on the extent and location of the organized thrombi, on the degree of PH, and on the presence of co-morbidities.	IIa	C
PAH-specific drug therapy may be indicated in selected CTEPH patients such as patients who are not candidates for surgery or patients with residual PH after pulmonary endarterectomy.	IIb	C

Table 2. Recommendations of the ESC/ERS guidelines for CTEPH [93].

measure the right-sided pressures at rest and after supine bicycle ergometry exercise. At rest, the pulmonary artery (PA) mean pressure and the pulmonary vascular resistance (PVR) were significantly higher in the heparin group compared with the thrombolytic group (22 vs. 17 mmHg, $p<0.05$, and 351 vs. 171 dynes s (-1) cm (-5), $p<0.02$, respectively). During exercise both parameters rose to a significantly higher level in the heparin group (from rest to exercise, PA: 22-32 mmHg, $p<0.01$; PVR: 351-437 dynes s (-1) cm 5, $p<0.01$, respectively), but not in the thrombolytic group (rest to exercise, PA: 17-19 mm Hg, p = NS; PVR: 171-179 dynes s (-1) cm (-5), p = NS). Thus, thrombolytic therapy preserves the normal hemodynamic response to exercise in the long-term and may prevent the development of pulmonary hypertension [34].

CTEPH may be related to a disorder of hemostasis such as elevated levels of factor VIII. The expression of plasminogen activator inhibitor (PAI-1) of type 1 was found to be higher in patients monitored for CTEPH [30, 35, 36]. Abnormalities in the structure of fibrinogen and function were also observed in other series. Traditional risk factors for venous thromboembolism (VTE) include antithrombin deficiency, protein C deficiency, protein S deficiency, factor V Leiden, plasminogen deficiency, and anticardiolipin antibodies [26]. However, in 147 consecutive patients with CTEPH, the prevalence of hereditary thrombotic risk factors was not increased when compared to 99 consecutive patients with IPAH or to 100 control patients.

Thrombophilia studies have shown that lupus anticoagulant may be found in 10% of CTEPH patients, and 20% carry antiphospholipid antibodies, lupus anticoagulant, or both. A recent study has demonstrated that the plasma level of factor VIII, a protein associated with both primary and recurrent VTE, is elevated in 39% of patients with CTEPH [12]. No abnormalities of fibrinolysis have been identified. Blood groups type A, B, and AB were found to be significantly more common in patients with CTEPH compared to patients with PAH (88% vs. 56%). Plasma lipoprotein levels (a) (Lp(a)), a subgroup of the low density lipoprotein with high atherogenic potency, were significantly higher in patients with CTEPH than in patients with PAH and control subjects, indicating an overlap of venous and arterial thrombotic risk factors. Antiphospholipid antibodies (APLA) have been documented in a significant proportion of patients followed for CTEPH [30, 37, 38]. There is also evidence that underlying genetic predisposition may be involved in the pathogenesis of CTEPH.

4. Natural history and pathogenesis of CTEPH

The pathophysiological basis of CTEPH is not yet well known. Despite progress in determining the pathophysiology and treatment of PH, CTEPH pathogenesis is complex and poorly understood [39]. The mechanisms by which acute pulmonary embolism evolves into chronic thromboembolic residues incorporated into the pulmonary vessel wall have been difficult to define [39,40]. The incomplete resolution of pulmonary emboli rather than in situ thrombosis of pulmonary arteries appears to be the main contributing factor [41]. Pulmonary hypertension in patients without preexisting cardiopulmonary disease occurs when at least 30% of the pulmonary vascular bed is obstructed [42]. Development of pulmonary hypertension is not simply related to a simple mechanical obstruction by chronic thromboembolic material, but rather the appearance of a secondary vasculopathy developed in regions injured by shear stresses caused by persistent thromboembolic lesions [43]. Vascular injury and shear stress eventually lead to the proliferation of endothelial cells and smooth muscle cells of the pulmonary arterial bed [42, 43, and 44]. These results were reported from pathological observations in patients examined for CTEPH who displayed an organization of the clot into fibrous tissue, but also vascular remodeling with disappearance of the intima and infiltration of the media arterial wall [45, 46, 47, 48, and 49]. This hypothesis was initially suggested by Moser and Braunwald in 1971 [4]. Indeed, they observed that the pulmonary arteries of small caliber located in the unobstructed territories had remodeling lesions similar to those described in idiopathic pulmonary arterial hypertension.

5. Clinical presentation

Generally, the clinical history is not helpful in the diagnosis of CTEPH.. Indeed, up to half of patients with CTEPH have no documented history of pulmonary embolism [50]. In one series, 63% of patients had no specific history of acute venous thromboembolism [51]. Therefore, the clinical index of suspicion has been clarified below. The Hispanic clinic has an important place in the diagnosis. It identifies clinical events that could be compatible with an unidentified acute venous thromboembolism [52, 53]. Symptoms of CTEPH are very similar to many other etiologies of pulmonary arterial hypertension. The majority of patients who displayed CTEPH were past the age of 60. The symptoms often occurred insidiously and were often attributed to other cardiac comorbidities, obesity or an underlying lung disease [54]. Dyspnea and fatigue were the symptoms most frequently encountered. Patients may present with exertional angina, presyncope, syncope and lower extremity edema. Chest pain may be caused by right ventricular ischemia. Syncope is an alarming symptom that raises concerns of advanced heart failure and should prompt urgent examination.

6. Physical examination

Physical signs vary depending on the severity of the pulmonary hypertension and associated right heart failure. Cardiac auscultation may be notable for accentuated pulmonic valve closure, tricuspid regurgitant murmur, or possibly bruit over the lung fields caused by turbulent blood flow through partially occluded pulmonary arteries [55, 56]. At a late stage, clinical signs of right ventricular failure may be present (jugular venous distension, hepatojugular reflux, lower limb edema, enlarged liver, and ascites). [56, 57].

7. Diagnostic approach

Patients with CTEPH have a higher mortality rate that may reach up to 10% to 20% among untreated patients [58, 59]. Thus, the most important step is the early detection of a population at risk, patients with a CTEPH and the accurate diagnosis of this pathology in order to adopt the best therapeutic strategy. Patients who experience acute symptomatic pulmonary embolism, persistent symptoms of dyspnea and chest pain may guide further diagnostic studies. Moreover, the persistence of pulmonary vascular perfusion defects are also common, 30% within 12 months after acute pulmonary embolism, and are associated with a higher prevalence of persistent symptoms, worse exercise capacity and pulmonary hypertension [60]. Thus, clinical and radiologic monitoring may detect patients with pulmonary embolism who have an increased risk of developing CTEPH.

It is important to acknowledge a history of deep vein thrombosis as an element that can guide the diagnosis, but it lacks sensitivity. Indeed, many patients with CTEPH have not had a documented DVT or PE [61, 62]. Patients monitored for pulmonary hypertension of another cause may exhibit symptoms similar to those of CTEPH [63]. V/Q scanning is an important tool for evaluation of all patients with pulmonary hypertension. It is essential because of the fact that CTEPH requires different therapies and may be amenable to surgical intervention. Thus, the objectives of the diagnostic processes are first to identify CTEPH, and then to define the stage of the disease and distribution of pulmonary arterial occlusion, with an assessment of the severity of pulmonary hypertension and other concomitant diseases, and finally determine eligibility for pulmonary endarterectomy (PEA) or medical treatment.

After a thorough history and physical exam, patients with suspicious symptoms or signs of pulmonary hypertension and a history of pulmonary embolism or pulmonary hypertension of unknown cause should be investigated to confirm or exclude the diagnosis of CTEPH [64]. Imaging is central to making the diagnosis and management of CTEPH, but which test do you use, and when? The imaging algorithm used at Papworth Hospital for CTEPH diagnosis is shown in Figure 1. Echocardiography is used in the initial assessment of suspected pulmonary hypertension. V/Q lung scanning may be used to differentiate chronic thromboembolic pulmonary hypertension from other causes of pulmonary hypertension.

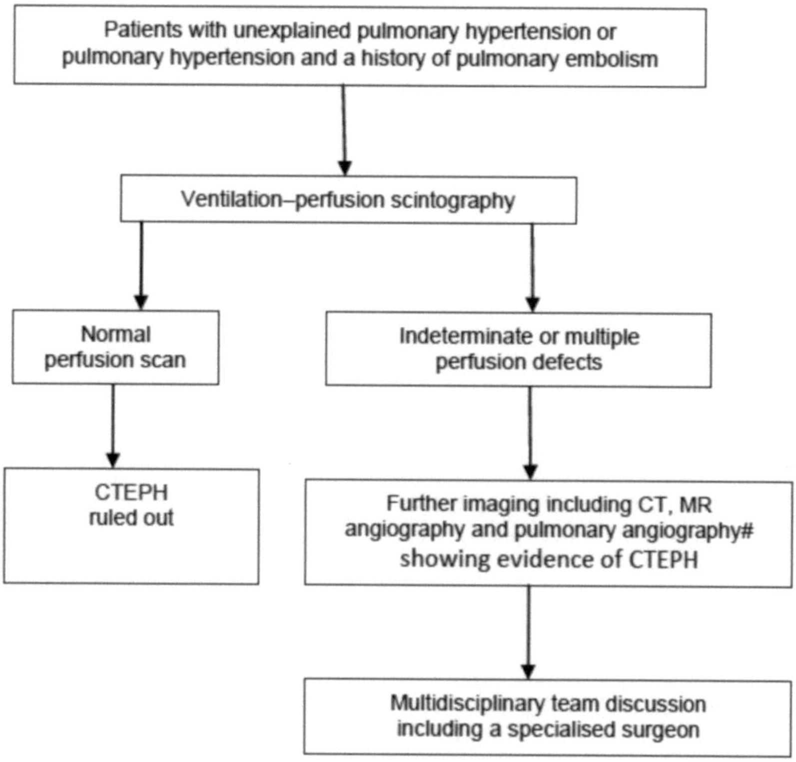

Figure 1. Diagnostic imaging algorithm for chronic thromboembolic pulmonary hypertension (CTEPH). CT: computed tomography; MR: magnetic resonance.: pulmonary angiography is usually performed in conjunction with right heart catheterisation and should be performed at centres experienced with CTEPH and pulmonary endarterectomy [20].

7.1. Echocardiography

Transthoracic echocardiography with Doppler imaging is a sensitive exam for the detection of pulmonary hypertension and right ventricular dysfunction, but it is not specific for the diagnosis of chronic thromboembolic pulmonary hypertension. [65] Common echocardiographic findings include right ventricular dilatation, hypertrophy, and hypokinesis; right atrial enlargement; right ventricular pressure overload as suggested by interventricular septal deviation toward the left ventricle during systole; and tricuspid regurgitation. The tricuspid regurgitant jet gradient provides an estimate of the pulmonary artery systolic pressure. In rare cases, transthoracic echocardiography shows proximal pulmonary artery thrombus. However, echocardiography cannot be used to reliably differentiate among acute, subacute, and chronic pulmonary embolism. Thus, all patients with pulmonary hypertension should be evaluated with a V/Q scan [66, 67] in addition to angiography.

7.2. Lung scan ventilation-perfusion

The V/Q lung scan should be performed in patients with PH to look for potentially treatable CTEPH. The V/Q scan remains the screening method of choice for CTEPH because of its higher sensitivity relative to CT scans. A normal- or low-probability V/Q scan effectively excludes CTEPH with a sensitivity of 90–100% and a specificity of 94–100% [68, 69, 76]. A recent study has shown that lung scintigraphy V/Q had a negative predictive value of 98.5% to exclude CTEPH, while CT pulmonary angiography had a negative predictive value of 79.7% compared with pulmonary angiography gold standard. Therefore, a negative pulmonary CT angiography does not formally exclude CTEPH [76].

In PAH the V/Q lung scan may be normal; it may also show small peripheral unmatched and nonsegmental perfusion defects. Contrast-enhanced CT may be used as a complementary investigation but does not replace the ventilation/perfusion (henceforth V/Q) scan or traditional pulmonary angiogram. One caveat is that unmatched perfusion defects are also seen in pulmonary veno-occlusive disease (PVOD). The V/Q scan in CTEPH typically shows multiple segmental or larger perfusion defects in areas of normal ventilation. Since there is often only partial vascular obstruction in CTEPH, there may be grey zones, and the lung perfusion scan can underestimate the degree of vascular obstruction. On the other hand, a normal or low probability V/Q scan virtually excludes the possibility of surgical intervention of CTEPH [70, 71].

7.3. Computed tomography

The spiral CT has the advantage of being non-invasive, with a spatial resolution close to pulmonary angiography. In patients with CTEPH, the spiral CT lung may reveal the presence of an organized thrombus lining the proximal pulmonary vessels and may better visualize thickening of the pulmonary arterial wall to identify a cleavage plane for endarterectomy. Conversely, it allows for the identification of atherosclerotic calcification of the arterial wall lung, which will increase the complexity of PEA. It also evokes rare differential diagnoses such as fibrous mediastinitis, arteritis, pulmonary emboli tumors or/and sarcomas [72]. The spiral CT lung is now considered the benchmark in acute pulmonary embolism and can accurately define the nature and extent of disease in CTEPH, and provide multi-planar reconstruction to produce a three-dimensional vascular tree [73]. The recent development of this method allows imaging to differentiate perfusion defects distal to those of proximal infusion [74]. The V/Q analysis does not distinguish between acute and chronic embolism. However, several studies have shown that acute pulmonary embolism disappears within 4 to 6 weeks in 90% of patients and within 6 months in all patients [75]. Therefore, symptomatic patients in whom perfusion defects persist despite adequate anticoagulation after 3 to 6 months should be referred to a specialist center for further evaluation, especially if there is direct or indirect evidence of pulmonary hypertension in the echocardiography. Sometimes, patients show symptoms at a later stage after the appearance of the signs of severe right ventricular dysfunction which might require urgent surgery or semi-urgent surgery, even if they have not yet completed 3 to 6 months of anticoagulation. Right heart catheterization and pulmonary angiography are generally required for definitive diagnosis of CTEPH. The spiral lung CT is also increasingly used to assess the extent of chronic thromboembolic disease. However, the spiral CT lung can sometimes fail to identify the presence of chronic thromboembolic disease.

7.4. Magnetic resonance imaging

This test is also useful for defining the anatomy and extent of obstruction in CTEPH. Currently, it is not routinely used in patients who can undergo conventional angiography, but in comparison with spiral CT, it seems to be equivalent for the identification of signs of CTEPH [77]. Both techniques provide a wealth of additional anatomical information, allowing the detection of other diagnoses that may be associated with pulmonary hypertension such as pulmonary vein stenosis and fibrosing mediastinitis.

7.5. Right heart catheterization and pulmonary angiography and angioscopy

7.5.1. Right heart catheterization

Preoperative evaluation of patients with CTEPH requires a battery of complementary examinations, starting with right heart catheterization and pulmonary angiography [78]. Right heart catheterization is necessary to confirm the diagnosis and severity of pulmonary hypertension and provide prognostic information. It allows precise measurement of pulmonary artery pressure and right atrial pressure, pulmonary artery occlusion pressure, and cardiac output. In patients with chronic thromboembolic obstruction, PH usually occurs with increased cardiac output; pulmonary artery pressure will rise in a nearly linear fashion and normal pulmonary vascular resistance will not occur [79]. In patients with CTEPH and risk factors for coronary artery disease, left heart catheterization with coronary angiography is performed before PEA.

7.5.2. Pulmonary angiography

Pulmonary angiography may confirm the diagnosis of chronic pulmonary thromboembolic disease. The angiographic appearance of CTEPH is distinct from that seen in acute pulmonary embolism, although the two processes can be seen simultaneously [80]. By defining the character of the proximal or distal lesions, pulmonary angiography is a determining factor in the use of PEA. The angiographic abnormalities related to CTEPH include intraluminal filling defects. A recently developed classification system for the anatomical location of thrombi is helpful in the selection of patients for PEA. Type I disease is characterised by a clear central thrombus; type II consists of the thickening of the intima and fibrous reticulum in a main or segmental bronchus, without thrombus in a main vessel; type III is limited to segmental or sub-segmental regions and type IV involves only peripheral vessels and is not an operable disease.[80, 81]. In addition, pulmonary angiography is not free of significant risk in the context of severe pulmonary hypertension. Therefore, some security measures should be taken [82, 83]. The biplane acquisition technique should be used whenever possible. The systematic use of the side view is extremely useful in determining the location and extent of anatomical proximal embolic obstruction and, therefore, surgical accessibility.

7.5.3. Pulmonary angioscopy

Pulmonary angioscopy is used as an adjunct to pulmonary angiography. In the early years of endarterectomy, pulmonary angioscopy was used more frequently. More recently, it has been replaced by other, less invasive imaging techniques [84]. The technique involves the introduction of the angioscope through an introducer, preferably in the right internal jugular vein, then through the right atrium and right ventricle and the right and left pulmonary arteries, where it can be guided in each lobe of the arteries. The distal balloon is inflated with carbon dioxide, which obstructs blood flow transiently and allows visualization of the vascular bed [84].

8. Treatment of CTEPH

Several therapies have been used for CTEPH patients since the initial discovery of this clinical entity [85, 86]. In recent years scientific societies have unanimously endorsed surgical intervention with PEA as the preferred treatment for CTEPH because of the significant improvement in survival for the majority of patients and long-term improved outcomes.

PAH specific medications have been investigated in CTEPH, though the number of patients studied is much smaller than those enrolled in PAH clinical trials. These studies have shown safety of several therapies, and varying degrees of benefit. Medical therapies are often considered for use in inoperable patients, or for patients who have residual pulmonary hypertension after surgery.

The decision to use a specific medication in patients with CTEPH who cannot undergo surgery or who present with residual PH after surgical intervention should be made after an evaluation by a referral center. In addition, these patients should remain under close clinical monitoring.

8.1. Surgical approach

8.1.1. Preparation of patients before pulmonary endarterectomy

After diagnostic evaluation, PEA is the treatment of choice for symptomatic patients with proximal CTEPH. The preoperative assessment of patients scheduled for PEA involves evaluating the presence of associated left heart disease with echocardiography to assess LV size and function as well as coronary angiography to exclude coronary artery disease in the appropriate patient [87]. Patients are also evaluated for significant concurrent disorders such as malignancy, using age-appropriate targeted screening, based on careful consideration of the symptoms presented. Patients are usually maintained on systemic anticoagulation immediately before surgery, although the actual protocol depends on local experience and preference of the expert center. Supplemental oxygen and diuretics are often administered to optimize the patient's oxygen and volume status. Thromboendarerectomy is the treatment of choice for symptomatic patients with CTEPH when surgically feasible. In some of these patients, particularly those with severe pulmonary hypertension and right ventricular failure, medical treatment pre-PEA with parenteral prostanoids (eg epoprostenol) may be initiated as a bridge to endarterectomy [87, 88, 89].

8.1.2. Pulmonary Endarterectomy (PEA)

Pulmonary endarterectomy is the preferred treatment for patients with CTEPH because of the potential for cure and complete resolution of PH and its complications. PEA has the potential to restore near normal cardiopulmonary function. Patient selection for surgery depends on the extent and location of the organized thrombus in relation to the degree of pulmonary hypertension. When the thrombus is situated in a proximal location, it represents the ideal condition for surgery, but if the thrombus is more distal, the intervention becomes more difficult.

8.1.2.1. Surgical strategy

PEA is performed during total circulatory arrest under conditions of profound hypothermia. This is required to enable visibility in the distal pulmonary arterial branches, which would otherwise be subject to back-bleeding during the endarterectomy due to the development of a systemic-to-pulmonary artery circulation at the precapillary level. A relatively recent technical advance is the introduction of video-assisted pulmonary endarterectomy, which uses a video camera connected to a rigid angioscope [90, 91]. Video technology is beneficial because it provides a source of light, allows visualization of the distal pulmonary vascular tree, and facilitates a close view of the surgery by the assistant surgeons.

8.1.2.2. Surgical procedure

After a median sternotomy, followed by a vertical pericardiotomy, the patient is placed on cardiopulmonary bypass with hypothermia at 18 to 20 ° C. Before the cardiopulmonary bypass the patient's head is wrapped in a blanket with circulating cold water at 4° C. [90, 91]. This blanket has a thermometer and a device for regulating the water circulation. After the cardiopulmonary bypass has been started vents are placed in the pulmonary artery and the right superior pulmonary vein. The right pulmonary artery is dissected between the aorta and the superior vena cava and is mobilised within the pericardial reflection. During a first period of circulatory arrest, the plane is circumferentially followed down to the segmental and sometimes subsegmental branches of each lobe using special suction dissectors, until a complete endartectomy is achieved. Once the field has been prepared, the endarterectomy precedes with the aid of a microscopic aspirator with a rounded tip. The surgical specimen often resembles the arborization of pulmonary arteries, sometimes containing a mixture of fresh and old clots. The pulmonary artery pressures are commonly reduced immediately after surgery. The patient is reperfused for approximately 15 min with cardiopulmonary bypass, while the arteriotomy is closed with a back-and-forth running suture. An arteriotomy is performed on the left pulmonary artery and the endarterectomy is repeated in the left lung within another period of circulatory arrest. The final stage comprises reperfusion during closure of the left pulmonary artery, de-airing of the cardiac chambers, unclamping of the aorta, and slow rewarming of the patient to 37°C. [92, 93].

8.1.3. PEA in patients with distal CTEPH

The potential benefits of PEA are uncertain in patients with distal arterial obstruction and associated CTEPH. Studies have focused specifically on this issue by comparing clinical and hemodynamic results of surgery in patients with CTEPH and proximal thrombosis or distal thrombosis [94]. In a study of patients evaluated for CTEPH, 83 patients were considered for thrombo-endarterectomy [95], 40 patients underwent the procedure of whom 14 had distal lesions affecting small vessels. In these 14 subjects, PEA was associated with improvement of the baseline dyspnea index. However, the distal thrombo-endarterectomy was associated with increased perioperative mortality and severe residual PH post-thrombo-endarterectomy. Currently, there is no clear consensus on optimal management of distal chronic thromboembolic disease with associated PH. [94].

8.1.4. Management of patients after surgery

This is a crucial element for the success of the pulmonary PEA. Although pulmonary hemodynamics improved immediately after surgery in most patients, the postoperative course may be complicated. Complications are usually not related to any specific aspect of the heart surgery (pericardial effusion, arrhythmia, atelectasis, wound infection), or specific to the pulmonary thromboendarterectomy [96]. The postoperative course is marked mainly by the risk of pulmonary edema-like lesionswhich may appear up to 72 hours after surgery in the areas where the thromboembolic obstruction was removed [96, 97]. This pulmonary edema is of varying severity, ranging from a simple acute hypoxemia transition to a fatal hemorrhagic complication sometimes requiring prolonged mechanical ventilation. Other complications encountered are right heart failure due to persistent PH, the dehiscence of an arteriotomy suture during an episode of PAH, nosocomial pneumonia, hemoptysis, which will be easily treated by embolization, or phrenic nerve paralysis which might prolong mechanical ventilation.

Reethrombosis in the region of the thromboendarterectomy is a rare but known complication, especially in unilateral obstruction, which justifies the initiation of anticoagulant therapy as early as possible after the operation. Patients often continue to improve functionally and hemodynamicly in the months after the operation.

http://dx.doi.org/10.5772/54749

8.1.5. Postoperative outcomes

Despite the potential for life-threatening complications, the perioperative mortality of patients undergoing lung PEA has improved in recent years. The first results of an international CTEPH registry, which included 386 consecutive patients with newly diagnosed CTEPH undergoing surgery showed a significant and sustained decrease in PVR from 736 to 248 dyn s cm-5, which was accompanied by substantial improvements in WHO functional class and exercise capacity at 1 year [97]. Reported rates of residual PH after PEA (mean PAP> 30 mmHg) were 16.7% and 31%, respectively. More recently, a greatly reduced surgical mortality rate of 2.2% was reported [98]. Perioperative mortality in patients undergoing pulmonary endarterectomy at the University of California at San Diego was 17% for the first 200 patients who underwent operation from 1970 to 1990 [98]. In a series from UCSD from 1998 until 2002, 500 patients underwent pulmonary endarterectomy, with a rate of hospital mortality of 4.4% [98]. The preoperative factors that may adversely affect surgical outcomes include age over 70 years, the presence of multiple comorbidities, preoperative pulmonary vascular resistance, severe heart failure with high right atrial pressure, and prolonged duration of pulmonary hypertension before surgery [99]. In order to detect persistent or recurrent pulmonary hypertension, systematic monitoring surveys are needed. Right heart catheterization is recommended for a period of 6 to 12 months after PEA.

The danger inherent in the initiation of specific medical treatment of pulmonary hypertension without consultation with a surgeon is that potentially operable patients are not referred to a center of expertise, and they do not respond to medical treatment or are sent to surgery at an advanced stage, which is associated with a significantly increased risk. Before starting treatment, it must be established that the patients are appropriate candidates for the surgical procedure [100].

8.1.6. Long-term outcomes

Changes in short and long term patient outcomes are generally favorable after PEA. Indeed, functional and hemodynamic results are very encouraging. Most patients who were New York Heart Association (NYHA) class III or IV preoperatively became class I or II after surgery and were able to resume normal activities. A significant reduction and standardization of both pulmonary artery pressure and resistance may also be affected. In the largest series to date, the mean pulmonary artery pressure decreased from 46 mm Hg to 28 mm Hg and the mean pulmonary vascular resistance decreased from 893 to 285 dyne/s-1, [98]. Similar improvements were observed in right ventricular function by echocardiography, exercise capacity, and quality of life [101].

8.2. Medical therapy

Pulmonary endarterectomy is the treatment of choice for patients with CTEPH; unfortunately, it cannot be performed in all CTEPH patients because of the inaccessibility of distal lesions or the presence of concomitant life-threatening diseases. [102]. In addition, patients with CTEPH who have undergone endarterectomy may experience a gradual hemodynamic and symptomatic decline related to a secondary hypertensive arteriopathy in the small precapillary pulmonary vessels. It has also been questioned what can be done to reduce risks from PEA surgery to improve outcomes in "high risk" patients with CTEPH with substantial impairment of pulmonary hemodynamics before surgery. Such patients may benefit from preoperative reduction of pulmonary vascular resistance by means of medical therapy. Conventional medical treatments, such as anticoagulation, diuretics, digitalis, and chronic oxygen therapy, show low efficacy in the treatment of CTEPH as they do not affect underlying disease processes. Over the last decade, several novel therapies have been developed for pulmonary arterial hypertension (PAH), including prostacyclin analogs (epoprostenol, beraprost, iloprost, treprostinil), endothelin receptor antagonists (bosentan, sitaxsentan, ambrisentan), and phosphodiesterase-5 inhibitors (sildenafil, tadalafil). Evidence of efficacy in PAH, coupled with studies showing histopathologic similarities between CTEPH and PAH, provides a rationale to extend the use of some of these medications to the treatment of CTEPH. However, direct evidence from clinical trials in CTEPH is limited to date [103, 104].

The BENEFiT (Bosentan Effects in iNopErable Forms of chronIc Thromboembolic pulmonary hypertension) study was a double-blind, randomized, placebo-controlled study in CTEPH including patients with either inoperable CTEPH or persistent/recurrent pulmonary hypertension after PEA (>6 months after PEA). Independent coprimary end points were change in PVR as a percentage of baseline and change from baseline in 6-min walk distance after 16 weeks of treatment [105]. This study demonstrated a positive treatment effect of bosentan on hemodynamics in this patient population. No improvement was observed in exercise capacity. Further trials are needed to define the role of medical therapy in patients with CTEPH. In a retrospective study, the authors analyzed the effects of long-term intravenous epoprostenol in 27 consecutive functional class III (n = 20) or IV (n = 7) patients with inoperable distal CTEPH. After three months of epoprostenol, NYHA functional class improved by one class in 11 of 23 surviving patients, 6-minute walk distance increased by 66 m (p 0.0001) and hemodynamics also improved. At the last evaluation (20 ± 8 months), functional class was improved in 9 of 18 surviving patients with sustained improvement in 6-minute walk distance (+46 m, p = 0.03) and hemodynamic parameters. Survival at one, two and three years was 73%, 59% and 41%, respectively [88]. Epoprostenol has also been shown to improve hemodynamics in CTEPH patients prior to pulmonary thromboendarterectomy. In an open-label uncontrolled study, the prostacyclin analog treprostinil has been used in patients with severe inoperable CTEPH. Treprostinil improves exercise capacity, hemodynamics and survival in patients with severe inoperable CTEPH. We speculate that the effects may be explained by a combined vasodilatory, platelet-antagonistic and potential antiproliferative action of the drug [106].

A double-blind, placebo-controlled, 12-week pilot study investigated the use of sildenafil, 40 mg three times daily, in 19 patients with inoperable CTEPH. Unfortunately, this study was inadequately powered to test the primary end-point (change in 6-min walk distance). Moreover, there was no significant difference between the sildenafil and placebo groups (17.5 m improvement). Nevertheless, there were significant improvements in WHO functional class (p=0.025) and pulmonary vascular resistance (p=0.044) for the sildenafil-treated [107].

8.3. Management of patients who are not candidates for endarterectomy

PEA remains the preferred approach for patients with CTEPH. Unfortunately, up to 50% of patients are not surgical candidates with the most common reasons for exclusion being distal chronic thromboembolic disease with surgical inaccessibility and significant comorbidities. Specific medical therapies for PAH in the future can be a real alternative for PEA CTEPH patients. Although the distinction between PAH and CTEPH is often clear, there are many similarities between the conditions, including the clinical presentation with progressive PH and RV failure, and overlapping pathophysiology. PAH and CTEPH may represent extremes of a continuum of disease based on several data sources such as the observation that microvascular arteriopathy with plexiform lesions may exist in the vascular bed of both obstructed and unobstructed patients with CTEPH [109]. The role of several medical therapies in these specific groups of patients with CTEPH has been explored in many small-uncontrolled studies.

Early indications are that medical therapies may have promise in all these subgroups of patients with CTEPH, but the precise role of medical treatment in each situation remains unclear. Studies to date have not demonstrated the same level of efficacy in CTEPH as for patients with PAH [110]. Other CTEPH patients who might receive PAH medications include those awaiting lung transplantation. The currently available data do not justify the continuation of medical treatment in these patients if the waiting time to lung transplantation is long.

8.4. Balloon angioplasty in patients with CTEPH

Some patients with CTEPH, despite proximal (main, lobar or segmental) pulmonary artery occlusion are not candidates for thromboendarterectomy or decline surgery. In these patients, balloon angioplasty is a therapeutic option to relieve the obstructed pulmonary artery and improve the degree of pulmonary hypertension. Uncontrolled case series [111] have demonstrated a short-term improvement in pulmonary hemodynamics, WHO functional class, and exercise capacity.

Although angioplasty may be beneficial, the long term results have not been thoroughly studied in CTEPH.

8.5. Review of transplantation in patients with CTEPH

Concerned patients with CTEPH in functional class III / IV who are inoperable or have residual pulmonary hypertension post-PEA are referred for lung transplantation to improve their clinical outcomes. Although no studies specifically addressing this medical issue have been identified, patients with CTEPH were included in studies of lung transplantation for pulmonary hypertension, and in reports from international transplant registries [112]. The average survival for patients with idiopathic pulmonary hypertension undergoing lung transplantation was 5.6 years. The absence of any direct evidence for lung transplantation compared to medical treatment, especially in patients with CTEPH, was noted. However, the health benefits of lung transplantation, and a high impact on morbidity and mortality in selected CTEPH patients was emphasized. The CTEPH patients who are inoperable or experience residual PH post-PEA and who remain in WHO functional class III or IV, despite optimal medical therapy, should be referred for lung transplantation evaluation. Because there can be significant delays until transplantation, early referral is important.

9. Conclusion

We believe that over the past decade, a paradigm shift has occurred in CTEPH. The disease is much more common than anticipated and it is imperative that patients with this condition be adequately diagnosed to have access to surgery and well designed clinical trials. Although CTEPH is one of the leading causes of severe PH, it remains underdiagnosed. These delays in diagnosis contribute to the poor prognosis associated with the disease. Diagnosis of CTEPH requires input from various imaging techniques. Echocardiography, V/Q scintigraphy and possibly CT angiography are all essential in the initial diagnosis of CTEPH. Pulmonary angiography remains the gold standard diagnostic technique for assessing operability but recent advances in CT and MRI angiography show great promise. Furthermore, haemodynamic evaluation by right heart catheterisation provides vital prognostic information and an estimate of the relative risk of PEA surgery. CTEPH should be considered in all patients with PH as early diagnosis helps to identify those patients suitable for PEA, a potentially curative treatment. All patients with suspected CTEPH should be referred to an expert centre for a proper diagnostic evaluation to exclude or confirm the diagnosis and assess operability.

Author details

Mehdi Badidi* and M'Barek Nazi

*Address all correspondence to: mehdibadidi@hotmail.com or m_nazzi@yahoo.com

Cardiology Department, Military hospital Moulay Ismail in Meknes, University Hospital Center Hassan II of Fes, Morocco

References

[1] Frachona I., Jaïs X., Leroyera C., Jobica Y. Diagnosis and care of postembolic pulmonary hypertension: The role of the pneumologist. *Revue de Pneumologie Clinique 2008*; 64: 316-324.

[2] Carroll D. Chronic obstruction of major pulmonary arteries. *American J Med* 1950; 9:175-85.

[3] Fedullo PF, Auger WR, Channick RN, et al. Chronic thromboembolic pulmonary hypertension. Clin Chest Med 1995; 16:353–74.

[4] Moser KM, Braunwald NS. Successful surgical intervention in severe chronic thromboembolic pulmonary hypertension. Chest 1973; 64:29-35.

[5] Fedullo PF, Auger WR, Kerr KM, Rubin LJ. Chronic thromboembolic pulmonary hypertension. N Engl J Med 2001; 345: 1465-72.

[6] Dartevelle P, Fadel E, Mussot S, Chapelier A, Hervé P, de Perrot M, et al. Chronic thromboembolic pulmonary hypertension. Eur Respir J 2004; 23:637-48.

[7] Petrucci L, Carlisi E, Ricotti S, et al. Pulmonary endarterectomy in chronic thromboembolic pulmonary hypertension: Short-term functional assessment in a longitudinal study. Europa Medicophysica. 2007; 43:147–53.

[8] Hagl C, Khaladj N, Peters T, et al. Technical advances in pulmonary thromboendarterectomy for chronic thromboembolic pulmonary hypertension. Eur J Cardiothorac Surg 2003; 23:776–81.

[9] Jamieson SW, Auger WR, Fedullo PF, et al. Experience and results with 150 pulmonary thromboendarterectomy operations over a 29-month period. J Thorac Cardiovasc Surg 1993; 106:116-27.

[10] Daily PO, Auger WR. Historical perspective: Surgery for chronic thromboembolic disease. Sem Thorac Cardiovasc Surg 1999; 11:143–51.

[11] Jamieson SW, Kapelanski DP. Pulmonary endarterectomy. Curr Probl Surg 2000; 37:165–252.

[12] Anderson FA, Jr, Wheeler HB, Goldberg RJ, et al. A population-based perspective of the hospital incidence and case-fatality rates of deep vein thrombosis and pulmonary embolism. The Worcester DVT Study. Arch Intern Med. 1991; 151:933–8.

[13] Hvid-Jacobsen K, Fogh J, Nielsen SL, et al Scintigraphic control of pulmonary embolism. Eur J Nucl Med 1988; 14, 71-72.

[14] Stevinson BG, Hernandez-Nino J, Rose G, Kline JA. Echocardiographic and functional cardiopulmonary problems 6 months after first-time pulmonary embolism in previously healthy patients. Eur Heart J. 2007; 28:2517–24.

[15] Pengo V, Lensing AW, Prins MH, Marchiori A, Davidson BL, Tiozzo F, Albanese P, Biasiolo A, Pegoraro C, Iliceto S, Prandoni P: Incidence of chronic thromboembolic pulmonary hypertension after pulmonary embolism. N Engl J Med 2004; 350: 2257-64.

[16] Dalen JE, Alpert JS. Natural history of pulmonary embolism. Prog Cardiovasc Dis. 1975; 17:259–70.

[17] Fedullo PF, Auger WR, Kerr KM, Rubin LJ. Chronic thromboembolic pulmonary hypertension. N Engl J Med. 2001; 345:1465–72.

[18] Becattini C, Agnelli G, Pesavento R, et al. Incidence of chronic thromboembolic pulmonary hypertension after a first episode of pulmonary embolism. Chest 2006; 130:172-5.

[19] Dentali F, Donadini M, Gianni M, et al. Incidence of chronic pulmonary hypertension in patients with previous pulmonary embolism. Thromb Res 2009; 124: 256-8.

[20] Hoeper MM, Albert Barbera J, Channick RN, et al. Diagnosis, assessment, and treatment of non-pulmonary arterial hypertension pulmonary hypertension. J Am Coll Cardiol 2009; 54: Suppl. 1, S85–S96

[21] Klok FA, Zondag W, van Kralingen KW, et al. Patient outcomes after acute pulmonary embolism. A pooled survival analysis of different adverse events. Am J Respir Crit Care Med. 2010; 181: 501–6.

[22] Klok FA, van Kralingen KW, van Dijk AP, Heyning FH, Vliegen HW, Huisman MV. Prospective cardiopulmonary screening program to detect chronic thromboembolic pulmonary hypertension in patients after acute pulmonary embolism. Haematologica. 2010; 95: 970–5.

[23] Pengo V, Lensing AW, Prins MH, et al. Incidence of chronic thromboembolic pulmonary hypertension after pulmonary embolism. N Engl J Med. 2004; 350:2257–64

[24] Becattini C, Agnelli G, Pesavento R, et al. Incidence of chronic thromboembolic pulmonary hypertension after a first episode of pulmonary embolism. Chest. 2006; 130:172–5.

[25] Jais X., Dartevelle P., Parent F., Sitbon O., Humberte M. al. Postembolic pulmonary hypertension. Rev Mal Respir 2007; 24: 497-508

[26] Wilkens H., Lang I., Behr J. Berghaus T. Chronic thromboembolic pulmonary hypertension (CTEPH): Updated Recommendations of the Cologne Consensus Conference 2011. International Journal of Cardiology 2011; 154S: S54–S60.

[27] Miniati M, Monti S, Bottai M, et al. Survival and restoration of pulmonary perfusion in a long-term follow-up of patients after pulmonary embolism. Medicine 2006; 85:253–262.

[28] Moser KM, Daily PO, Peterson K, et al. Thromboendarterectomy for chronic, major-vessel thromboembolic pulmonary hypertension. Immediate and long-term results in 42 patients. Ann Intern Med. 1987; 107:560–5.

[29] Moser KM, Auger WR, Fedullo PF. Chronic major-vessel thromboembolic pulmonary hypertension. Circulation 1990; 81: 1735-43.

[30] Kim N.H, Lang I.M. Risk factors for chronic thromboembolic pulmonary hypertension. Eur Respir Rev 2012; 21: 123, 27–31

[31] Ribeiro A, Lindmarker P, Johnsson H, et al. Pulmonary embolism: A follow-up study of the relation between the degree of right ventricular overload and the extent of perfusion defects. J Intern Med 1999; 245:601–10.

[32] Ribeiro A, Lindmarker P, Johnsson H, Juhlin-Dannfelt A, Jorfeldt L. Pulmonary embolism: One-year follow-up with echocardiography doppler and five-year survival analysis. Circulation.1999; 99:1325–30.

[33] Lund O, Nielsen TT, Ronne K, Schifter S. Pulmonary embolism: Long-term follow-up after treatment with full-dose heparin, streptokinase or embolectomy. Acta Med Scand. 1987; 221:61–71.

[34] Sharma GV, Folland ED, McIntyre KM, Sasahara AA. Long-term benefit of thrombolytic therapy in patients with pulmonary embolism. Vasc Med. 2000; 5:91–5.

[35] Lund O, Nielsen TT, Schifter S, Roenne K. Treatment of pulmonary embolism with full-dose heparin, streptokinase or embolectomy – results and indications. Thorac Cardiovasc Surg. 1986; 34:240–6.

[36] Remy-Jardin M, Louvegny S, Remy J, et al. Acute central thromboembolic disease: Posttherapeutic follow-up with spiral CT angiography. Radiology. 1997; 203:173–80.

[37] Colorio CC, Martinuzzo ME, Forastiero RR, Pombo G, Adamczuk Y, Carreras LO. Thrombophilic factors in chronic thromboembolic pulmonary hypertension. Blood Coagul Fibrinolysis. 2001; 12: 427–32.

[38] Bonderman D, Turecek PL, Jakowitsch J, et al. High prevalence of elevated clotting factor VIII in chronic thromboembolic pulmonary hypertension. Thromb Haemost. 2003; 90:372–6.

[39] Jais X, Dartevelle P, Parent F, Sitbon O, Humbert M, Fadel E, et al. Postembolic pulmonary hypertension. Rev Mal Respir 2007; 24(4 Pt 1): 497—508.

[40] Dalen JE, Alpert JS. Natural history of pulmonary embolism. Prog Cardiovasc Dis 1975; 17:259–70.

[41] Nijkeuter M, Hovens MM, Davidson BL, Huisman MV. Resolution of thromboemboli in patients with acute pulmonary embolism: A systematic review. Chest. 2006; 129:192–7.

[42] Stevinson BG, Hernandez-Nino J, Rose G, Kline JA. Echocardiographic and functional cardiopulmonary problems 6 months after first-time pulmonary embolism in previously healthy patients. Eur Heart J. 2007; 28:2517–24.

[43] Lang IM. Chronic thromboembolic pulmonary hypertension – not so rare after all. N Engl J Med 2004; 350:2236–8.

[44] Wolfe MW, Lee RT, Feldstein ML, et al. Prognostic significance of right ventricular hypokinesis and perfusion lung scan defects in pulmonary embolism. Am Heart J 1994; 127:1371–5.

[45] Moser KM, Bloor CM: Pulmonary vascular lesions occurring in patients with chronic major vessel thromboembolic pulmonary hypertension. Chest 1993; 103: 685-92.

[46] Azarian R, Wartski M, Collignon MA, Parent F, Herve P, Sors H, Simonneau G: Lung perfusion scans and hemodynamics in acute and chronic pulmonary embolism. J Nucl Med 1997; 38: 980-3.

[47] Blauwet LA, Edwards WD, Tazelaar HD, McGregor CG: Surgical pathology of pulmonary thromboendarterectomy: a study of 54 cases from 1990 to 2001. Hum Pathol 2003; 34: 1290-8.

[48] Puthenkalam S, Jakowitsch J, Panzenboeck A, et al. Angiogenesis in chronic thromboembolic pulmonary hypertension (CTEPH). Am J Respir Crit Care Med 2011; 183: A2424.

[49] de Perrot M, Fadel E, McRae K, Tan K, Slinger P, Paul N, Mak S, Granton JT. Evaluation of persistent pulmonary hypertension after acute pulmonary embolism. Chest 2007 Sep; 132(3): 780-5.

[50] Rubin LJ, Badesch DB. Evaluation and management of the patient with pulmonary arterial hypertension. Ann Intern Med 2005; 143: 282–292.

[51] Pepke-Zaba J, Delcroix M, Lang I, et al. Chronic thromboembolic pulmonary hypertension (CTEPH): results from an international prospective registry. Circulation 2011; 124: 1973–1981.

[52] Azarian R, Brenot F, Sitbon O, Musset D, Grimon G, Boyer-Neumann C et al. Hypertension artérielle pulmonaire d'origine thrombo-embolique chronique. Presse Med 1994; 23: 1017-22.

[53] Dartevelle P, Fadel E, Mussot S, Cerrina J, Leroy Ladurie F, Lehouerou D, Parquin F, Paul JF, Musset D,: Traitement chirurgical de la maladie thromboembolique pulmonaire chronique. Presse Med 2005; 34: 1475-86.

[54] Ribeiro A, Lindmarker P, Johnsson H, et al. Pulmonary embolism: A follow-up study of the relation between the degree of right ventricular overload and the extent of perfusion defects. J Intern Med 1999; 245:601–10.

[55] Meignan M, Rosso J, Gauthier H, et al. Systematic lung scans reveal a high frequency of silent pulmonary embolism in patients with proximal deep venous thrombosis. Arch Intern Med 2000; 160:159–64.

[56] ZuWallack RL, Liss JP, Lahiri B: Acquired continuous murmur associated with acute pulmonary thromboembolism. Chest 1976; 70: 557-9.

[57] Hoeper MM, Mayer E, Simonneau G, et al. Chronic thromboembolic pulmonary hypertension. Circulation 2006; 113: 2011–2020.

[58] Lewczuk J, Piszko P, Jagas J, et al. Prognostic factors in medically treated patients with chronic pulmonary embolism. Chest. 2001; 119:818–23.

[59] Riedel M, Stanek V, Widimsky J, Prerovsky I. Longterm follow-up of patients with pulmonary thromboembolism. Late prognosis and evolution of hemodynamic and respiratory data. Chest.1982; 81:151–8.

[60] Sanchez O, Helley D, Couchon S, et al. Perfusion defects after pulmonary embolism: Risk factors and clinical significance. J Thromb Haemost. 2010; 8:1248–55.

[61] Bonderman D, Jakowitsch J, Adlbrecht C, et al. Medical conditions increasing the risk of chronic thromboembolic pulmonary hypertension. Thromb Haemost. 2005; 93:512–6.

[62] Dartevelle P, Fadel E, Mussot S, et al. Chronic thromboembolic pulmonary hypertension. Eur Respir J. 2004; 23:637–48.

[63] McLaughlin VV, Presberg KW, Doyle RL, et al. Prognosis of pulmonary arterial hypertension: ACCP evidence-based clinical practice guidelines. Chest. 2004; 126:78S-92S.

[64] D'Alonzo GE, Bower JS, Dantzker DR: Differentiation of patients with primary and thromboembolic pulmonary hypertension. Chest 1984; 85: 457-61.

[65] Badidi M., Belhachmi H., Lakhal Z., Nazzi M. post embolic pulmonary hypertension revealed with floating thrombosis in the vena cava inferior. Sang Thrombose Vaisseaux 2010; 22 (8): 1-2.

[66] Kapitan KS, Buchbinder M, Wagner PD, et al. Mechanisms of hypoxemia in chronic thromboembolic pulmonary hypertension. Am Rev Respir Dis 1989; 139:1149–54.

[67] Galie` N, Hoeper MM, Humbert M, et al. Guidelines for the diagnosis and treatment of pulmonary hypertension. Eur Respir J 2009; 34: 1219–1263.

[68] Lisbona R, Kreisman H, Novales-Diaz J, et al. Perfusion lung scanning: differentiation of primary from thromboembolic pulmonary hypertension. Am J Roentgenol 1985; 144:27–30.

[69] Powe JE, Palevsky HI, McCarthy KE, et al. Pulmonary arterial hypertension: value of perfusion scintigraphy. Radiology 1987; 164:727–730.

[70] Tunariu N, Gibbs SJR, Win Z, et al. Ventilation-perfusion scintigraphy is more sensitive than multidetector CTPA in detecting chronic thromboembolic pulmonary disease as a treatable cause of pulmonary hypertension. J Nucl Med 2007; 48:680–684.

[71] Silversides CK, Granton JT, Konen E, et al. Pulmonary thrombosis in adults with Eisenmenger syndrome. J Am Coll Cardiol 2003; 42:1982–1987.

[72] Lisbona R, Kreisman H, Novales-Diaz J, et al. Perfusion lung scanning: Differentiation of primary from thromboembolic pulmonary hypertension. Am J Roentgenol 1985; 144:27–30.

[73] Coulden R. State-of-the-art imaging techniques in chronic thromboembolic pulmonary hypertension. Proc Am Thorac Soc. 2006; 3:577–83.

[74] Reichelt A, Hoeper MM, Galanski M, et al. Chronic thromboembolic pulmonary hypertension: evaluation with 64-detector row CT versus digital substraction angiography. Eur J Radiol 2009; 71:49–54.

[75] Hoeper MM, Mayer E, Simonneau G, Rubin LJ. Chronic thromboembolic pulmonary hypertension. Circulation 2006 Apr 25; 113(16): 2011-20.

[76] Tunariu N, Gibbs SJ, Win Z, Gin-Sing W, Graham A, Gishen P, Al-Nahhas A. Ventilation-perfusion scintigraphy is more sensitive than multidetector CTPA in detecting chronic thromboembolic pulmonary disease as a treatable cause of pulmonary hypertension. J Nucl Med 2007 May; 48(5): 680-4.

[77] Kruger S, Haage P, Hoffmann R, et al. Diagnosis of pulmonary arterial hypertension and pulmonary embolism with magnetic resonance angiography. Chest. 2001; 120:1556–61.

[78] Hoeper MM, Lee SH, Voswinckel R, et al. Complications of right heart catheterization procedures in patients with pulmonary hypertension in experienced centers. J Am Coll Cardiol 2006; 48:2546–52.

[79] Auger WR, Fedullo PF, Moser KM, et al. Chronic major-vessel chronic thromboembolic pulmonary artery obstruction: Appearance of angiography. Radiology 1992; 182:393–8.

[80] Fishman AJ, Moser KM, Fedullo PF. Perfusion lung scans vs pulmonary angiography in evaluation of suspected primary pulmonary hypertension. Chest 1983; 84:679–83.

[81] Coulden R. State-of-the-art imaging techniques in chronic thromboembolic pulmonary hypertension. Proc Am Thorac Soc. 2006; 3:577–83.

[82] Ryan KL, Fedullo PF, Davis GB, et al. Perfusion scan findings understate the severity of angiographic and hemodynamic compromise in chronic thromboembolic pulmonary hypertension. Chest 1988; 93:1180–5.

[83] Sompradeekul S, Fedullo PF, Kerr KM, et al. The role of pulmonary angioscopy in the preoperative assessment of patients with thromboembolic pulmonary hypertension (CTEPH). Am J Respir Crit Care Med 1999; 159:A-456.

[84] de Perrot M, McRae K, Shargall Y, Thenganatt J, Moric J, Mak S, Granton JT. Early postoperative pulmonary vascular compliance predicts outcome after pulmonary endarterectomy for chronic thromboembolic pulmonary hypertension. Chest 2011 Jul; 140(1): 34-41.

[85] Mayer E, Kramm T, Dahm M, et al. Early results of pulmonary thromboendarterectomy in chronic thromboembolic pulmonary hypertension. Z Kardiol 1997; 86:920–7.

[86] Hagl C, Khaladj N, Peters T, et al. Technical advances in pulmonary thromboendarterectomy for chronic thromboembolic pulmonary hypertension. Eur J Cardiothorac Surg 2003; 23:776–81.

[87] Thistlethwaite PA, Kaneko K, Madani MM, Jamieson SW. Technique and outcomes of pulmonary endarterectomy surgery. Ann Thorac Cardiovasc Surg 2008; 14:274–82.

[88] Cabrol S, Souza R, Jais X, Fadel E, Ali RH, et al. Intravenous epoprostenol in inoperable chronic thromboembolic pulmonary hypertension. J Heart Lung Transplant. 2007 Apr; 26(4): 357-62.

[89] Kim M. Kerr, MD, FCCP; Lewis J. Rubin. Epoprostenol Therapy as a Bridge to Pulmonary Thromboendarterectomy for Chronic Thromboembolic Pulmonary Hypertension. CHEST.2003; 123(2): 319-320.

[90] D'Armini AM, Cattadori B, Monterroso C, et al. Pulmonary thromboendarterectomy in patients with chronic thromboembolic pulmonary hypertension: Hemodynamic characteristics and changes. Eur J Cardiothoracic Surg. 2000; 18:696–702

[91] Jamieson SW. Historical perspective: Surgery for chronic thromboembolic disease. Semin Thorac Cardiovasc Surg. 2006; 18:218–22.

[92] Mehta S, Helmersen D, Provencher S, Hirani N, Rubens FD, et al. for the Canadian Thoracic Society Pulmonary Vascular Disease - CTEPH CPG Development Committee; and the Canadian Thoracic Society Canadian Respiratory Guidelines Committee. Diagnostic evaluation and management of chronic thromboembolic pulmonary hypertension: A clinical practice guideline. Can Respir J 2010 November/December; 17(6): 301-334.

[93] Galiè N, Hoeper MM, Humbert M, et al. Guidelines for the diagnosis and treatment of pulmonary hypertension: The Task Force for the Diagnosis and Treatment of Pulmonary Hypertension of the European Society of Cardiology (ESC) and the European Respiratory Society (ERS), endorsed by the International Society of Heart and Lung Transplantation (ISHLT). Eur Heart J 2009; 30:2493–2537.

[94] Jamieson SW. Pulmonary endarterectomy. In: Current problems in surgery. New-York: Mosby, 2000, 165-252.

[95] Yoshimi S, Tanabe N, Masuda M, et al. Survival and quality of life for patients with peripheral type chronic thromboembolic pulmonary hypertension. Circ J. 2008; 72:958–65.

[96] Nakajima N, Masuda M, Mogi K. The surgical treatment for chronicp ulmonary thromboembolism. Our experience and current review of the literature. Ann Thorac Cardiovasc Surg 1997; 3:15–21.

[97] Mayer E, Jenkins D, Lindner J, D'Armini A, Kloek J, Meyns B, Ilkjaer LB, Klepetko W, Delcroix M, Lang I, Pepke-Zaba J, Simonneau G, Dartevelle P. Surgical management and outcome of patients with chronic thromboembolic pulmonary hypertension: re-

sults from an international prospective registry. J Thorac Cardiovasc Surg 2011 Mar; 141(3):702-10.

[98] Freed DH, Thomson BM, Berman M, et al. Survival after pulmonary thrombendarterectomy: Effect of residual pulmonary hypertension. J Thorac Cardiovasc Surg 2011; 141:383–7.

[99] Mares P, Gilbert TB, Tschernko EM, et al. Pulmonary artery thromboendarterectomy: A comparison of two different postoperative treatment strategies. Anesth Analg 2000; 90:267–73.

[100] Thistlethwaite PA, Auger WR, Madani MM, et al. Pulmonary thromboendarterectomy combined with other cardiac operations: Indications, surgical approach, and outcome. Ann Thorac Surg 2001; 72:13–9.

[101] Tscholl D, Langer F, Wendler O, et al. Pulmonary thromboendarterectomy— Risk factors for early survival and hemodynamic improvement. Eur J Cardiothorac Surg 2001; 19:771–6.

[102] Jamieson SW, Kapelanski DP, Sakakibara N, Manecke GR, Thistlethwaite PA, Kerr KM, Channick RN, Fedullo PF, Auger WR. Pulmonary endarterectomy: experience and lessons learned in 1,500 cases. Ann Thorac Surg 2003; 76:1457–1462.

[103] Bresser. P, Pepke-Zaba J., Jais X., Humbert M., Therapies for Chronic Thromboembolic Pulmonary Hypertension, An Evolving Treatment Paradigm, Proc Am Thorac Soc Vol 3. pp 594–600, 2006.

[104] Jensen KW, Kerr KM, Fedullo PF, Kim NH, Test VJ, Ben-Yehuda O, Auger WR. Pulmonary hypertensive medical therapy in chronic thromboembolic pulmonary hypertension before pulmonary thromboendarterectomy. Circulation 2009; 120:1248–54.

[105] Ulrich S, Speich R, Domenighetti G, et al. Bosentan therapy for chronic thromboembolic pulmonary hypertension. A national open label study assessing the effect of Bosentan on haemodynamics, exercise capacity, quality of life, safety and tolerability in patients with chronic thromboembolic pulmonary hypertension (BOCTEPH-Study) Swiss Med Wkly. 2007;137:573–80.

[106] Skoro-Sajer N, Bonderman D, Wiesbauer F, Harja E, Jakowitsch J, Klepetko W, Kneussl MP, Lang IM. Treprostinil for severe inoperable chronic thromboembolic pulmonary hypertension. J Thromb Haemost 2007; 5: 483–9.

[107] Suntharalingam J, Treacy CM, Doughty NJ, Goldsmith K, Soon E, Toshner MR, Sheares KK, Hughes R, Morrell NW, Pepke-Zaba J. Long-term use of sildenafil in inoperable chronic thromboembolic pulmonary hypertension. Chest. 2008 Aug; 134(2): 229-36.

[108] Vizza CD, Badagliacca R, Sciomer S, Poscia R, Battagliese A, Schina M, Agati L, Fedele F. Mid-term efficacy of beraprost, an oral prostacyclin analog, in the treatment

of distal CTEPH: a case control study. Cardiology. 2006; 106(3): 168-73. Epub 2006 Apr 26.

[109] Peacock A, Simonneau G, Rubin L. Controversies, uncertainties and future research on the treatment of chronic thromboembolic pulmonary hypertension. Proc Am Thorac Soc. 2006; 3:608–14.

[110] Galie N, Manes A, Negro L, Palazzini M, Bacchi-Reggiani ML, Branzi A. A meta-analysis of randomized controlled trials in pulmonary arterial hypertension. Eur Heart J. 2009; 30:394–403.

[111] Feinstein JA, Goldhaber SZ, Lock JE, Ferndandes SM, Landzberg MJ. Balloon pulmonary angioplasty for treatment of chronic thromboembolic pulmonary hypertension. Circulation.2001; 103:10–13.

[112] Christie JD, Edwards LB, Aurora P, et al. The Registry of the International Society for Heart and Lung Transplantation: Twenty-sixth Official Adult Lung and Heart-Lung Transplantation Report – 2009. J Heart Lung Transplant. 2009; 28:1031–49.

Chapter 8

Assessment of Diagnostic Testing to Guide the Surgical Management of Chronic Thromboembolic Pulmonary Hypertension

Juan C Grignola, María José Ruiz-Cano, Juan Pablo Salisbury, Gabriela Pascal, Pablo Curbelo and Pilar Escribano-Subías

Additional information is available at the end of the chapter

http://dx.doi.org/10.5772/55687

1. Introduction

Chronic thromboembolic pulmonary hypertension (CTEPH) is caused by organizing thrombotic obstructions in the pulmonary arteries by nonresolving thromboemboli, formation of fibrosis and remodeling of pulmonary blood vessels. It is defined as precapillary PH as assessed by right heart catheterization (mean pulmonary arterial pressure, mPAP ≥ 25 mmHg with a pulmonary arterial occlusion pressure, (PAOP) ≤ 15 mmHg and pulmonary vascular resistance (PVR) > 3 wood units, in the presence of one or more mismatched segmental or larger perfusion defects by ventilation-perfusion lung scintigraphy, computerized tomography, and/or pulmonary angiography after at least 3 months of effective anticoagulation (Lang, 2010) (Table 1).

Although the incidence and prevalence of CTEPH have been a matter of debate, it represents one of the most prevalent forms of PH. Current data derived from registries suggest that CTEPH occurs at an incidence of 3-30 cases per million in the general population. Classical estimates of disease frequency refer to the number of CTEPH cases per survived pulmonary thromboembolic events and report cumulative incidences between 0.1% and 9.1% after a single episode of pulmonary embolism (median follow-up of 4-8 years) and 13.4% after recurrent venous thromboembolism. However, 25 to 40% of patients with CTEPH do not have a documented antecedent venous thromboembolic event (depending on prospective versus retrospective reports, respectively) (Pengo et al., 2004; Bonderman et al., 2009; Pepke-Zaba et al., 2011). Finally, CTEPH can be diagnosed if organized thrombi in main, lobar, segmental or subsegmental pulmonary arteries can be visualized in a patient with precapillary pulmonary hypertension.

The final diagnosis of CTEPH is based on the presence of:
1. Symptomatic PH
2. mPAP ≥ 25 mmHg, PAOP ≤ 15 mmHg
3. With chronic/organized thrombi/emboli in the elastic pulmonary arteries (main, lobar, segmental, or subsegmental level)
4. After at least three months of effective anticoagulation.

Table 1. Diagnostic criteria in CTEPH.

Hemodynamic failure and death occur in 20% of patients within 1 hour of acute pulmonary embolism (massive pulmonary embolism). Among the survivors, the natural evolution, in most cases, is the reabsorption of blood clots by local fibrinolysis with complete restoration of the pulmonary arterial bed. In some patients, reabsorption does not occur and the emboli evolves from an organized clot into fibrous tissue inside the pulmonary artery (PA). A latency period ("honeymoon") between the acute pulmonary embolus and the occurrence of symptoms of PH is common. The occurrence of dyspnoea after a symptom-free interval of several years is not due to recurrent emboli, but to development of local thrombosis and small vessels arteriopathy (Dartevelle et al., 2004).

Management decisions for patients with CTEPH should be made at an expert center based upon interdisciplinary discussion among internists, subspecialists, radiologists, and expert surgeons. Surgical pulmonary endarterectomy (PEA) is the therapy of choice for patients with CTEPH as it is a potentially curative treatment option, leading to a profound improvement in hemodynamics, functional class and survival (Wilkens et al., 2011; Pepke-Zaba, 2010). Selecting the candidates who will benefit from surgery is still a challenging task. Detailed pre-operative patient evaluation and selection, surgical technique and experience, and meticulous post-operative management are essential prerequisites for success after this intervention (Pepke-Zaba et al., 2011). Criteria for surgical suitability have been described but the decision to proceed with surgical intervention remains subjective (Jamieson et al., 2003; Condliffe et al., 2009; Skoro-Sajer et al., 2009; Freed et al., 2011). This is in agreement with a recent prospective CTEPH international registry, which showed a wide variation in non operability amongst participating countries (from 12 to 61%) (Mayer et al., 2011).

The aims of the present chapter are to evaluate the different preoperative diagnostic tools to assess the relative contribution of the extent of mechanical obstructions by organized thrombi and the distal small vessel disease. In addition, we analyze these tools to predict the hemodynamic improvement and early mortality after PEA.

http://dx.doi.org/10.5772/55687

2. Pathogenesis of CTEPH

The pathogenesis of CTEPH is complex and is not fully understood. The most important pathobiological process is non-resolution of acute embolic thrombi which later undergo endothelialization and fibrosis, thus leading to narrowed or even obstructed pulmonary arteries.

Incomplete resolution occurs in a significant proportion of patients despite appropriate treatment, placing them at risk of developing CTEPH. Several studies have evaluated the resolution rate of acute PE and report divergent data. A meta-analysis of four prospective imaging studies found that more than 50% of patients with PE still have pulmonary perfusion defects 6 months after the primary diagnosis. A history of acute thromboembolism is not present in approximately 30% of patients presenting with CTEPH. Factors that appear to predispose to the development of CTEPH include recurrent embolic events, estimated systolic pulmonary pressure > 50 mmHg (on echocardiogram) at presentation of an acute pulmonary embolic event, and greater than 50% occlusion of the pulmonary vascular bed after a "single" embolic occurrence. Although CTEPH is commonly conceptualized as a thromboembolic disorder, neither coagulation cascade risk factors for venous thromboembolism nor defects in the fibrinolytic system have been identified in affected patients (Bonderman & Lang, 2012). For example, a deficiency of protein C, protein S, or antithrombin III, or the presence of factor V Leiden and factor II mutations, do not appear to be associated with a higher risk of CTEPH. Only the presence of a lupus anticoagulant (10%), elevated levels of antiphospholipid antibodies (20%), and elevated levels of factor VIII (39%), all well-known prothrombotic risk factors for venous thromboembolism, have been found in a significant proportion of CTEPH patients in a majority of studies (Wong et al., 2010). Other factors such as immunologic, inflammatory, or infectious mechanisms trigger pathological remodeling of major and small pulmonary vessels as a response to deranged thrombus resolution. Certain conditions are associated with an increased risk for CTEPH, including previous splenectomy, ventriculo-atrial shunt or pacemakers recipients with a history of device infection, and individuals with inflammatory bowel disease, myeloproliferative disorders, cancer, hypothyroidism treated with thyroid hormone replacement, non-0 blood types, and carriers of the fibrinogen Aα Thr312Ala polymorphism (Bonderman et al., 2009; Bonderman & Lang, 2012; Kim & Lang, 2012).

There are two main hypotheses explaining the pathologic process in CTEPH. In the classical *embolic hypothesis*, acute (single or recurrent) pulmonary emboli arising from sites of venous thrombosis are the initial event in developing CTEPH, but disease progression probably results from progressive vascular remodeling of the small vessels (Salisbury et al., 2011). The alternative *thrombotic hypothesis*, states that pulmonary vascular occlusions are caused by a primary arteriopathy and endothelial dysfunction and secondary *in situ* (local) thrombosis. Once vessel obliteration is sufficient to cause an increase in the pulmonary arterial pressure, self-perpetuated pulmonary vascular remodeling occurs and culminates in the development of PH (Jenkins et al., 2012b). This is supported by the fact that 1) unlike acute PE, there is no linear correlation between a compromised hemodynamic state and the mechanical obstruction of pulmonary arteries; 2) PH progresses in the absence of recurrent thromboembolic events; and 3) PVR is still significantly higher in CTEPH patients than in acute PE patients with a similar percentage of vascular bed obstruction (Sacks et al., 2006).

Several lines of evidence suggest that increased pulmonary arterial pressures in CTEPH are caused by both vascular obstruction by organized thrombi tightly attached to the pulmonary arterial medial layer in the elastic PA, replacing the normal intima, and remodeling of small distal pulmonary arterioles in non-occluded areas (including plexiform lesions), a pulmonary arteriopathy indistinguishable from idiopathic pulmonary arterial hypertension (Lang & Klepetko, 2008; Auger et al., 2010). Therefore, as proposed by Moser and Braunwald, CTEPH is considered a 'dual' pulmonary vascular disorder, consisting of a large vessel vascular remodeling process of thrombus organization combined with a small vessel vascular disease secondary to redistribution of blood flow within the pulmonary vasculature causing the development of overflow and postobstructive vasculopathy (Moser & Braunwald, 1973; Hoeper et al., 2006) (Fig. 1).

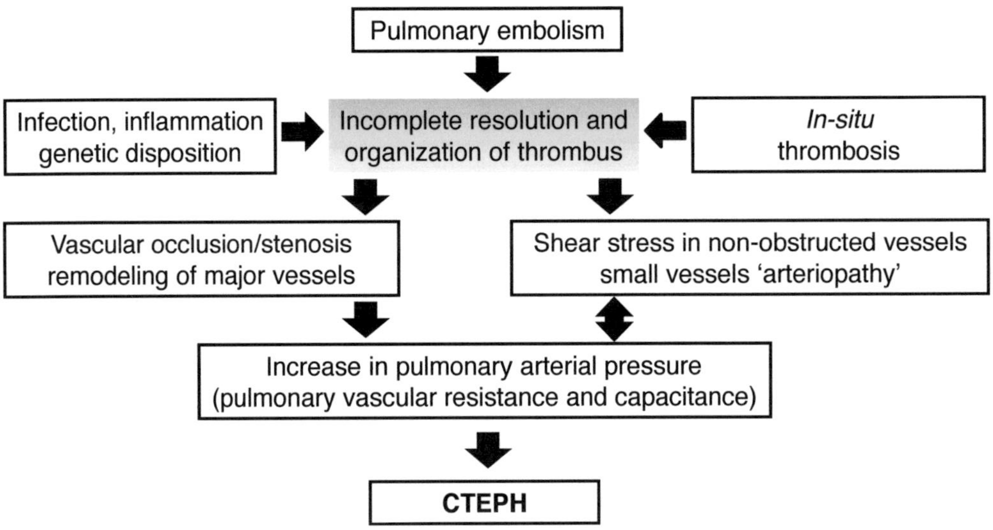

Figure 1. Current hypothesis for the pathogenesis of CTEPH.

Many fundamental questions persist about the risk factors and pathogenesis of CTEPH: 1) why many patients with PE do not develop CTEPH; 2) why many CTEPH patients have postoperative residual PH and; 3) whether patients with CTEPH who have poor postoperative outcome have cellular, molecular, and genetic abnormalities in the pulmonary vasculature similar to those in idiopathic PAH patients. Answering these questions poses a challenge for years ahead. However, a growing body of evidence suggests that in affected patients, minor o major thromboemboli do not resolve under conditions of concomitant inflammation, infection or malignancy, leading to fibrotic transformation of thrombus tissue (major vessel fibrosis) and small-vessel remodeling (Bonderman & Lang, 2012).

http://dx.doi.org/10.5772/55687

3. Diagnostic evaluation

The diagnosis of CTEPH is often delayed because the onset of symptoms is insidious and the symptoms themselves are nonspecific. Like patients with other forms of PH, CTEPH patients suffer from symptoms of progressive right ventricular failure. At early stages, exertional dyspnoea, fatigue and rapid exhaustion are typical. At more advanced stages, signs and symptoms (resting dyspnoea and fluid retention) of overt right heart failure are predominant. In contrast to a progressive course of disease in PAH, CTEPH progresses episodically. Episodes of desaturation and deterioration occur, interrupting apparent health (so-called honeymoon period). Thus a high degree of suspicion is required to detect CTEPH. Symptoms are related to impaired cardiac output and RV failure due to obstruction of the PA by unresolved thrombus and associated vasculopathy (Hoeper et al., 2006). The 1-year untreated mortality rate in CTEPH ranges from 12-24% and is predicted by the PA pressure at diagnosis (Condliffe et al., 2008). In contrast to other subtypes of pre-capillary PH, CTEPH is amenable to surgery. With PEA, patient survival improves to 89% and 75% at 5 and 6 years, respectively. Therefore, the main goal of the diagnostic evaluation of patients with an established diagnosis of pre-capillary PH is to test for the presence of thrombotic obstructions in major PA and refer patients to specialized expert centres for this life-saving surgery (Ryan et al., 2011).

All patients with unexplained PH should be evaluated for the presence of CTEPH. Suspicion should be high when the patient presents with a history of previous venous thromboembolism. Patients who survive an episode of acute PE are treated with anticoagulants for at least 3 months as secondary prevention to avoid recurrence (Kearon et al., 2012). However, the optimal duration of anticoagulant therapy is still unclear. After a first episode of PE, three major problems need to be considered: the risk of recurrence when anticoagulation is stopped, the risk of bleeding when anticoagulation is continued, and the risk of CTEPH. CTEPH is a rare complication of PE but it is associated with severe morbidity and mortality. There is no generally accepted strategy of follow-up of acute PE survivors. This is related to the relatively low incidence of clinically relevant CTEPH after an embolic episode (1 to 4%) which is diagnosed early and adequately treated. Echocardiographic follow-up after discharge (usually 3-6 months) is certainly advisable in all survivors of acute PE who remain symptomatic or develop exercise limitation due to dyspnoea at any time during their hospital stay to determine whether or not PH has resolved (Torbicki, 2010). Few prospective data are available on the incidence of CTEPH after a first episode of PE (Table 2) (Poli et al., 2010).

The initial diagnosis of CTEPH is established by echocardiography and ventilation/perfusion (V/Q) scan. Evidence of PH on echocardiography associated with mismatched segmental perfusion defects on the V/Q scan provides enough information to warrant referral to a centre with expertise in PEA (Fig. 2). A V/Q lung scan is recommended to exclude CTEPH; it is more sensitive than pulmonary computed angiotomography (CT). A normal V/Q lung scan virtually excludes CTEPH, with few exceptions (Skoro-Sajer et al., 2004), while unmatched perfusion defects can also occur in other conditions, such as mediastinal fibrosis, pulmonary artery sarcoma, schistosomiasis, and non-thrombotic embolism. In clinical practice, an abnormal perfusion study alone is diagnostic for CTEPH, if pulmonary parenchymal disease is absent.

Author (year)	Patients (n)	Screening method for CTEPH	Diagnostic method for CTEPH	Median follow-up (months)	Incidence of CTEPH (%)
Pengo et al. (2004)	223	Transthoracic echocardiography	V/Q lung scan. Pulmonary angiography	94.3	3.8
Miniati et al. (2006)	320	Perfusion lung scanning, TTx echocardiography	Right heart catheterization	25.2	1.3
Becattini et al. (2006)	259	Transthoracic echocardiography	Perfusion lung scan. Pulmonary angiography	46	0.8
Dentali et al. (2009)	91	Transthoracic echocardiography	Perfusion lung scan. TTx echocardiography	12	8.8
Klok et al. (2010)	866	Transthoracic echocardiography	Perfusion lung scintigraphy and right heart catheterization	34	0.57

Table 2. Summary of studies examining the incidence of CTPH after pulmonary embolism

Recent data from a CTEPH registry showed that 98.7% of patients had abnormal perfusion scans and 19% had abnormal ventilation scans (Pepke-Zaba et al., 2011). Such findings should be followed by further diagnostic studies since V/Q scanning might underestimate the burden of vascular obstruction. Furthermore, although V/Q scanning is a functional technique, it has limited spatial resolution.

The confirmation of the diagnosis and the determination of the best therapeutic options rely on the hemodynamics and morphological data provided by invasive pulmonary angiography and computed tomography pulmonary angiography (Pepke-Zaba, 2010). CT pulmonary angiography can accurately define the nature and extent of disease in CTEPH, and provide multi-planar and three-dimensional reconstructions of the vascular tree. It may reveal organised thrombi lining the proximal pulmonary vessels, abrupt tapering or amputation of vessels or subtle intraluminal fibrous webs (Castañer, 2009). Enlarged bronchial artery collaterals may be also seen and are considered a good prognostic sign in operable patients. Other findings include pouch defects, bands, scarring and a mosaic perfusion pattern (Willemink et al., 2012).

Pulmonary angiography is still considered to be the gold standard diagnostic procedure for defining the extent and distribution of disease in CTEPH with a relatively good safety profile. Findings typically include dilatation of the pulmonary artery, vascular obstructions, vascular webs, post-obstructive dilatations and poorly perfused areas of the lung. Pulmonary angiography is often performed in conjunction with right heart catheterisation that provides accurate prognostic information (Jenkins et al., 2012b).

http://dx.doi.org/10.5772/55687

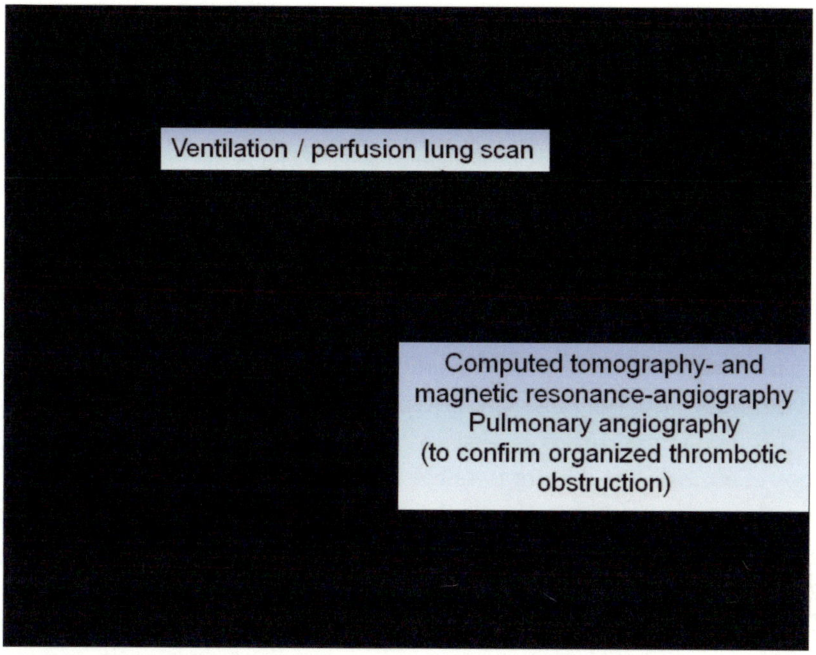

Figure 2. Diagnostic algorithm for CTEPH (modified from Hoeper M et al., 2006).

In summary, the reference standard for the diagnosis and determination of surgical accessibility remains combined right heart catheterization (to quantify the hemodynamic impairment) and conventional pulmonary angiography (to determine the extent and proximal location of chronic thromboembolic obstruction) (Fedullo et al., 2011). Vasodilator testing does not appear to be useful or necessary in determining operability, although preliminary data in a small cohort of patients suggest that preoperative vasodilator responsiveness (> 10.4% reduction in mPAP) is associated with an improved long-term hemodynamic outcome in patients who subsequently undergo PEA (Skoro-Sajer et al., 2009).

4. Surgical selection

Ultimately, the evaluation of patients with suspected CTEPH culminates in a decision regarding candidacy for PEA, since it is a realistic option for cure. Left untreated, CTEPH has a poor prognosis, proportional to the severity of PH. The 5-year survival is estimated to be approximately 30% if the mPA is greater than 30 mmHg and 10% if the Pm is greater than 50 mmHg (Riedel et al., 1982). When PH is established, the disease will progress despite adequate anticoagulation and eventually lead to right heart failure and death. Despite a strong rationale to administer vasodilator drugs in affected patients, current evidence from randomised controlled trials does not support the use of PAH-targeted pharmacotherapy. Still, compassionate use may be justified in cases considered inoperable, as a therapeutic bridge to PEA, in patients with persistent or recurrent PH after PEA, or when surgery is contra-indicated due to comorbid conditions (Wilkens et al., 2011). Despite disappointing study results, a significant proportion of real world CTEPH patients are managed with vasodilator treatment. In a recent international prospective registry, 37.9% initiated at least one PAH-targeted therapy (28% of operable and 54% of inoperable patients) including prostanoids, endothelin receptor antagonists, and phosphodiesterase type-5 inhibitors (Pepke-Zaba et al., 2011).

With experience and optimal patient selection, experienced centres may achieve a PEA operative mortality as low as of 4%. However, these results, are difficult to reproduce in different institutions, in part due to a long peri-operative and surgical management learning curve. Recent calculations based on delegates to the CTEPH association Cambridge meeting in June 2011 indicated that there were currently about 26 PEA centres worldwide, but many have a low volume of cases (Jenkins et al., 2012a). A centre can be considered to have sufficient expertise in this field if it performs at least 20 PEA operations per year with a mortality rate < 10% (Wilkens et al., 2011). If it were possible to organise treatment facilities, the ideal plan might be one centre geographically situated within a catchment area of 50 million individuals and performing > 75-100 cases per year (perhaps with a minimum of 50 cases per year) to achieve optimal outcomes. Exact prediction of operative risk and functional result is therefore, essential. PEA of major, lobar, and segmental pulmonary arterial branches is recognized as the standard treatment for CTEPH in most patients. The procedure involves the removal of fibrous obstructive tissue from the pulmonary arteries during circulatory arrest under deep hypothermia. The subsequent degree of relief of PH is variable, but in many cases may be total with restoration of pulmonary hemodynamics to normal or near normal (Wilkens et al., 2011). However, it has been recognized that the disorder may be accompanied by small-vessel pulmonary arteriopathy that is associated with perioperative death, postoperative persistent PH, or recurrence of disease. The decision whether PEA is feasible for specific patients must be made at a specialized centre. Operability is clearly a centre-specific assessment with large centre-to-centre variability. CTEPH is considered inoperable in 20-40% of cases, with the proportion of patients deemed inoperable differing between countries and specialist centres. The number of patients rejected from surgery due to distal obstructive disease decreases significantly with increasing expertise of the surgical centre (Mayer et al., 2011). In a contemporary registry, inoperability (37%) was due to surgical inaccessibility of the occlusions in almost half of patients, imbalance between PVR and the amount of accessible occlusions in 10%, PVR greater than 1500 dyn.s.cm^{-5} in 2.5%, advanced age in 2%, comorbidities in 13.4% and other reasons in 23% of patients. (Pepke-Zaba et al., 2011). The majority of patients selected for surgery are in New York Heart Association (NYHA) functional class III or IV and have dyspnea at low levels of exertion or at rest. Surgery may also be considered in patients in NYHA functional class II and with close to normal PVR at rest, if PVR increases significantly with exertion. In these patients, PEA will improve the ventilation-perfusion balance. Treatment of the disease at a relatively mild stage may, in time, help to minimise the development of secondary pulmonary arteriopathy. In 5-30% of patients with CTEPH, PEA may not be successful, because of residual PH (formal definition: mPAP ≥ 25 mmHg and PVR ≥ 240 dynes.s.cm^{-5}) Which is also the most common cause of perioperative mortality at many centres (Freed et al., 2011).

http://dx.doi.org/10.5772/55687

Selecting the candidates who will benefit from surgery is still a challenging task, and currently there is no reliable preoperative risk stratification classification system. Some functional and hemodynamic variables have been associated with perioperative survival. A PVR > 1200 dyn.s.cm^{-5}, mPAP > 50 mmHg, transfer coefficient of the lung for carbon monoxide < 70% and a low fractional pulse pressure (fPp) have a higher likelihood of operative mortality, while higher CI and six minute walk distance, and a decrease of mPAP by at least 10% after administration of inhaled nitric oxide have been associated with better perioperative survival (Skoro-Sajer et al., 2009). Expert opinion consensus (Cambridge meeting, 2011) has concluded that major factors for any risk score system should include PVR, NYHA class, 6 min walk distance, presence of indwelling catheters, medical pretreatment and the amount of disease on imaging studies. The only risk factors that affected in-hospital mortality in the European CTEPH registry were presence of PH specific drug treatment, time from last PE, PVR value at diagnosis, 6 min walk distance at diagnosis, and PVR at discharge from the ICU (Pepke-Zaba et al., 2011).

At the time of operation, the major predictors of outcome after PEA are the endarterectomy specimens categorized according to location and property of thrombus and vessel wall pathology (Jamieson et al., 2003). Type I refers to clot burden in the proximal main and lobar branches with evidence of fresh or subacute thromboembolic material (about 25% of cases). Type II refers to more chronic and fibrotic disease in the proximal branches with no fresh clot (about 40% of cases). Patients with type III present with disease in the segmental and subsegmental branches only, making the procedure much more challenging, as the plane of the dissection has to be developed individually in each of the segmental and subsegmental branches. It may represent CTEPH with reabsorption of the proximal clot burden (about 30% of cases). Type IV refers to distal arteriolar vasculopathy with no visible thromboembolic disease (<5% of cases) (Thistlethwaite et al., 2002; Jamieson et al., 2003). Because this classification is based upon the operative determination of lesions as proximal or distal, it is not useful before PEA.

To improve outcomes after PEA, accurate predictors of operative success and surgical mortality should be established. The optimal characterization of the contribution of large vessel and small vessel disease to the increase in right ventricular afterload and severity of hemodynamic derangement is crucial for the preoperative assessment and outcome prediction of PEA. Different methods to analyze the various components contributing to pulmonary vascular afterload have been investigated. We will discuss first possible preoperative hemodynamic, angiographic, and echocardiographic predictors for PEA success, and finally we will review efforts to partition pulmonary vascular afterload in order to predict outcome after PEA.

4.1. Classical hemodynamic features

Among the criteria defining patient operability, the pre-operative assessment of the relative contribution between proximal and distal small-vessel disease is crucial. Both processes determine a wide spectrum increase of dynamic (steady and pulsatile) afterload in CTEPH patients. The extent of vascular obstruction and associated vasculopathy are the major determinants of PVR. However, a more proximal occlusive site causes greater PA stiffness and an earlier and bigger wave reflection (pulsatile afterload) with a lower pulmonary vascular capacitance (Cp).

It is well known that high preoperative PVR is associated with higher short- and long-term postoperative mortality, especially in the absence of substantial chronic thromboembolic disease on the angiogram. This was supported by Dartevelle et al., and Condliffe et al. (Dartevelle et al., 2004; Condliffe et al., 2008) (Fig. 3). Dartevelle and colleagues reported that when the PVR was <900 dyn.s.cm^{-5}, the mortality rate was 4%, and increased to 10% in patients with PVR between 900-1200 dyn.s.cm^{-5}, and to 20% for PVR >1200 dyn.s.cm^{-5}. Condliffe and coworkers reported that total PVR (tPVR = input impedance) ≥900 dyn.s.cm^{-5} was associated with a PEA mortality above 10%, reaching 30% when total PVR was ≥1500 dyn.s.cm^{-5}. Patients with PVR in the range of 700 to 1100 dynes.sec.cm^{-5} are typically referred to surgical centres and many of these individuals will still benefit from surgical endarterectomy (Grignola, 2011). More detailed analysis revealed that the mortality is related to the degree of anatomic obstruction rather than to the resistance. Indeed, a patient with very high PVR and a low anatomic obstruction is at high risk, whereas one with the same PVR but with proximal anatomic obstruction presents with a low risk (Dartevelle et al., 2004).

Recent studies suggest that Cp, measured by stroke volume over pulse pressure (pPAP), may be a better prognostic marker of outcome than PVR in patients with idiopathic PAH. This observation may be of particular importance in CTEPH because the disease may predominantly affect the Cp rather than the resistance of the pulmonary vascular system (Naeije & Huez, 2007). De Perrot et al, have demonstrated that Cp is severely and rapidly affected in patients with CTEPH and does not always normalize three months after PEA despite a reduction in tPVR to <500 dynes.s.cm^{-5}. Cp improvement after PEA correlated with improvement in functional and exercise capacity, suggesting that Cp is an important parameter of the hemodynamic severity of CTEPH (De Perrot et al., 2011).

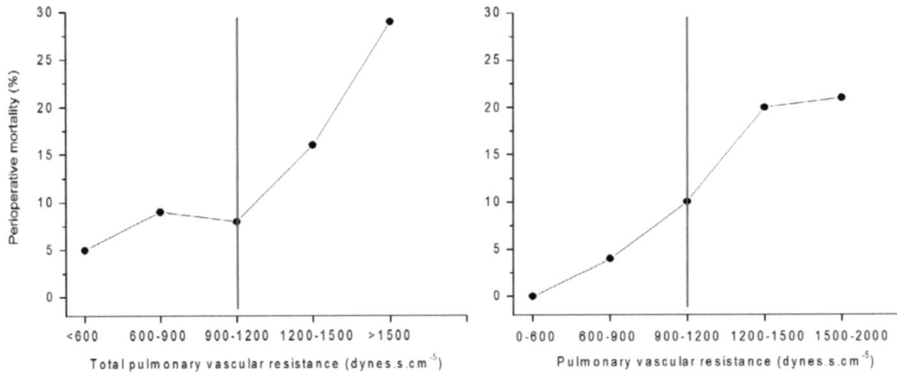

Figure 3. Perioperative mortality according to the pulmonary resistance (modified from Dartevelle et al, 2004 and Condliffe et al, 2009).

We also demonstrated that PEA improves long-term dynamic RV afterload. It is noteworthy that the postoperative increase of Cp is accompanied by a higher slope of the relationship between Cp and Pm with respect to preoperative values (Fig. 4). This observation allowed us to consider an improvement of the arterial cushioning function irrespective of mPAP decrease. However, some patients had persistent PH one year after PEA. These patients showed a significant lower improvement of Cp (2.0±0.8 vs. 3.9±1.1 ml/mmHg) and pPAP (38±11 vs. 18±6 mmHg), despite similar preoperative values (1.02±0.6 vs. 1.07±0.4 ml/mmHg and 58±15 vs. 58±16 mmHg). This lower increase in Cp at the expense of a reduced decrease in pPAP, associated with persistent PH could be related to a persistent impairment of the vessel wall viscoelastic properties secondary to vascular remodeling distal of the occluded major pulmonary artery and in vascular territories free of clot (Grignola et al., 2009a).

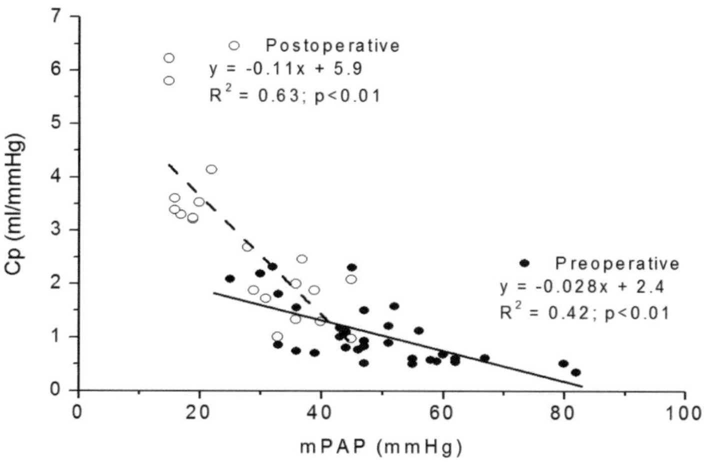

Figure 4. Correlation between mean PAP and Cp preoperative and one year post PEA.

In order to correlate functional hemodynamics with the anatomical lesions of CTEPH, we compared the multidetector pulmonary computed tomography angiography (MDCT) findings and the steady and pulsatile components of RV afterload in ten operable CTEPH patients (6 men; 50±11 years) who underwent PEA. Right-side catheterization and MDCT were performed preoperatively and one year after PEA. PVR and tPVR as steady components and Cp as the pulsatile component (viscoelastic properties of pulmonary arteries) were calculated. MDCT vascular (PA score), parenchymal (mosaic attenuation pattern score, MPP) and main PA diameter changes were evaluated. PA score was obtained by assigning every affected lobar or segmental PA n points (×2 if completely obstructed) according to the number of branches that originate from it (max score = 40). MPP was quantified (0-20) by giving 1 point to every parenchyma segment with a mosaic pattern (Ruiz-Cano et al., 2009). There was a significant improvement in the steady (PVR, tPVR) and pulsatile (Cp) components of the hemodynamic RV afterload after PEA along with a significant improvement of the parameters that assess the anatomical (PA score, PA diameter) and functional (MPP) changes in the lungs (Table 3).

	mPAP (mmHg)	PVR (dyn.s.cm^{-5})	tPVR (dyn.s.cm^{-5})	Cp (ml/mmHg)	PA diameter (mm)	PA score (%)	MPP
Preoperative	47±13	683±121	874±198	1.1±0.4	41±4.6	44±19	9.2±5
Postoperative	26±10§	323±210*	437±203*	2.6±1.1*	35±4.6§	24±18§	3.3±4*

Mean ± SD. *p<0.01; §p<0.001

Table 3. Preoperative and postoperative pulmonary hemodynamic (functional) and computed angio-tomography (anatomical) data.

Linear regression analysis demonstrated a significant correlation between changes in Cp and PA diameter (r = -0.63), between PVR and PA score (r = 0.58) and between PVR and MPP score (r = 0.6) (Fig. 5).

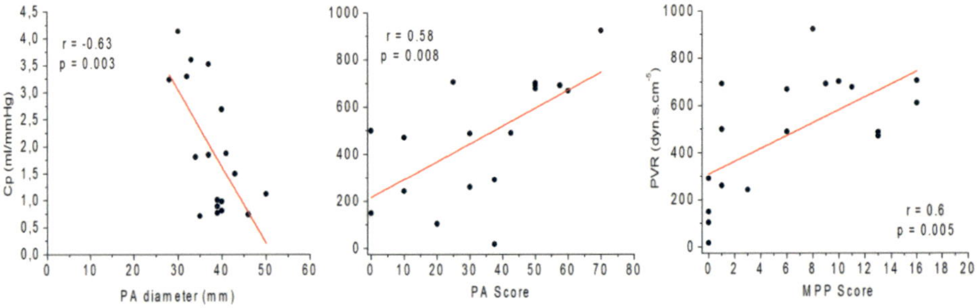

Figure 5. Correlations between pulmonary capacitance (Cp) and pulmonary arterial (PA) diameter and pulmonary vascular resistance (PVR) with PA score and mosaic attenuation pattern (MPP) score.

Further studies will be necessary to demonstrate that, vascular and parenchymal radiologic changes after PEA reflect the modification of the steady and pulsatile components of RV afterload.

Nakayama et al. showed that fPp (pPAP/mPAP) was useful for the differential diagnosis between CTEPH and idiopathic PAH (Nakayama et al., 1997). Accordingly, Tanabe et al. reported that fPp was higher in operable CTEPH than in idiopathic PAH and that it might be useful in predicting for the outcome of surgery, especially in patients with severe hemodynamic impairment (Tanabe et al., 2001). They proposed that both, increased characteristic impedance of PA and early and increased reflection wave could accentuate pPAP and fPp in CTEPH. Therefore, the assessment of fPp as well as the angiographic findings could be useful to determine the surgical accessibility to thrombi: high PVR with low fPp might be related to secondary PH change and/or distal thrombi, resulting in high operative mortality.

4.2. Echocardiographic findings

Patients with PH present with a pulmonary pressure wave with a huge pulse pressure, and a flow wave with a shortened time to peak velocity and a late or midsystolic deceleration (pulmonary flow systolic notch) secondary to systolic partial closure of the pulmonary valve. This midsystolic notching is caused by the negative effect of an early returned reflected wave on the forward wave. Wave reflection also explains a shorter time to notching on pulmonary arterial flow waves in embolic PH when compared with PAH. Clinical and experimental studies have provided evidence that an early notch signifies a proximal obstruction to pulmonary flow, whereas a late notch suggests that the obstruction site is more distal. All these changes are largely determined by wave reflections (Naeije & Huez, 2007). While a proximal site of reflection is an obvious determinant for an earlier return of a reflected wave, this can also be caused by an increased pulse wave velocity (PWV). PA wall distension with decreased compliance as a consequence of high pressures increases PWV. This explains why we also see a midsystolic deceleration of pulmonary flow in patients with severe PAH, in spite of the peripheral site of resistance in the PA tree and wave reflection. Recently, Hardziyenka et al. proposed that the so-called pulmonary flow systolic notch may distinguish proximally located obstruction in the pulmonary vascular bed. They defined a time to notching expressed as a notch ratio (NR), or the ratio of time from the onset of flow to maximum flow deceleration to time from maximum flow deceleration to end of flow (Fig. 6) (Hardziyenka et al., 2007).

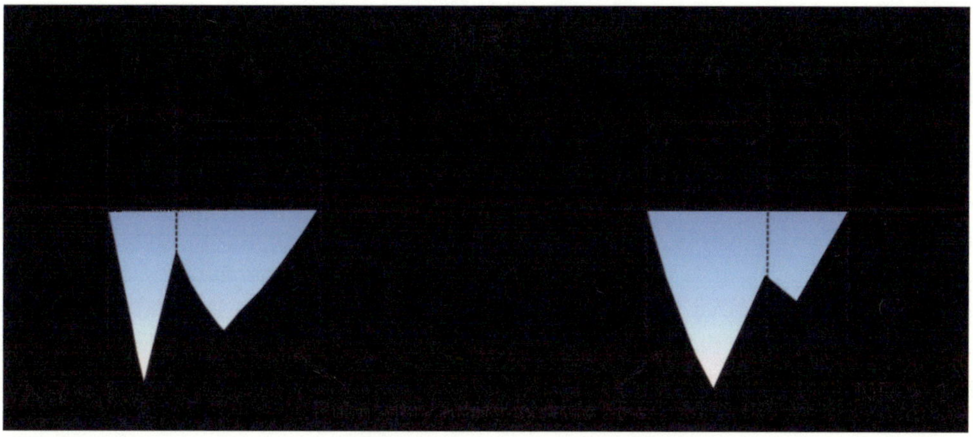

Figure 6. Schematic illustration of the method to calculate pulmonary flow systolic notch ratio (NR).

The timing of such a notch within the cardiac cycle is an excellent predictor of peri-operative mortality and functional improvement after PEA, with a lower mortality risk in patients with NR < 1. This optimal cutoff point (NR = 1) showed a sensitivity of 100% but a relative low specificity of 77% (confidence interval, 65-88%). Unfortunately, a preoperative notch was not observed in up to 12% of patients (Hardziyenka et al., 2007).

4.3. Angiographic assessment

As we mentioned before, the anatomic classification into proximal and distal lesions proposed by Jamieson et al is based on intraoperative findings and thus not useful to facilitate a decision before PEA. Also, interest should be focused on which patients with peripheral disease may still benefit from surgical intervention. Thus, the need for more detailed interpretation of angiographic findings of the peripheral pulmonary vascular tree appears evident. The typical angiographic findings of CTEPH are characterized as irregular intimal surface, vascular webs or bandlike narrowings, pouch-like termination of segmental branches, abrupt and angular narrowing of the central vessels, and obstruction of pulmonary vessels (Castañer, 2009). Recently, Kunihara et al, proposed a quantitative analysis of the pulmonary angiogram in conjunction with hemodynamic data to predict mortality and hemodynamic improvements after PEA (Kunihara et al., 2010). The proximal 2 cm of a segmental artery was classified into three categories: A, occlusion; B, pouch or membrane but preserved distal perfusion or C, delayed perfusion. They showed that the extent of angiographically involved segments played an important role in conjunction with preoperative hemodynamic severity of the disease in estimating postoperative outcome. Above all, segments with obstruction but preserved peripheral perfusion (type B lesion) seemed to have a higher impact on postoperative improvement after PEA than occluded segments (Kunihara et al., 2010). These novel findings may greatly help to identify suitable candidates with CTEPH for PEA.

4.4. Composite hemodynamic method of pulsatile and steady right ventricular afterload assessment

An approach to identify distal vasculopathy in CTEPH is the analysis of pressure decay curves after pulmonary arterial occlusion (between the moment of occlusion and the pulmonary artery occluded pressure, PAOP). Such curves consist of an initial fast component, which corresponds to the reduction of flow through arterial resistance, and a subsequent lower component, which corresponds to the emptying of compliant capillaries through a venous resistance. This biexponential fitting of the pressure decay curve allows identification of an inflection point (Poccl), from which one calculates an upstream resistance (Rup), essentially determined by the resistive properties of the large pulmonary arteries, and a downstream resistance determined by the cumulated resistance of small arterioles, capillaries and venules. Rup is calculated as follows: Rup (%) = 100×(mPAP-Poccl)/(mPAP-PAOP). A study on a small series of CTEPH patients referred for PEA showed excellent predictive values of residual PH and associated mortality by a relative increase in Rup (Kim et al., 2004). Patients with CTEPH and Rup value < 60% appear to be at the greatest risk for significant distal, small-vessel disease.

Some concerns can be made about the validity of this technique: the size of vessel that partitioning segregates, and the reliability of a single flow-directed measurement in a heterogeneous disease. To test the hypothesis that the occlusion technique is able to discriminate large vessel organized thrombus from distal vasculopathy, Toshner et al. performed occlusion pressures on patients with operable CTEPH, distal inoperable CTEPH and post-PEA residual CTEPH (Toshner et al., 2012). They also undertook measurements in patients with idiopathic or connective tissue associated PAH, where distal vasculopathy is traditionally accepted as the predominant process. The authors found that Rup measured by the occlusion technique is increased in operable predominantly proximal CTEPH when compared with inoperable CTEPH and idiopathic PAH. It is noteworthy they determined a higher Rup cutoff value compared to Kim et al: 79% (sensitivity 100%, specificity 57%) versus 60% (sensitivity and specificity 100%). They proposed that the occlusion technique would not interrogate the correct range of vessel caliber and would mislabel a significant portion of resistance in these small vessels as upstream. They did not explain the differences in the Rup values, including the values of the two patients who died postoperatively (68 and 73%). This is supported by the fact that the idiopathic PAH and inoperable CTEPH cohorts had a much higher Rup than would be expected if resistance had been accurately partitioned into clinically relevant small and large vessels (Toshner et al., 2012). Finally, they proposed multiple measurements using a wire directed catheter in conjunction with the flow-directed one, in order to provide additional information on disease heterogeneity in CTEPH.

Surgical operability depends on surgical accessibility rather than the extent of small vessel arteriopathy. Surgical accessibility depends on the presence of distal obstructions which are defined by the surgeon's technical ability and experience. The best surgical results are achieved with complete endarterectomy and early postoperative reduction of PVR to < 500 dynes.s.cm^{-5} (6.25 wood units). A more proximal occlusive site of the pulmonary circulation causes a higher PA stiffness and an earlier and greater wave reflection which increases systolic PAP (sPAP) and especially decreases diastolic PAP (dPAP), so called "ventricularization" of the PAP curve, with non-significant changes in mPAP and PAOP (Wittine & Auger, 2010). Cp a component of pulsatile afterload, is inversely proportional to pPAP (pPAP = sPAP-dPAP). Considering that mPAP = (sPAP+2dPAP)/3, then mPAP-dPAP is proportional to 1/Cp. Furthermore, the difference between mPAP and PAOP (transpulmonary gradient) is proportional to PVR (steady component of afterload).

We studied Zup, a novel hemodynamic index that is calculated by (mPAP-dPAP) x100/(mPAP-PAOP) (Fig. 7). mPAP is the time-averaged PA pressure throughout cardiac cycle length and it is accurately described by cardiac output, tPVR and right atrial pressure. Previous studies have established a link between the steady and pulsatile component of PA pressure by estimating mPAP from sPAP and dPAP ('two-pressure model') (Kind et al., 2010; Saouti et al., 2010). The geometric mean of sPAP and dPAP was the most precise estimate of mPAP ($mPAP^2 = sPAP \times dPAP$). sPAP and dPAP mainly depend on tPVR and PA stiffness and wave reflection. Increasing tPVR causes both sPAP and dPAP to increase while increasing PA stiffness and wave reflection generate a wider pPAP without significant mPAP change. The negative contribution of arterial stiffness to sPAP and dPAP may have been canceled when one multiplies sPAP by dPAP, thus unmasking the remaining influence of tPVR (Chemla et al, 2009). The extent of vascular obstruction and associated vasculopathy are the major determinants of mPAP. A more proximal occlusive site by the fibrotic organized thromboembolic material incorporated into the native vascular intima causes a higher PA stiffness. Stiffening of proximal PAs could increase characteristic impedance and wave reflection (higher upstream afterload), increasing tPVR but with a lower dPAP, a faster pressure decay profile and Zup increase. The balance between mPAP and dPAP provides a rapid tool to describe the functional afterload status of CTEPH patient, since their absolute contributions on Zup value are higher than PAOP.

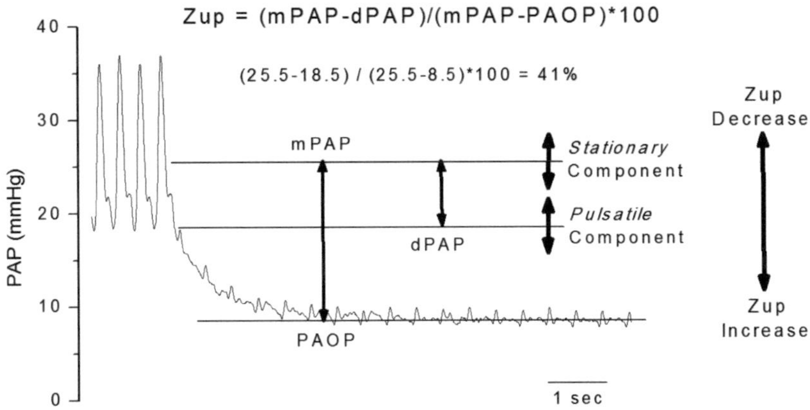

Figure 7. Example of the pulmonary artery decay curve showing the calculus of Zup index (mPAP and dPAP: mean and diastolic pulmonary arterial pressure, respectively; PAOP: pulmonary arterial occluded pressure).

Unlike the partition method described by Kim et al, (Kim et al., 2004) Zup index can be obtained directly from hemodynamic data without assumptions or fitting, and is affected by the extent and localization of anatomic obstruction, vascular remodeling and microvascular disease, setting a wide spectrum of dynamic afterload (steady and pulsatile components) (Ruiz-Cano et al., 2012).

Zup is inversely proportional to Cp, heart rate and PVR and it evaluates pulsatile and steady afterload components simultaneously (Fig. 7). A more important 'ventricularization' of PA pressure curve due to a higher proximal component of the afterload due to the lower dPAP and faster pressure decay profile would determine a higher Zup. Inversely, we hypothesized that preoperative Zup might be low in patients with CTEPH with inaccessible distal thrombi and/or secondary pulmonary hypertensive changes, resulting in a high operative mortality (Ruiz-Cano et al., 2010, 2012).

Total in-hospital mortality was 9.8% (6/61). According to the univariate analysis, lower preoperative Zup (OR 0.90, 95%CI 0.84–0.98, p=0.04) and CI (OR 0.004, 95%CI 0.001–0.67, p=0.03), and higher preoperative PVR (OR 1.3, 95%CI 1.08–1.64, p=0.007) had a significant association with early mortality after PEA. A low Zup value (cut-off point < 47%) predicted mortality after PEA with a sensitivity of 100% and a specificity of 78% [area under the curve (AUC)=0.86, p=0.006]. The AUC of ROC curves obtained for Zup and PVR showed no differences (p=0.4). When we analyzed the subgroup of 23 patients with higher preoperative PVR (>9 wood units, median of the cohort) Zup was a mortality risk predictor with sensitivity of 100% and specificity of 86% [AUC=0.86, p=0.013] for a cut-off point of 46.5%. On the other hand, PVR lost its capacity to predict mortality in this group [AUC=0.66, p=0.25]. Interestingly, in the population with the highest mortality risk according to the preoperative PVR (>9 wood units), Zup <46.5% could identify non-survivors more accurately with a sensitivity of 100% and a specificity of 86%. In this population, Zup >46.5% identified 7 patients who had successfully PEA operations even though they were very high risk based upon their pre-operative PVR (>15 wood units). The PVR and Cp of these patients were similar to the values of the patients who died. Thus, Zup might be an index of PA pressure 'ventricularization', that distinguishes proximal from distal disease in patients with the same pulmonary vascular RC constant. Concomitantly, PVR lost its ability to predict mortality in this population (Ruiz-Cano et al., 2012).

Finally, while it is likely that the functional adaptation of the pulmonary circulation to disease processes is generally monotonous (any change in PVR is associated with proportional changes in compliance and wave reflections), CTEPH is characterized by more predominant wave reflection as a cause of a disproportionate increase of sPAP and decrease of dPAP. We analyzed the behavior of Zup, fPp and Cp between idiopathic PAH and operable CTEPH in age and sex-matched cohort of patients with isobaric steady component of RV load and its effect on RV remodeling (Table 4) (Grignola et al., 2009b).

CTEPH patients were 53±14 years old and 58% were men, and IPAH patients were 56±5 years and 57% were men. Cardiac index and heart rate were similar in both groups. Isobaric steady component analysis permitted differentiation of the pulsatile component of IPAH and CTEPH cohorts, Table 4. The dynamic RV afterload in CTEPH patients was higher than in the IPAH patients. The lower Cp and fPp of operable CTEPH would be related to different vascular wall remodeling (thrombus organization and small vessel arteriopathy) and would explain the higher RV diastolic diameter (RVDd). The lower Zup in IPAH patients is in agreement with a more homogeneous distribution of the RV afterload.

	sPAP (mmHg)	dPAP (mmHg)	mPAP (mmHg)	pPAP (mmHg)	PVR (dyn.s.cm^{-5})	Cp (ml/mmHg)	fPp	Zup (%)	RVDd (mm)
CTEPH (n = 40)	83±21	27±8	48±12	56±18	744±350	1.17±0.6	1.19±0.2	57±15	49±7
IPAH (n = 44)	73±15*	32±10*	47±10	42±10§	760±370	1.5±0.7*	0.9±0.2§	43±15§	42±9§

Mean ± SD. *p<0.05; §p<0.01. (sPAP, dPAP, mPAP, pPAP: systolic, diastolic, mean and pulse pulmonary arterial pressure, respectively; PVR: pulmonary vascular resistance; Cp: pulmonary vascular capacitance; fPp: fractional pulse pressure; RVDd: right ventricle diastolic diameter).

Table 4. Steady (PVR) and pulsatile (Cp) afterload, hemodynamic data, Zup and RV diastolic diameter in idiopathic PAH and CTEPH patients.

To understand the hemodynamics of the pulmonary circulation in PAH, PVR and Cp have been measured. Lankhaar et al. showed that resistance and compliance in the pulmonary circulation are inversely related by a hyperbolic function (Lankhaar et al., 2008). They also showed, that the product, *i.e.* the RC-time, in the pulmonary circulation remains the same in healthy individuals and in patients with PAH. Clinical consequences of the constant RC-time are that CO can be increased more when a resistance decrease is accompanied by a compliance increase, than when resistance alone decreases with only a very small increase in compliance. Even when they included ten CTEPH patients in the analysis, six of them had inoperable CTEPH and they had different PVR.

Figure 8 shows the RC curve of our IPAH and CTEPH patients. The data show an inverse Cp-PVR relationship which reflects the coupling of these two components of RV afterload. However, the CTEPH curve is displaced down and leftward with respect to the IPAH curve. For patients with the same PVR (isobaric steady afterload), preoperative operable CTEPH showed a lower Cp, reflecting a higher pulsatile afterload component. These results disagree with the findings of Lankhaar et al and might expose a different RC coupling in operable CTEPH (Grignola et al., 2009b).

Finally, we analyzed Zup in operable and inoperable CTEPH patients (Ruiz-Cano et al., 2010). Among operable patients with good outcomes one year after PEA, lower Zup is predictive of persistent PH (PVR ≥ 240 dyn.s.cm^{-5}), which is associated with a lower improvement of Cp and pPAP. The lower Zup in inoperable CTEPH patients is in agreement with a more diffuse distribution of RV afterload seen in IPAH and would be related to different vascular wall remodeling (thrombus organization and small vessel arteriopathy).

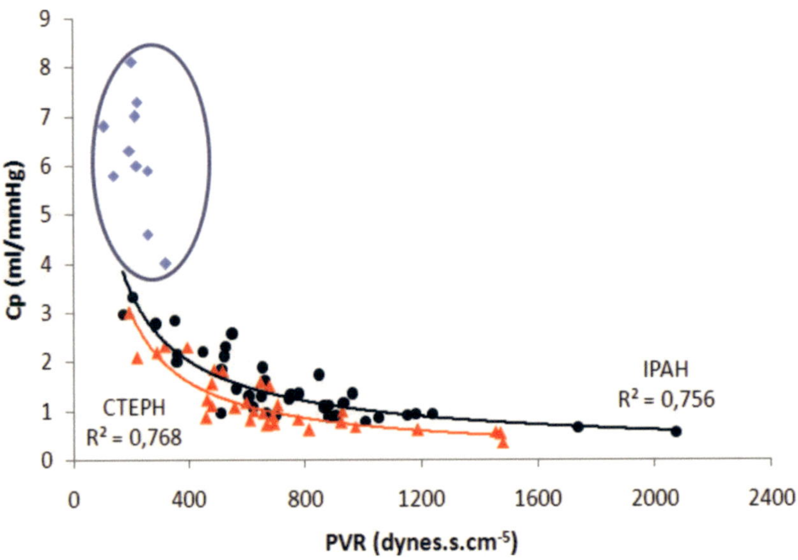

Figure 8. PVR-Cp (pulmonary vascular resistance-capacitance) plot of CTEPH and idiopathic PAH patients (fill diamonds represent ten normal subject without pulmonary hypertension) (Grignola et al., 2009b).

5. Conclusions

Substantial advances have occurred over the past quarter century in the diagnostic and therapeutic approach to CTEPH. In terms of management, surgery (PEA) is likely to remain the mainstay of therapy for patients with CTEPH. Further studies are necessary to obtain reliable long-term data on the effect of medical therapies in patients with CTEPH. It would be beneficial to have more objective definitions of what is considered to be operable and inoperable disease based on anatomic and functional variables. At the present time, this is a purely subjective determination made at centres with varying levels of experience, surgical expertise, and postoperative hemodynamic expectations. Recent data would suggest that the risk of some element of persistent postoperative PH should not serve as a contraindication to PEA (Freed et al., 2011). However, criteria have not been defined to determine when the risk of PEA outweighs its potential benefit. This determination requires the development of diagnostic techniques or algorithms capable of more objectively partitioning the central, surgically correctable component of the PVR from the peripheral component. The relative contribution of large vessel and small distal vessel disease to the elevation of RV afterload remains part of the art of the PEA evaluation. We propose a novel hemodynamic index, Zup, that considers both steady (PVR) and pulsatile (Cp) components of the RV afterload simultaneously and would predict mortality shortly after PEA as accurately as PVR for the global population with CTEPH who are suitable for surgery. In patients with higher PVR, Zup < 47% provided better identification of the population with the highest risk for early postoperative mortality. Zup could therefore be a complementary tool to improve risk assessment for PEA in patients with CTEPH. Larger and prospective studies will be necessary to validate the different predictors that have been presented as indexes to evaluate operative risk in CTEPH patients.

Acknowledgements

Juan C Grignola is supported by CSIC (Comisión Sectorial de Investigación Científica) and is a member of ANII (Agencia Nacional de Investigación e Innovación). María J Ruiz-Cano and Pilar Escribano are members of the REDINSCOR cardiovascular research network, which is supported by the Spanish Ministry of Health through the Instituto de Salud Carlos III.

Author details

Juan C Grignola[1], María José Ruiz-Cano[2], Juan Pablo Salisbury[3], Gabriela Pascal[4], Pablo Curbelo[3] and Pilar Escribano-Subías[2]

1 Department of Pathophysiology, Hospital de Clínicas, Universidad de la República, Montevideo, Uruguay

2 Heart Failure, Heart Transplantation and Pulmonary Hypertension Unit, Department of Cardiology, de Octubre University Hospital, Madrid, Spain

3 Department of Pulmonary Medicine, Hospital Maciel, Ministerio de Salud Pública, Montevideo, Uruguay

4 Department of Cardiology, Hospital Maciel, Ministerio de Salud Pública, Montevideo, Uruguay

References

[1] Auger, W.R., Kim, N.H. & Trow, T.K. (2010). Chronic thromboembolic pulmonary hypertension. *Clinics in Chest Medicine* Vol. 31, pp. 741-58, ISSN 0272-5231.

[2] Becattini, C., Agnelli, G., Pesavento, R., Silingardi, M., Poggio, R., Taliani, M.R. & Ageno, W. (2006). Incidence of chronic thromboembolic pulmonary hypertension after a first episode of pulmonary embolism. *Chest* Vol. 130, pp. 172–175, ISSN 0012-3692.

[3] Bonderman, D., Wilkens, H., Wakounig, S., Schafers, H-J., Jansa, P., Lindner, J., Simkova, I., Martischnig, A.M., Dudczak, J., Sadushi, R., Skoro-Sajer, N., Klepetko, W. & Lang, I.M. (2009). Risk factors for chronic thromboembolic pulmonary hypertension. *European Respiratory Journal* Vol. 33, pp. 325-31, ISSN 0903-1936.

[4] Bonderman, D. & Lang, I.,M. (2012). Chronic thromboembolic pulmonary hypertension. *European Respiratory Monography* Vol. 57, pp. 108-18, ISSN 2075-6674.

[5] Castañer, E. (2009). CT diagnosis of chronic thromboembolic pulmonary embolism. *RadioGraphics* Vol. 29, pp. 31-53, ISSN 0271-5333.

[6] Condliffe, R., Kiely, D.G., Gibbs, J.S.R., Corris, P.A., Peacock, A.J., Jenkins, D.P., Hodgkins, D., Goldsmith, K., Hughes, R.J., Sheares, K., Tsui, S.S.L., Armstrong, I.J., Torpy, C., Crackett, R., Carlin, C.M., Das, C., Coghlan, J.G., & Pepke-Zaba, J. (2008). Improved outcomes in medically and surgically treated chronic thromboembolic pulmonary hypertension. *American Journal of Respiratory Critical Care Medicine* Vol. 177, pp. 1122-1127. ISSN 1073-449X.

[7] Condliffe, R., Kiely, D.G., Gibbs, J.S.R., Corris, P.A., Peacock, A.J., Jenkins, D.P., Goldsmith, K., Coghlan, J.G., & Pepke-Zaba, J. (2009). Prognostic and aetiological factors in chronic thromboembolic pulmonary hypertension. *European Respiratory Journal* Vol. 33, pp. 332-7, ISSN 0903-1936.

[8] Dartevelle, P., Fadel, E., Mussot, S., Chapelier, A., Hervé, P., de Perrot, M., Cerrina, J., Ladurie, F.L., Lehouerou, D., Humbert, M., Sitbon, O. & Simonneau, G. (2004). Chronic thromboembolic pulmonary hypertension. *European Respiratory Journal* Vol. 23, pp. 637-48, ISSN 0903-1936.

[9] Dentali, F., Donadini, M., Gianni, M., Bertolini, A., Squizzato, A., Venco, A. & Ageno, W. (2009). Incidence of chronic pulmonary hypertension in patients with previous pulmonary embolism. *Thrombosis Research* Vol. 124, pp. 256–258, ISSN 0049-3848.

[10] De Perrot, M., McRae, K., Shargall, Y., Thenganatt, J., Moric, J., Mak, S. & Granton, J.T. (2011). Early postoperative pulmonary vascular compliance predicts outcome after pulmonary endarterectomy for chronic thromboembolic pulmonary hypertension. *Chest* Vol. 140, pp. 34-41, ISSN 0012-3692.

[11] Fedullo, P., Kerr, K.M., Kim. N.H. & Auger, R. (2011). Chronic thromboembolic pulmonary hypertension. *American Journal of Respiratory and Critical Care Medicine* Vol. 183, pp. 1605-13, ISSN 1073-449X.

[12] Freed, D., Thomson, B.M., Berman, M., Tsui, S.S.L., Dunning, J., Sheares, K.K., Pepke-Zaba, J. & Jenkins, D.P. (2011). Survival after pulmonary thromboendarterectomy: effect of residual pulmonary hypertension. *Journal of Thoracic and Cardiovascular Surgery* Vol. 141, pp. 303-7, ISSN 0022-5223.

[13] Grignola, J.C. (2011). Hemodynamic assessment of pulmonary hypertension. *World Journal of Cardiology* Vol. 3, pp. 10-17, ISSN 1949-8462.

[14] Grignola, J.C., Ruiz-Cano, M.J, Escribano, P., Cortina, J., Velázquez, T., Gómez-Sánchez, M.A., Delgado, J. & Saenz de la Calzada C. (2009a). Impaired pulmonary compliance in patients with long term residual pulmonary hypertension after endarterectomy for chronic thromboembolic pulmonary hypertension. *European Heart Journal* Vol 30(Suppl), pp. 108, ISSN 1520-765X.

[15] Grignola, J.C., Ruiz-Cano, M.J, Escribano, P., Tello de Meneses, R., Gómez-Sánchez, M.A., Delgado, J., Jiménez, C. & Saenz de la Calzada C. (2009b). Isobaric analysis of pulmonary arterial compliance of idiopathic and CTEPH: correlation with right ventricular remodeling. *European Heart Journal* Vol 30(Suppl), pp. 108, ISSN 1520-765X.

[16] Hardziyenka, M., Reesink, H.J., Bouma, B.J., Rianne de Bruin-Bon, H.A.C.M., Campian, M.E., Tanck, M.W.T., van den Brink, R.B.A., Kloek, J.J., Tan, H.L. & Bresser, P. (2007). A novel echocardiographic predictor of in-hospital mortality and mid-term haemodynamic improvement after pulmonary endarterectomy for chronic thromboembolic pulmonary hypertension. *European Heart Journal* Vol. 28, pp. 842-49, ISSN 1520-765X.

[17] Hoeper, M.M., Mayer, E., Simonneau, G. & Rubin, L.J. (2006). Chronic thromboembolic pulmonary hypertension. *Circulation* Vol. 113, pp. 2011-20, ISSN 0009-7322.

[18] Jamieson, S.W., Kapelanski, D.P., Sakakibara, N., Manecke, G.R., Thistlethwaite, P.A., Kerr, K.M., Channick, R.N., Fedullo, P.F. & Augeret W.R. (2003). Pulmonary endarterectomy: experience and lessons learned in 1500 cases. *Annals of Thoracic Surgery* Vol. 76, pp. 1457-62, ISSN 0003-4975.

[19] Jenkins, D., Madani, M., Mayer, E., Kerr, K., Kim, N., Klepetko, W., Morsolini, M. & Dartevelle, P. (2012a). Surgical treatment of CTEPH. *European Respiratory Journal* doi: 10.1183/09031936.00058112, ISSN 0903-1936.

[20] Jenkins, D., Mayer, E., Screaton, N. & Madani, M. (2012b). State-of-the-art chronic thromboembolic pulmonary hypertension diagnosis and management. *European Respiratory Review* Vol. 21, pp. 32-39, ISSN 0905-9180.

[21] Kearon, C., Akl, E.A., Comerota, A.J., Prandoni, P., Bounameaux, H., Goldhaber, S.Z., Nelson, M.E., Wells, P.S., Gould, M.K., Dentali, F., Crowther, M. & Kahn, S.R. (2012).

Antithrombotic therapy for VTE disease. *Chest* Vol. 141(Suppl), pp. 419S-494S, ISSN 0012-3692.

[22] Kim, N.H.S., Fesler, P., Channick, R.N., Knowlton, K.U., Ben-Yehuda, O., Lee, S.H., Naeije, R. & Rubin, L.J. (2004). Preoperative partitioning of pulmonary vascular resistance correlates with early outcome after thromboendarterectomy for chronic thromboembolic pulmonary hypertension. *Circulation* Vol. 109, pp. 18-22, ISSN 0009-7322.

[23] Kim, N.H.S. & Lang, I.M. (2012). Risk factors for chronic thromboembolic pulmonary hypertension. European Respiratory Review Vol. 21, pp. 27-31, ISSN 0905-9180.

[24] Kind, T., Faes, T.J.C., Vonk-Noordegraaf, A. & Westerhof, N. (2010). Proportional relations between systolic, diastolic and mean pulmonary artery pressure are explained by vascular properties. *Cardiovascular Engineering and Technology* Vol. 2, pp. 15-23, ISSN 1869-408X.

[25] Klok, F., van Kralingen, K., van Dijk, A., Heyning, F., Vliegen, H. & Huisman, M. (2011). Prospective cardiopulmonary screening program to detect chronic thromboembolic pulmonary hypertension in patients after acute pulmonary embolism. *Haematologica* Vol. 96, pp. 331-52, ISSN 0390-6078.

[26] Kunihara, T., Moller, M., Langer, F., Sata, F., Tscholl, D., Aicher, D. & Schafers, H-J. (2010). Angiographic predictors of hemodynamic improvement after pulmonary endarterectomy. *Annals of Thoracic Surgery* Vol. 90, pp. 957-64, ISSN 0003-4975.

[27] Kunihara, T., Gerdts, J., Groesdonk, H., Sata, F., Langer, F., Tscholl, D., Aicher, D. & Schafers, H-J (2011). Predictors of postoperative outcome after pulmonary endarterectomy from a 14-year experience with 279 patients. *European Journal of Cardio-thoracic Surgery* Vol. 40, pp. 154-161, ISSN 1010-7940.

[28] Lang, I.M. (2010). Advances in understanding the pathogenesis of chronic thromboembolic pulmonary hypertension. *British Journal of Haematology* Vol. 149, pp. 478-83, ISSN 0007-1048.

[29] Lang, I.M. & Klepetko, W. (2008). Chronic thromboembolic pulmonary hypertension: an update review. *Current Opinion in Cardiology* Vol. 23, pp. 555-59, ISSN 0268-4705.

[30] Lankhaar, J-W., Westerhof, N., Faes, T.J.C., Gan, T.J., Marques, K.M., Boonstra, A., van den Berg, F.G., Postmus, P.E. & Vonk-Noordegraaf, A. (2008). Pulmonary vascular resistance and compliance stay inversely related during treatment of pulmonary hypertension. *European Heart Journal* Vol. 29, pp. 1688-95, ISSN 1520-765X.

[31] Mayer, E. (2010). Surgical and post-operative treatment of chronic thromboembolic pulmonary hypertension. *European Respiratory Review* Vol. 19, pp. 64-67, ISSN 0905-9180.

[32] Mayer, E., Jenkins, D., Lindner, J., D'Armini, A., Kloek, J., Meyns, B., Bollkjaer, L., Klepetko, W., Delcroix, M., Lang, I.M., Pepke-Zaba, J., Simonneau, G. & Dartevelle P.

(2011). Surgical management and outcome of patients with chronic thromboembolic pulmonary hypertension: results from an international prospective registry. *Journal of Thoracic and Cardiovascular Surgery* Vol. 141, pp. 702-10, ISSN 0022-5223.

[33] Miniati, M., Monti, S., Bottai, M., Scoscia, E., Bauleo, C., Tonelli, L., Dainelli, A. & Giuntini, C. (2006). Survival and restoration of pulmonary perfusion in a long-term follow-up of patients after acute pulmonary embolism. *Medicine* Vol. 85, pp. 253–262, ISSN 0025-7974.

[34] Moser, K.M. & Braunwald, N.S. (1973). Successful surgical intervention in severe chronic thromboembolic pulmonary hypertension. *Chest* Vol. 64, pp. 29-35, ISSN 0012-3692.

[35] Nakayama, Y., Nakanishi, N., Sugimachi, M., Takaki, H., Kyotani, S., Satoh, T., Okeno, Y., Kunieda, T. & Sunagawa, K. (1997). Characteristics of pulmonary artery pressure waveform for differential diagnosis of chronic pulmonary thromboembolism and primary pulmonary hypertension. *Journal of the American College of Cardiology* Vol. 29, pp. 1311-16. ISSN 0735-1097.

[36] Naeije, R. & Huez, S. (2007). Reflections on wave reflections in chronic thromboembolic pulmonary hypertension. *European Heart Journal* Vol. 28, pp. 785-87, ISSN 1520-765X.

[37] Pengo, V., Lensing, A.W., Prins, M.H., Marchiori, A., Davidson, B.L., Tiozzo, F., Albanese, P., Biasiolo, A., Pegoraro, C., Iliceto, S. & Prandoni, P. (2004). Incidence of chronic thromboembolic pulmonary hypertension after pulmonary embolism. *New England Journal of Medicine* Vol. 350, pp. 2257–2264, ISSN 0028-4793.

[38] Pepke-Zaba, J. (2010). Diagnostic testing to guide the management of chronic thromboembolic pulmonary hypertension: state of the art. *European Respiratory Review* Vol. 19, pp. 55-58, ISSN 0905-9180.

[39] Pepke-Zaba, J., Delcroix, M., Lang, I., Mayer, E., Jansa, P., Ambroz, D., Morsolini, M., Snijder, R., Bresser, P., Torbicki, A., Kristensen, B., Lewczuk, J., Simkova, I., Barberà, J.A., de Perrot, M., Hoeper, M.M., Gaine, S., Speich, R., Gomez-Sanchez, M.A., Kovacs, G., Hamid, A.M., Jaïs, X., & Simonneau G. (2011). Chronic thromboembolic pulmonary hypertension (CTEPH). Results from an International Prospective Registry. *Circulation* Vol. 124, pp. 1973-81, ISSN 0009-7322.

[40] Poli, P., Grifoni, E., Antonucci, E., Arcangeli, C., Prisco, D., Abbate, R. & Miniati, M. (2010). Incidence of recurrent venous thromboembolism and of chronic thromboembolic pulmonary hypertension in patients after a first episode of pulmonary embolism. *Journal of Thrombosis and Thrombolysis* Vol. 30, pp. 294-299, ISSN 0929-5305.

[41] Riedel, M., Stanek, V., Widimsky, J. & Prerovsky, I. (1982). Long term follow-up of patients with pulmonary thromboembolism. Late prognosis and evolution of hemodynamic and respiratory data. *Chest* Vol. 81, pp.151-158, ISSN 0012-3692.

[42] Ruiz-Cano, M.J., Grignola, J.C., Escribano, P., Sanchez Nistal, A., Díaz, P., Velázquez, T., Gómez-Sánchez MA., Delgado, J. & Sáenz de la Calzada, C. (2009). Correlation between a novel multislice-computed tomography score and dynamic pulmonary afterload in patients with chronic thromboembolic pulmonary hypertension. *European Heart Journal* Vol 30(Suppl), pp. 748, ISSN 1520-765X.

[43] Ruiz-Cano, M.J., Grignola, J.C., Escribano, P., Cortina, J., Velázquez, T., Gómez-Sánchez, M.A., Delgado, J. & Sáenz de la Calzada, C. (2010). Preoperative partitioning of pulmonary vascular impedance: a novel hemodynamic index for operable and inoperable chronic thromboembolic pulmonary hypertension. *Journal of the American College of Cardiology* Vol. 55(Suppl1), A361, ISSN 0735-1097.

[44] Ruiz-Cano, M.J., Grignola, J.C., Cortina, J., Jiménez, C., Velázquez, M.T., Gómez-Sánchez, M.A., Delgado, J., & Escribano, P. (2012). Composite hemodynamic method of pulsatile and steady right ventricular afterload predicts early outcome after pulmonary endarterectomy for chronic thromboembolic pulmonary hypertension. *International Journal of Cardiology* Vol. 158, pp.475-476, ISSN 0167-5273.

[45] Ryan, J.J., Rich, S. & Archer, S.L. (2011). Pulmonary endarterectomy surgery: a technically demanding cure for WHO group IV pulmonary hypertension, requirements for centres of excellence and availability in Canada. *Canadian Journal of Cardiology* Vol. 27, pp. 671-74, ISSN 0828-282X.

[46] Sacks, R.S., Remillard C.V., Agange, N., Auger, W.R., Thistlethwaite, P.A. & Yuan, J.X-J. (2006). Molecular biology of chronic thromboembolic pulmonary hypertension. *Seminars in Thoracic and Cardiovascular Surgery* Vol. 18, pp. 265-76, ISSN 1043-0679.

[47] Salisbury, J.P., Curbelo, P., Arcaus, M. & Caneva, J. (2011). [Hipertensión pulmonar tromboembólica crónica]. *Revista Médica del Uruguay* Vol. 27, pp. 166-74, ISSN 1688-0390.

[48] Saouti, N., Weterhof, N., Postmus, P.E. & Vonk-Noordegraf A. (2010). The arterial load in pulmonary hypertension. *European Respiratory Review* Vol. 19, pp. 197-203, ISSN 0905-9180.

[49] Skoro-Sajer, N., Becherer, A., Klepetko, W., Kneussl, M.P., Maurer, G. & Lang, I.M. (2004). Longitudinal analysis of perfusion lung scintigrams of patients with unoperated chronic thromboembolic pulmonary hypertension. *Thrombosis & Haemostasis* Vol. 92, pp. 201-7. ISSN 0340-6245.

[50] Skoro-Sajer, N., Hack, N., Sadushi-Kolici, R., Bonderman, D., Jakowitsch, J., Klepetko, W., Reza Hoda, M.A., Kneussl, M.P., Fedullo, P. & Lang, I.M. (2009). Pulmonary vascular reactivity and prognosis in patients with chronic thromboembolic pulmonary hypertension. *Circulation* Vol. 119, pp. 298-305, ISSN 0009-7322.

[51] Tanabe, N., Okada, O., Abe, Y., Masuda, M., Nakajima, N. & Kuriyama, T. (2001). The influence of fractional pulse pressure on the outcome of pulmonary thromboendarterctomy. *European Respiratory Journal* Vol. 17, pp. 653-59, ISSN 0903-1936.

[52] Thistlethwaite, P.A., Mo, M., Madani, M., Deutsch, R., Blanchard, D., Kapelanski, D.P. & Jamieson, S.W. (2002). Operative classification of thromboembolic disease determines outcome after pulmonary endarterectomy. *Journal of the Thoracic and Cardiovascular Surgery* Vol. 124, pp. 1203-11, ISSN 0022-5223.

[53] Torbicki, A. (2010). Acute and long term management of pulmonary embolism. *Heart* Vol.96 , pp. 1418-24, ISSN 1355-6037.

[54] Toshner, M., Suntharalingam, J., Fesler, P., Soon, E., Sheares, K.K., Jenkins, D., White, P., Morrell, N.W., Naeije, R. & Pepke-Zaba, J. (2012). Occlusion pressure analysis role in partitioning of pulmonary vascular resistance in CTEPH. *European Respiratory Journal* ISSN 0903-1936, 40, 612-617.

[55] Wilkens, H., Lang, I., Behr, J., Berghaus, T., Grohe, C., Guth, S., Hoeper, M.M., Kramm, T., Kruger, U., Langer, F., Rosenkranz, S., Schafers, H-J., Schmidt, M., Seyfarth, H-J., Thorsten, W., Worth, H & Mayer E. (2011). Chronic thromboembolic pulmonary hypertension (CTEPH): updated recommendations of the Cologne Consensus Conference 2011. *International Journal of Cardiology* Suppl. Vol. 154, pp. S54-S60, ISSN 0167-5273.

[56] Willemink, M.J., van Es, H.W., Koobsa, L., Morshuisb, W.J., Snijderc, R.J. & van Heesewijk, J.P.M. (2012). CT evaluation of chronic thromboembolic pulmonary hypertension. *Clinical Radiology* Vol. 67, pp. 277-285, ISSN 0009-9260.

[57] Wittine, L.M. & Auger, W.R. Chronic thromboembolic pulmonary hypertension. (2010). *Current Treatment Options in Cardiovascular Medicine* Vol. 12, pp. 131-41, ISSN 1092-8464.

[58] Wong, C.L., Szydlo, R., Gibbs, J.S. & Laffan, M. Hereditary and acquired thrombotic risk factors for chronic thromboembolic pulmonary hypertension (2010). *Blood Coagulation & Fibrinolysis* Vol. 21, pp. 201-6, ISSN 1473-5733.

Chapter 9

Perioperative Considerations of Patients with Pulmonary Hypertension

Henry Liu, Philip L. Kalarickal, Yiru Tong, Daisuke Inui, Michael J. Yarborough, Kavitha A. Mathew, Amanda Gelineau, Alan D. Kaye and Charles Fox

Additional information is available at the end of the chapter

http://dx.doi.org/10.5772/56056

1. Introduction

Pulmonary hypertension (PH) is a devastating and potentially life-threatening condition that results from a heterogeneous group of diseases. PH is characterized by a sustained increase of mean pulmonary artery pressure (PAP) of 25 mmHg or greater due to any etiology [1]. PH is the manifestation of abnormal pulmonary vascular bed anatomy, abnormal vasoconstrictive status, and pulmonary parenchymal abnormalities which result in obstruction to pulmonary blood flow, cardiac diseases which may impede venous return from the lungs, or a combination of the above. Although many different causes exist, hypertension in the pulmonary circulation is the result of increased vascular resistance, increased vascular bed flow, or a coexistence of both. Initially the signs and symptoms of PH are usually subtle and nonspecific, often ignored by the patients. If left untreated, however, these patients with PH will develop progressive symptoms of dyspnea, fatigue, poor exercise tolerance and right heart failure culminating in a markedly shortened survival [2]. The mechanism for the pathogenesis of pulmonary arterial hypertension (PAH) is not completely understood. There is a conceptual transition in recent decades from the traditional view of mechanical obstruction of blood flow leading to elevated pressure in the pulmonary circulation to cellular growth and vascular remodeling causing increased resistance in pulmonary vasculature resistance [3][4]. Though uncommon, there are patients with PH scheduled for various surgical procedures and requiring anesthetic care perioperatively. In recent years some emerging strategies in the management of PH are potentially applicable to anesthesia practice intraoperatively. From the clinical anesthesia standpoint, although mild or transient PH won't considerably complicate anesthetic management, moderate or severe PH surely can dramatically deteriorate intraoperatively or postoperatively and potentially lead to acute right heart failure (RHF), cardiogenic shock and even death. The perioperative management of patients with PH varies depending upon the pathological features present, functional clinical classification, hemodynamic status, and success of current medical therapy. This chapter will review the epidemiology, etiologies, the mechanisms, especially cellular growth-related remodeling mechanisms, preoperative evaluation, intraoperative considerations and anesthetic management strategies, and postoperative management of patients with PH.

2. Definition and classifications of pulmonary hypertension

During the 4th World Symposium on Pulmonary Hypertension held in Dana Point, California in 2008, the thresholds for the diagnosis of PH were introduced: an mPAP ≥ 25 mm Hg was designated as manifest PH, while mPAP < 21 mm Hg was defined as normal, and mPAP from 21 to 25 mmHg was categorized as borderline. Correspondingly, echocardiographic systolic tricuspid regurgitation (TR) velocity thresholds < 2.5 m/s is defined as normal, 2.5 to 2.8 m/s as borderline, and > 2.8 m/s is highly indicative for manifest PH [1], as in Table-1.

	Invasive (mPAP)	**Non-invasive (systolic TR velocity)**
Normal	<21 mmHg	<2.5 m/s
Borderline	21-25 mmHg	2.5-2.8 m/s
Manifest PH	"/>25 mmHg	"/>2.8 m/s

mPAP: mean pulmonary artery pressure; TR: Tricuspid regurgitation; m/s: meter/second

Table 1. Definition of pulmonary hypertension [1]

The earliest PH Classification was introduced during a meeting sponsored by World Health Organization in 1973, basically this classification separated PH into two broad categories: primary or idiopathic (no identifiable causes can be found) and secondary (cause can be identified). Then in 1983 the Evian classification was proposed based on pathophysiological mechanism, clinical presentation and therapeutic options. PH Classification underwent two major modifications in Venice, Italy in 2003: the term idiopathic pulmonary arterial hypertension (IPAH) replaced the term primary pulmonary hypertension and, combined pulmonary veno-occlusive disease (PVOD) and pulmonary capillary hemangiomatosis (PCH) from separate categories into a single subcategory of pulmonary arterial hypertension (PAH) [5] [6]. The latest classification (Dana Point classification) became available in 2008 during the 4th World Symposium on Pulmonary Hypertension, in which PH is categorized into five groups: Group I: Pulmonary arterial hypertension (PAH); Group II: PH owing to left heart diseases; Group III: PH owing to lung diseases and/or hypoxeia; Group IV: Chronic thromboembolic pulmonary hypertension; Group V: Others (Tumor obstruction, fibrosing mediastinitis, chronic renal failure on dialysis). [5] [6], and is presented in Table-2.

	Subcategory of pulmonary hypertension	Hemodynamics
I	Pulmonary arterial hypertension (PAH): idiopathic or inheritable PAH A. Idiopathic B. Infectious C. Connective tissue disorders D. Congenital heart diseases	Pre-capillary mPAP ≥25 mmHg PCWP ≤15 mmHg CO normal or reduced^{+}
II	Pulmonary (venous) hypertension because of left-heart disease (PH with left-heart diseases)	Post-capillary, mPAP ≥25 mmHg PCWP "/>15 mmHg CO normal or reduced^{+}
III	Pulmonary hypertension associated with lung diseases and/or hypoxemia (PH with lung diseases)	Pre-capillary mPAP ≥25 mmHg PCWP≤15 mmHg CO normal or reduced^{+} Passive: TPG≤12 mmHg Reactive: TPG"/>12 mmHg
IV	Pulmonary hypertension associated with chronic thrombotic and/or embolic disease (PH with thromboembolic diseases)	Pre- capillary mPAP ≥25 mmHg PCWP ≤15 mmHg CO normal or reduced^{+}
V	Pulmonary hypertension associated with unclear and/or multifactorial mechanisms. Functional versus pathophysiologic considerations are important issue in classification. A more detailed description of PH Classification is available in other chapters of the book	Pre-capillary mPAP ≥25 mmHg PCWP ≤15 mmHg CO normal or reduced^{+}

PAH: Pulmonary arterial hypertension; PH: Pulmonary hypertension; mPAP: mean pulmonary artery pressure; PCWP: pulmonary artery wedge pressure; TPG: transpulmonary pressure gradient ($\bar{P}$pa - $\bar{P}$pcw). #: all values measured at rest; +: high CO can be present in cases of hyperkinetic conditions such as systemic-to-pulmonary shunts (only in the pulmonary circulation), anemia, hyperthyroidism, etc.

Table 2. DANA POINT Classification of Pulmonary Hypertension [5] [6]

3. Epidemiology of pulmonary hypertension

A review of a large U.S. database by Memtsoudis *et al* was undertaken to identify mortality in patients undergoing total hip arthroplasty (THA) and total knee arthroplasty (TKA).[7] The authors studied 1359 THA and 2184 TKA patients who also carried the diagnosis of PH. In comparison to a demographically-matched group of patients without PH, the THA patients demonstrated a 4-fold increased adjusted risk of in-hospital mortality and the TKA patients demonstrated a 4.5-fold increase (p<.001) [7]. Lai *et al* analyzed 62 patients with PH who underwent non-cardiac, non-local anesthetic surgery; they found that PH is an important predictor of adverse cardiopulmonary outcome in non-cardiac surgery as reflected by markedly increased postoperative complications, especially in patients with coexistent high-risk clinical and surgical characteristics [8]. Their results are listed in Table-3.

	Control (N=62)	PH (N=62)	P value
Morbidity %	2 (3.2)	15 (24.2)	0.002
Heart failure %	0(0)	6 (9.7)	0.028
Delayed extubation"/>24 hours %	2(3.2)	13(21)	0.004
Stroke %	0(0)	1(1.6)	NS
Myocardial ischemia/infarct %	0(0)	1(1.6)	NS
Major dysrhythmia %	0(0)	2(3.2)	NS
Mortality(in hospital death %)	0(0)	6(9.7)	0.028

PH= Pulmonary Hypertension

Table 3. Postoperative morbidity in patients with Pulmonary Hypertension [8]

Strange *et al* estimated community-based prevalence of PH in a district in Australia. They studied 10,314 individuals (6.2% of the surrounding Armadale community population) between 2003 and 2009 and they had 15,633 echocardiographic studies performed, 3,320 patients (32%) had insufficient tricuspid regurgitant (TR) or echocardiographic pulmonary artery systolic pressure (ePASP, echocardiographical calculation of PASP requires the measurement of regurgitant flow's Doppler velocity) and 936 individuals (9.1%) identified having PH regardless of etiology (defined as ePASP > 40 mmHg). Their minimum 'indicative' prevalence for all forms of PH is 326 cases/100,000 inhabitants of the local population, with left heart disease-associated PH being the most common cause (250 cases/100,000); these patients with PH secondary to left heart disease also had the worst prognosis. They identified 15 cases of pulmonary arterial hypertension/100,000 inhabitants and an additional 144 individuals (15% of all patients with PH) with no identifiable cause for their PH. The mean time to death for those with ePASP >40 mmHg (calculated from the first recorded ePASP) was 4.1 years. PH increased mortality regardless of the underlying causes, with those with idiopathic pulmonary arterial hypertension (IPAH) receiving disease-specific treatment having the best prognoses. Risk of death increased with PH severity: severe PH shortened the lifespan by an average of 1.1 years compared with mild PH [9]. Recent hemodynamic studies performed in large cohorts of adult patients with sickle cell disease have estimated the prevalence of PH in this disease group to be about 6 to 10% [10]. Over half of these patients have postcapillary PH. Precapilliary arterial PH seems to be a relatively infrequent complication of sickle cell disease. It is characterized by a different hemodynamic profile from IPAH with lower levels of PAP and PVR. However, pulmonary vascular disease appears to have a significant impact on the functional status and vital prognosis of patients with sickle cell disease. The predictive value of echocardiography to detect PH in this patient population is low (25-32%) when the threshold of tricuspid regurgitation velocity of 2.5m/s is used. At present, no specific treatment is currently approved for the treatment of PH associated with sickle cell disease due to lack of data in this specific population [10].

PH frequently accompanies childhood congenital heart disease (CHD) and may persist into adult life. The advent of specific therapies for PH prompted formation of a national Australia and New Zealand registry in 2010 to record the incidence, demographics, presentation and outcomes for these patients. They established a multicenter, prospective, web-based registry which enrolls patients with CHD-associated PH who are being followed at a tertiary medical center. The inclusion criteria stipulate patient age >16 years, a measured mPAP >25mmHg at rest or echocardiographic evidence of PH or a diagnosis of Eisenmenger's syndrome, and these patients have been followed since 1/1/2000. The investigators obtained the following results: of the first 50 patients enrolled, 30 (60%) are female, the mean age [Standard Deviation (SD)] at the time of PH diagnosis or confirmation in an adult center was 27.23 years (SD=10.07) and 32 patients (64%) are currently aged >30 years. Fourteen (28%) patients were in WHO functional Class (Table-4) II and 36 (72%) in Class III at the time of diagnosis. Forty-seven of 50 (94%) had congenital systemic-pulmonary shunts and 36 (72%) never underwent intervention. 13 (26%) had Down's syndrome. Confirmation of PH by recent cardiac catheterization was available in 30 (60%) subjects. During follow-up a total of 32 (64%) patients received a PH specific therapy. They concluded that CHD-associated PH in adult life has resulted in a new population with unique needs. This registry will allow documentation of clinical courses and long-term outcomes for these patients [11].

Class	Functional status of patients with pulmonary hypertension
I	Patients with pulmonary hypertension but without resulting limitation of physical activity. Ordinary physical activity does not cause undue dyspnea or fatigue, chest pain or near syncope.
II	Patients with pulmonary hypertension resulting in slight limitation of physical activity. These patients are comfortable at rest, but ordinary physical activity causes undue dyspnea or fatigue, chest pain or near syncope.
III	Patients with pulmonary hypertension resulting in marked limitation of physical activity. These patients are comfortable at rest, but less than ordinary physical activity causes undue dyspnea or fatigue, chest pain or near syncope.
IV	Patients with pulmonary hypertension resulting in inability to perform any physical activity without symptoms. These patients manifest signs of right heart failure. Dyspnea and/or fatigue may be present at rest, and discomfort is increased by any physical activity.

*--Modified from the New York Heart Association classification of patients with cardiac disease. Adapted with permission from Rich S., ed. Executive summary from the World symposium on Primary Pulmonary Hypertension 1998, Evian, France, September 6-10, 1998, cosponsored by the World health Organization. Retrieved April 14, 2000, from the World Wide Web: http://www.who.int/ncd/cvd/pph.html.

Table 4. WHO Functional Assessment of Patients with Pulmonary Hypertension*

PH can complicate interstitial lung disease (ILD). Anderson *et al* evaluated 212 ILD patients and found that PH occurred in 14% of a cohort of patients with ILD and was associated with lower lung function parameters. Mortality was markedly higher in ILD patients with PH, and the presence of PH reduced 6 Minutes Walk Test (MWT) independently of lung function. The present results emphasize the need for intensified treatment of patients with ILD and PH [12].

4. Etiologies of pulmonary hypertension

1. Causes of pulmonary arterial hypertension(PAH) [1]:

a. Idiopathic PAH (IPAH): No identifiable cause for the PH;

b. Familial PAH: A family history can be reported.

c. PAH associated with other diseases (APAH): Patient's PH can be associated with other co-existing diseases such as connective tissue diseases, infectious diseases as HIV infection,

d. Portal hypertension: like in many end-stage liver disease patient, they often have increased pressure in pulmonary artery;

e. Drugs & toxins: many decongestants containing ephedrine, pseudoephedrine, propylhexedrine, or oxymetazoline may lead to PAH. Other agents as NSAIDS, sodium and caffeine can also cause PAH [13]

f. Pulmonary veno-occlusive or capillary hemangiomatosis.

g. Regarding the pathogenesis of PAH, there is a conceptual transition in recent decades from the traditional view of mechanical obstruction of blood flow leading to elevated pressure in the pulmonary circulation to cellular growth and vascular remodeling causing increased pulmonary vasculature resistance [3][4].

2. PH with left-heart diseases: Congenital systemic-to-pulmonary shuts or left-sided atrial or ventricular diseases. Any congenital abnormality which leads blood circulating from high-pressure side to the low-pressure pulmonary circulation will have PAH;

3. PH with lung diseases and/or hypoxemia can be caused by following diseases:

a. Chronic obstructive pulmonary diseases

b. Interstitial pulmonary diseases

c. Sleep apnea or other sleep disorders with breathing problems;

d. Alveolar hypoventilation or other causes related hypoxemia

e. Developmental abnormalities.

4. PH caused by thrombotic and/or embolic diseases.

http://dx.doi.org/10.5772/56056

5. Miscellaneous: sarcoidosis, histocytosis X, lymphangiomatosis, pulmonary vascular compression by various pathologies.

5. Pathophysiology of pulmonary hypertension

Though a small percentage of patients have idiopathic PH [14], most perioperative patients with PH acquired PH secondary to either cardiac or pulmonary disease processes or both. Left sided ventricular or atrial disease and left sided valvular heart disease are common causes of PH. Both of these conditions increase left atrial pressure and elevate pulmonary venous pressure (PVP) and lead subsequently to increased PAP. Multiple respiratory diseases can lead to the development of PH via hypoxia-induced pulmonary vasoconstriction (HPV) or elevated PVR due to pulmonary fibrosis [15]. Regardless of the cause, all pathways may lead to an altered vascular endothelium and smooth muscle function through cellular remodeling and growth [16] [17]. This results in increased vascular contractility or lack of vascular relaxation in response to various endogenous vasodilator substances. Morphological abnormalities of the vascular wall are present in all three layers of the pulmonary arteries of patients with PH, and medial hypertrophy due to overproliferation of smooth muscle cells is a constant feature of all forms of PH. The classical mechanical concepts of pressure, flow, shear stress, RV wall stress and impedance have been gradually complemented with the new concepts of cell injury, repair/remodeling and interactions of complex multi-cellular systems [17]. Integrating these recent concepts will become critically important in completely understanding the mechanisms of PH, as we develop new interventions in order to change the prognosis of the patients with this devastating condition. Since PH can develop in association with many different diseases and with multiple risk factors, it is believed that the multi-factorial interplay may very likely be responsible for the pathogenesis of PH. The right ventricle (RV) is a crescent shaped, thin walled and compliant muscle chamber intended for volume work, not pressure work. Chronic PH leads to right ventricular hypertrophy (RVH) as a compensatory mechanism. However, the ability of the RV to adapt is finite and may eventually lead to RV failure. Unlike the muscular left ventricular chamber, a hypertrophied RV may not tolerate the acute rises in PVR that are associated with pain, surgical stimulation and positive pressure ventilation. RV failure and dilatation can lead to left ventricular compression and diminished cardiac output. This in turn leads to decreased coronary blood flow and perfusion pressure and can become a viscous cycle that can be difficult for the patient to overcome. The mechanisms for the pathogenesis of PH can be simply outlined as one or more of the following aspects: vascular remodeling with narrowness of vascular lumen and increased resistance, abnormal vascular reactivity leading to persistent vasoconstriction and loss of relaxation, left-side cardiac diseases impeding pulmonary venous return and various lung diseases compromising the pulmonary vascular bed leading to increased PVR. Here we discuss the pathophysiological changes of PH:

5.1. Pulmonary vascular inflammation and immune responses

The presence of antinuclear and antiphospholipid antibodies in the serum of patients with PH has been documented for many years [18]. There is more evidence that lymphoid neogenesis occurs in IPAH. Macrophages, mast cells, T- and B- lymphocytes, plasma cells and anti-endothelial cell antibodies are all present in and around the complex pulmonary vascular lesions in IPAH patients. Serum levels of IL-1 and IL-6 are high in IPAH patients, and serum IL-6 levels negatively predict patient survival. However, whether inflammation and aberrant immune responses in IPAH are cause or consequence remains unknown. Likely PH occurs when an inflammatory pulmonary arteriolar injury is not resolved by (normally) protective, innate anti-inflammatory mechanisms. Regulatory T-cells (Tregs) control not only other T-cells but also regulate monocytes, macrophages, dendritic cells, natural killer cells and B-cells, and recent evidence suggests that decreased Treg cell number or function may favor the development of PH. For example, conditions associated with PH, such as HIV, systemic sclerosis, systemic lupus erythematosus (SLE), Hashimoto's thyroiditis, Sjogren's Syndrome and the antiphospholipid syndrome are characterized by abnormal CD4+ T-cell number and function. Athymic rats lacking T-cells, develop pronounced PH after vascular injury with a vascular endothelial growth factor receptor blocker. The lungs in these animals are populated by infiltrating macrophages, mast cells and B cells, similar to human PH lesions. Most importantly, PH is prevented by immune reconstitution of Tregs prior to the induction of vascular injury. Putting these together all points to a possibility that aberrant Treg-cell function in the face of vascular injury can result in heightened innate and adaptive immune responses that could initiate and/or worsen the development of PH [19]. There is increasing evidence suggesting a role for immune deregulation in PH.

PH can potentially respond to immunosuppresive therapy (glucocorticoids or targeted B cell depletion) [20]. Sanchez *et al* reported on treatment of patients with mixed connective tissue disease or SLE– associated PH, where corticosteroid and cyclophosphamide has been used as first-line drugs, they found that PAH associated with SLE or mixed connective tissue disease may respond to a treatment combining glucocorticosteroids and cyclophosphamide and improve pulmonary hemodynamics. [21]. The effectiveness of B cell depletion is currently being examined in an NIH-trial studying the effectiveness of rituximab–a chimeric monoclonal antibody against the protein CD20, primarily expressed by B-cells – for systemic sclerosis-associated PAH. It is becoming clear that circulating factors can potentially amplify pulmonary vascular injury, attract immune cells and/or repair cells which respond to a variety of chemotactic stimulations, suggesting a systemic disease component contributing to the development or progression of PAH. In the "modern era" of PAH treatments, where standard vasodilation therapies have failed to reverse or stop the progression of PAH, novel targets such as discrete immune pathways hold promising alternatives [20][21]. Nevertheless, new drugs and clinical trials will all require assessing which patients may respond to anti-inflammatory or immune-modulating treatment strategies.

Several clinical studies indicated that obesity is a risk factor for the development of PH [22]. [23]; however, the mechanisms leading to this association are unknown. It is a well known fact that adipocytes secrete multiple bioactive mediators that can influence inflammation and tissue remodeling, suggesting that adipose tissue may per se directly influence the pathogenesis of PH. One of these mediators by adipocytes is adiponectin which is a protein with a wide range of metabolic, anti-inflammatory, and anti-proliferative activities. Adiponectin is present in high concentration in the serum of lean healthy individuals, but decreased level in obesity. There are studies suggesting that relative adiponectin-deficiency may contribute to the development of inflammatory diseases in obesity, and recent animal studies implicate adiponectin in the pathogenesis of pulmonary hypertension. Experimental studies showed that adiponectin can reduce lung vascular remodeling in response to inflammation and hypoxia. Moreover, mice lacking adiponectin can develop a spontaneous lung vascular phenotype characterized by age-dependent increases in perivascular inflammatory cells and elevated PAP. Some emerging evidence indicates adiponectin's effects are mediated through anti-inflammatory and anti-proliferative actions on cells in the lung [22]. PH has been associated with autoimmune disorders [18] [24]. Cell-free hemoglobin (Hb) exposure alone can be a pathogenic mediator in the development of PH and when combined with chronic hypoxia, the potential for exacerbation of PH and vascular remodeling can be significantly more profound. Buehler *et al* found this Hb-exposure related PH is also largely mediated by inflammatory process [25].

5.2. Pulmonary vascular endothelial injury, cellular growth and remodeling

Endothelial injury is central to the development of PH, a proliferative vasculopathy of the pulmonary circulation. Pulmonary vascular remodeling plays an important role in the sustained development of PH. Platelet-derived growth factor (PDGF) signaling has been demonstrated to be a major mediator of vascular remodeling implicated in PH. Xing *et al* investigated cigarette smoking (CS)-induced PH in rats and the expression of PDGF and PDGF receptor (PDGFR) in pulmonary artery, they established the association of PDGF signaling with CS-induced PH. Forty male rats were randomly divided into control group and three experimental groups that were exposed to CS for 1, 2, and 3 months, respectively. CS significantly increased right ventricular systolic pressure (RVSP) and right ventricular hypertrophy index (RVHI). Histology staining demonstrated that CS significantly increased the thickness of pulmonary artery wall and collagen deposition. The expression of PDGFR isoform B (PDGFR-B) and PDGFR-β were significantly increased at both protein and mRNA levels in pulmonary artery of rats with CS exposure. Furthermore, Cigarette smoke extract significantly increased rat pulmonary artery smooth muscle cell (PASMC) proliferation, which was inhibited by PDGFR inhibitor Imatinib. Thus, their results indicated PDGF signaling is also implicated in CS-induced PH [26].

PH is a condition for which no disease-modifying therapies exist for the time being. PH is recognized as proliferative disease of the pulmonary artery (PA). In the experimental new-born calf model of hypoxia-induced PH, adventitial fibroblasts in the PA wall exhibit heightened replication index. Because elevated PDGFR-β signaling is associated with PH, Panzhinskiy *et al* tested the hypothesis that activation of PDGFR-β contributes to fibroblast proliferation and adventitial remodeling in PH. In their study, newborn calves were exposed to either ambient air (P(B) = 640 mm Hg) (Neo-C) or high altitude (P(B) = 445 mm Hg) (Neo-PH) for 2 weeks. PDGFR-β phosphorylation was markedly elevated in PA adventitia of Neo-PH calves as well as in cultured PA fibroblasts isolated from Neo-PH animals. PDGFR-β activation with PDGF-BB stimulated higher replication in Neo-PH cells compared to that of control fibroblasts. PDGF-BB-induced proliferation was dependent on reactive oxygen species (ROS) generation and extracellular signal regulated kinase1/2 (ERK1/2) activation in both cell populations, however only Neo-PH cell division via PDGFR-β activation displayed a unique dependence on c-Jun N-terminal kinase1 (JNK1) stimulation as the blockade of JNK1 with SP600125, a pharmacological antagonist of JNK pathway, and JNK1-targeted siRNA blunted selectively Neo-PH cell proliferation. These data strongly suggest that hypoxia-induced modified cells engage PDGFR-β-JNK1 axis to confer distinctively heightened proliferation and adventitial remodeling in PH [27].

It is also known that 15-lipoxygenase (15-LO) plays an important role in chronic PH. Accumulating evidence for its down-stream participants in the vasoconstriction and remodeling processes of pulmonary arteries. Zhang *et al* investigated how hypoxia regulates 15-LO/15-hydroxyeicosatetraenoic acid (15-HETE) to mediate hypoxic PH, whether hypoxia advances the pulmonary vascular remodeling through the PDGF/15-LO/15-HETE pathway. What they found is pulmonary arterial medial thickening caused by hypoxia could be alleviated by treatment of the hypoxic rats with Imatinib, which was associated with down-regulations of 15-LO-2 expression and 15-HETE production. Moreover, the increases in cell proliferation and endogenous 15-HETE content by hypoxia were attenuated by the inhibitors of PDGFR-β in pulmonary artery smooth muscle cells (PASMCs). The effects of PDGF-BB on cell proliferation and survival were weakened after the administration of 15-LO inhibitors or 15-LO RNA interference. These results suggest that hypoxia promotes PASMCs proliferation and survival, contributing to pulmonary vascular medial hypertrophy, which is likely to be mediated via the PDGF-BB/15-LO-2/15-HETE pathway [28].

5.3. Pulmonary parenchymal diseases/fibrosis

The pathophysiology of PH in parenchymal lung diseases is partially related to hypoxic pulmonary vasoconstriction (HPV). This category is also called group III PH, namely PH attributable to lung diseases and/or hypoxia. Group III PH includes chronic obstructive pulmonary disease (COPD) and interstitial lung diseases (ILD); the most common parenchymal lung diseases associated with PH. Group III PH also includes sleep-disordered breathing and hypoventilation from any cause. Other parenchymal lung diseases associated with PH include sarcoidosis and systemic vasculitis (group V). There are controversies in terms of managing this group of patients [29].

5.4. Genetics and pharmacogenomics

Genetic factors may predispose some patients to the development or progression of severe PH. Mutations of the Bone Morphogenetic Type II Receptor (BMPR2) gene and a member of the transforming growth factor (TGF-β) superfamily were the first described in patients with familial/hereditary PH [30],[31][32]. Although BMPR2 mutations in PH have a high prevalence (70%), limited numbers of patients with PH have mutations, and only 20% of the carriers ever develop PH during their lifetime. BMPR2 mutation carriers at the time of PH diagnosis are younger and less likely to have a vasoreactive component [33][34]. A large number of mutations have been reported and the majority cause a loss of function or reduced BMPR2 expression. It has been reported that the disease appears to be more severe when patients carry a truncating BMPR2 mutation. However, this appears not to be the case in the French patients. Mechanistic studies indicate that BMPR2 mutations are permissive but not necessary for the development of severe PH. BMPR2 may be one of the guardians of lung vessel homeostasis, as gene knockout and silencing experiments have clearly demonstrated that both apoptosis and cell proliferation of PASMCs and endothelial cells are controlled by BMPR2. Intact BMPR2 signaling may be necessary for the execution of a normal lung vascular wound-healing program, preventing apoptosis-induced compensatory cell proliferation. BMPR2 loss makes cells more susceptible to apoptosis, however, vascular cell-apoptosis alone, is insufficient for angioproliferation to occur. BMPR2 signaling appears to define the cellular identity during reparative responses. BMP signaling is regulated at many different levels and each level could potentially contribute to abnormal BMPR-2 function, without necessarily involving a mutation in the BMPR2 gene. For example, mutations in the type I TGF-receptor, ALK-1, have been observed in patients with severe PAH occurring in families with hereditary hemorrhagic telangiectasia. Moreover, although infrequent, mutations in the BMPR-2-downstream mediators, the smad proteins, have also been described in PH patients. Their data also indicated that BMP/TGF-β signaling plays an important role in the maintenance of the normal lung arteriolar structure [30][31]. Epigenetic mechanisms influence gene expression via modifications of the chromatin, histones and regulatory micro RNAs. At present, there is no firm evidence that PH has an epigenetic component. Downregulation of BMPR2 expression has been explained by activation of a 5 STAT3/miRNA-17-92 microRNA axis in normal human lung endothelial cells after interleukin-6 exposure. Interestingly, mice overexpressing IL-6 develop severe pulmonary hypertension and, unlike other PH mice models, also develop angioobliterative vascular remodelling and robust RV hypertrophy. Overexpression of miR-17 also increases proliferation of human PASMCs and inhibition with a specific miR-17 antagonist ameliorated PH in two experimental models [35] [36]. Another microRNA, miR204, has been found downregulated in pulmonary artery smooth muscle cells isolated from patients with PH. Upregulation of miR204 seems to induce an apoptosis-resistant phenotype in smooth muscle cells [37].

PAH is an uncommon disease in the general population, but a disease with significant morbidity and mortality. The prevalence of heritable PH remains unknown. The reason for incomplete penetrance of heritable PAH is not well understood. A patient's clinical response to disease-specific therapy is complicated with potential involvement of the disease severity, comorbidities, appropriateness of the prescribed therapy, and patient compliance. Dempsie *et al* studied the effects of gender on development of PH in mice with over-expressing Mts1 (Mts1+ mice) by measuring pulmonary arterial remodeling, systolic right ventricular pressure (sRVP) and RVH. Gender differences in pulmonary arterial Mts1 and the receptor for advanced glycosylation end products (RAGE) expression were assessed by qRT-PCR and immunohistochemistry. Western blotting and cell counts were applied to investigate interactions between 17β-estradiol, Mts1 and RAGE on proliferation of human PASMCs. Statistical analysis methods used were one-way analysis of variance with Dunnetts post test or two-way analysis of variance with Bonferronis post test, as appropriate. Their results showed that female Mts1+ mice developed increased sRVP and pulmonary vascular remodeling, whereas male Mts1+ mice remained unaffected, and the development of plexiform-like lesions in Mts1+ mice was specific to females. These changes stained positive for both Mts1 and RAGE in the endothelial and adventitial layers. Expression of pulmonary arterial Mts1 was greater in female than male

Mts1+ mice, and was localized to the medial and adventitial layers in non plexiform-like pulmonary arteries. RAGE gene expression and immunoreactivity were similar between male and female Mts1+ mice and RAGE staining was localized to the endothelial layer in non plexiform-like pulmonary arteries adjacent to airways. In non-plexiform like pulmonary arteries not associated with airways RAGE staining was present in the medial and adventitial layers. Physiological concentrations of 17β-estradiol increased Mts1 expression in PASMCs, while 17β-estradiol-induced hPASMC proliferation was inhibited by soluble RAGE, which antagonizes the membrane bound form of RAGE. Authors believe Mts1 over-expression combined with female gender is permissive to the development of experimental PAH in mice. Up-regulation of Mts1 and subsequent activation of RAGE may contribute to 17β-estradiol-induced proliferation of hPASMCs [38].

5.5. Chronic pulmonary thromboembolic events

Chronic thromboembolic events may lead to PH. Long-standing thromboembolic obstruction of pulmonary arterial vasculature by acute or recurrent thromboemboli with subsequent organization can cause progressive PH and RVF. Advances in diagnostic modalities and surgical pulmonary endarterectomy techniques have made this PH induced by these chronic thromboembolization treatable and even potentially preventable and/or curable. Although published guidelines are available, in the absence of randomized controlled trials regarding chronic thromboembolic PH, there is a lack of standardization, and treatment options have to be individualized [39].

5.6. Exercise-induced pulmonary hypertension

Though exercise-induced increase in pulmonary arterial pressure has been removed fromn current PH Classification, exercise stress tests of the pulmonary circulation can potentially help detect early or latent pulmonary vascular disease and may help understand the clinical evolution and effects of treatments in patients with established PH. Exercise stresses the pulmonary circulation through increases in cardiac output and left atrial pressure. Recent studies have shown that exercise-induced increase in PAP is associated with dyspnea-fatigue symptomatology, validating the notion of exercise-induced PH. Exercise in established PH has no diagnostic relevance, but may help in the understanding of changes in functional state and the effects of therapies [40] [41].

5.7. Chronic hypoxemia

Chronic hypoxic lung diseases can lead to PH which subsequently increases patients' morbidity and mortality. Since the identification of heterozygous morphogenetic protein (BMP) receptor mutations as the underlying factor in the rare heritable form of pulmonary arterial hypertension, the important role of altered BMP signaling in PH was then significantly more appreciated [42] [43]. Later studies demonstrated that BMP signaling was also reduced in other more common forms of PH. The mechanism of the BMP signaling reduction was recently elucidated by Cahill and associates. They found that expression of 2 BMP antagonists, Gremlin 1 and Gremlin 2 was significantly higher in the lung than in other organ systems. And Gremlin

1 was further increased in the walls of small intrapulmonary vessels of mice during the development of hypoxic PH. In vitro studies showed that hypoxia stimulated cultured human pulmonary microvascular endothelial cells to secrete Gremlin secretion which inhibited endothelial BMP signaling and BMP-stimulated endothelial repair. Haplodeficiency of Gremlin 1 augmented BMP signaling in the hypoxic mouse lung and reduced PVR by attenuating vascular remodeling. Furthermore, Gremlin was increased in the walls of small intrapulmonary vessels in IPAH and the rare heritable form of PAH in a distribution suggesting endothelial localization. Their findings demonstrated the central role for increased Gremlin in hypoxia-induced pulmonary vascular remodeling and the increased PVR in hypoxic PH. High levels of basal Gremlin expression in the lung may account for the unique vulnerability of the pulmonary circulation to heterozygous mutations of BMP type 2 receptor in PAH [42]. Interestingly, digoxin was found to inhibit the development of hypoxemia-induced PH in an animal model [43]. One of the mechanisms involved in the development of hypoxic PH is hypoxia-inducible factor 1 (HIF-1)-dependent transactivation of genes controlling pulmonary arterial smooth muscle cells (PASMC) intracellular calcium concentration ([Ca(2+)](i)) and pH. Digoxin was shown to inhibit HIF-1 transcriptional activity, and potentially prevent and reverse the development of PH. And digoxin can attenuate the hypoxia-induced increases in RV pressure and PASMC pH and [Ca(2+)](i) [42].

The etiologies and mechanisms of PH are illustrated in Figure-1.

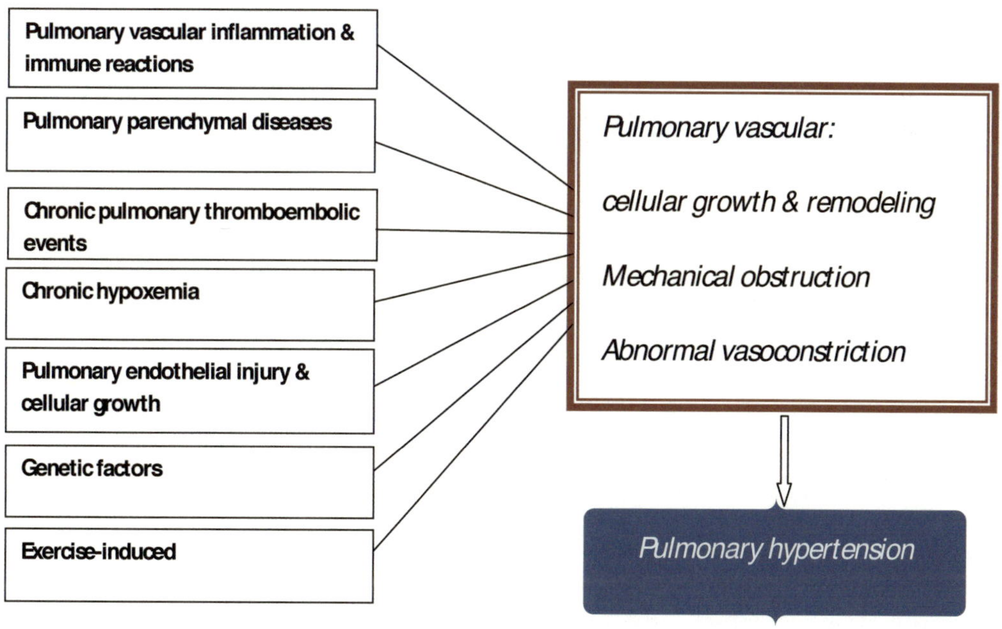

Figure 1. Etiologies and mechanisms of pulmonary hypertension (Illustrated by Henry Liu, MD)

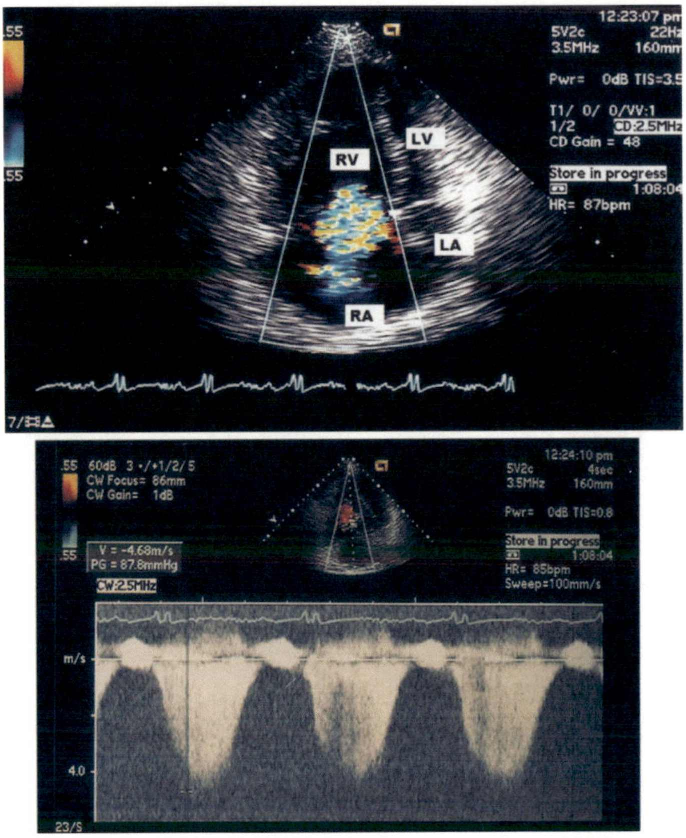

Figure 2. Top: Apical four-chamber view (systole) showing enlarged right-side chambers with compressed and geometric distortion of an intrinsically normal LV secondary to marked RV pressure overload; severe TR. RA-right atrium; LA- left atrium. Bottom: Peak TR velocity of 4.68 m/s, with a peak gradient of 87.8 mm Hg indicating severe PH.

6. Perioperative management of pulmonary hypertension

6.1. Preoperative assessment

Patients with PH undergo surgical procedures with significantly higher risks for morbidity and mortality regardless of the etiologies of the PH, the types of surgery and the anesthetic technique [44] [45] [46] [47] [48] [49]. The clinical outcome is especially worse for those with Eisenmenger's syndrome. Kahn reported that patients with Eisenmenger's syndrome undergoing cesarean section had mortality as high as 70% [50]. Although there is not an overabundance of literature regarding the development of postoperative pulmonary complications following noncardiac surgery, the few available studies demonstrate the increased risk associated with these surgical procedures. Preoperative medical optimization is therefore necessary. During preoperative risk assessment, one should take into account the type of surgery, the patient's functional status, the severity of the PH, the function of the right ventricle and any other co-morbidities. Generally superficial procedures and non-orthopedic procedures are associated with less hemodynamic and sympathetic nervous system perturbations than more invasive/traumatizing procedures. Orthopedic procedures with bony involvement can be quite stimulating for the patients and will increase the risk of elevating PVR and RV failure. Thoracic surgery is associated with significant changes in intrathoracic pressures, lung volumes and oxygenation, which may cause acute increases in PVR and decreased RV function [51]. Laparoscopic surgery requires pneumoperitoneum which may be poorly tolerated because it can decrease preload and increase afterload. Surgical procedures associated with rapid or massive blood loss will be poorly tolerated by patients with severe PH. WHO standardized the functional status definition as shown in Table-4.

History and Physical Exam: Preoperative evaluation should include a thorough history and physical examination with special attention to signs and symptoms of respiratory insufficiency and right ventricular dysfunction. Symptoms are typically nonspecific with the most frequent being progressive dyspnea. The signs depend on disease severity and include dyspnea at rest, low cardiac output with metabolic acidosis, hypoxemia, evidence of right heart failure (large V wave on jugular vein, peripheral edema, hepatomegaly), and syncope [52]. Laboratory studies and special tests should be determined by the surgical procedure that the patient is undergoing and the medication profile of the patient. Routine preoperative tests include electrocardiography (EKG), chest radiographs (CXR), complete blood counts (CBC), electrolytes, baseline arterial blood gas analysis (ABG), room air oxygen saturation. Although ECG changes alone cannot determine disease severity or prognosis of PH [53] [54], the ECG may show signs of right ventricular hypertrophy, such as tall right precordial R waves, right axis deviation and right ventricular strain [55]. The chest radiography may show evidence of right ventricular hypertrophy (decreased retrosternal space, cardiomegaly, enlarged cardiac silhouette) or prominent pulmonary vasculature. CBC will help decide the necessity of preoperatively optimizing the hematocrit of the patients or not. Plasma electrolytes assess baseline electrolytes and acid-base disturbances.

Delayed post-exercise heart rate recovery (HRR) has been associated with disability and poor prognosis in chronic cardiopulmonary diseases. Ramos *et al* investigated the usefulness of HRR to predict exercise impairment and mortality in patients with PH. They studied 72 PH patients with varied etiologies [New York Heart Association (NYHA) classes' I-IV] and 21 age- and gender-matched controls. Both groups underwent a maximal incremental cardiopulmonary exercise test (CPET) with heart rate being recorded up to the fifth minute of recovery. Their results revealed that HRR was consistently lower in the patients compared with the controls ($P < 0.05$). The best cutoff for HRR in 1 minute (HRR (1 min)) to discriminate the patients from the controls was 18 beats. Compared with patients with HRR (1 min) ≤ 18 (n = 40), those with HRR (1 min) >18 (n = 32) had better NYHA scores, resting hemodynamics and 6-minute walking distance (6MWD). In fact, HRR (1 min) >18 was associated with a range of maximal and submaximal CPET variables indicative of less severe exercise impairment ($P < 0.05$). The single independent predictor of HRR (1 min) ≤ 18 was the 6MWD (odds ratio 0.99, $P < 0.05$). On a multiple regression analysis that considered only CPET-independent variables, HRR (1 min) ≤ 18 was the single predictor of mortality (hazard ratio 1.19, $P < 0.05$). Thus they concluded preserved HRR(1 min) (>18 beats) is associated with less impaired responses to incremental exercise in patients with PH. To the contrary, a delayed HRR (1 min) response has negative prognostic implications, a finding likely to be clinically useful when more complicated (and costlier) analyses provided by a full CPET are not available [56]. Minai *et al* had a similar finding: they evaluate the association between HRR at 1 minute of rest (HRR1) after 6-min walk test (6MW test) and clinical worsening in patients with IPAH. HRR (1 min) was defined as the difference in heart rate at the end of 6MW test and at 1 minute after completion of the 6MW test. Seventy-five consecutive patients with IPAH underwent 6MW test and were included in the analysis. The results showed those patients with HRR1 less than 16 ($n = 30$) were more likely to have clinical worsening (odds ratio, 9.7, $P < 0.001$) and shorter time to first clinical worsening event (TCW) (6.7 mo vs. 13 mo; $P < 0.001$) during follow-up. With multivariable analysis, the best predictors of clinical worsening were HRR (1 min) less than 16 (hazard ratio, 5.2, $P = 0.002$) and mean PAP (hazard ratio, 1.04, $P = 0.02$). Compared with the distance walked during the 6MW test (6MW test), HRR (1 min) less than 16 was a better predictor of clinical worsening and TCW. The addition of HRR (1 min) increased the ability of 6MWD to predict clinical worsening events. HRR (1 min) after 6MW test is a strong predictor of clinical worsening and TCW in patients with IPAH. The addition of HRR (1 min) to 6MWD increases the capacity of 6MWD to predict clinical worsening and TCW in patients with IPAH [56].

Additional tests which can potentially benefit patients include echocardiography, right heart catheterization, pulmonary function testing, ventilation/perfusion (V/Q) scanning, pulmonary angiography, spiral computed tomography, serologic testing, liver function testing, and N-terminal pro-B-type natriuretic peptide (NT-proBNP). Among these available tests, echocardiography is probably the best screening study. Echocardiography is used to assess right ventricular (RV) size, function and estimate pulmonary artery pressures [52]. Echocardiography is a useful tool for both assessment and monitoring of disease progression in PH. Although transthoracic echocardiography is the most widely used modality for this purpose, especially for the initial PH evaluation, transesophageal echocardiography (TEE) can be a more useful technology for patients with poor acoustic windows and for intraoperative monitoring. Compared to other monitoring modalities, TEE can be particularly useful in narrowing the differential diagnoses for intraoperative hemodynamic instability (hypovolemia, hypervolemia, right or left ventricular ischemia/failure) and in formulating a therapeutic plan. Multiple echocardiographic methods, M-mode, 2D and real-time 3D have been utilized to assess PH. The usual echocardiographic findings associated with PH include the following: 1). enlarged right atrial or right ventricular (RV) chambers; 2) mid-systolic closure or notching of the pulmonary valve; 3) diminished or absent atrial wave of the pulmonary valve; 4) intraventricular septal flattening; 5) paradoxical systolic motion of the intraventricular septum (IVS) toward the left ventricle; 6) a dilated inferior vena cava with reduced respiratory variability; 7) increased IVS/posterior left ventricular (LV) wall ratio (>1); 8) increased RV end-diastolic volume index; 9) increased RV endsystolic volume index, and 10) decreased RV ejection fraction [58] [59] [60]. 11). right ventricular enlargement with tricuspid regurgitation, small left ventricle with an asymmetric hypetrophic wall, with ventricular stiffness and diastolic incompetence [61]. Methods used to determine PAP by echocardiography include: measurement of the tricuspid annular plane systolic excursion (TAPSE), two-dimensional strain, tissue

Doppler echocardiography, the speckle tracking method, acceleration time across the pulmonic valve, the pulmonary artery regurgitant jet method and the tricuspid regurgitant jet method [62]. The tricuspid regurgitant jet method is most commonly used for determination of the pulmonary artery systolic pressure (PASP). The simplified Bernoulli equation, Pressure gradient (P1 – P2) = $4V^2$, where V is the peak velocity, is used to approximate the PASP by continuous wave Doppler across the tricuspid valve regurgitant jet. In this case, RVSP ≈ PASP = $4V^2$ + RAP, where RVSP is the right ventricular systolic pressure and RAP is the right atrial pressure. The RVSP approximates PASP when no pulmonary valve stenosis or right ventricular outflow obstruction exists [62]. Although right heart catheterization (RHC) remains the gold standard for assessment of hemodynamic parameters in PH, advantages of echocardiography include wide availability, noninvasive modality, and lower costs. Intraoperatively, TEE allows dynamic interpretation and assessment of the therapeutic management of PH. Disadvantages include the need for specialized training for interpretation, modest diagnostic accuracy and the correlation to PH as compared to RHC [62] [63]. Janda *et al* revealed that the correlation coefficient of systolic pulmonary artery pressure (PASP) by echocardiography as compared with PASP by RHC to be 0.70 (95% CI 0.67 to 0.73) as well as a summary sensitivity and specificity of 83% (95% CI 73 to 90) and 72% (95% CI 53 to 85), respectively for diagnostic accuracy of echocardiography for pulmonary hypertension [62]. The variability of echocardiography to correlate to RHC is in part related to the underlying disease, lung conditions, time of the examination, and the skills of the echocardiographer [51] [64] [65]. Underestimation of PASP by echocardiography resulting in improper classification of PH (mild, moderate, severe) is more likely than overestimation, however inaccuracy in both under and overestimation occur with similar frequency [64]. Improvement in obtaining the tricuspid regurgitant jet peak velocity has been found with the use of an intravenous bolus of agitated saline [58] [59] [66]. Despite the technical challenges and inaccuracies associated with echocardiography, it remains a useful tool, especially for perioperative management of patients with PH. For the initial evaluation, monitoring, and management of PH. Takatsuki *et al* evaluated the usefulness of tissue Doppler imaging (TDI) in assessment of disease severity and prognostic value in children with IPAH. The authors studied TDI velocities (systolic myocardial velocity, early diastolic myocardial relaxation velocity [Em], late diastolic myocardial velocity associated with atrial contraction), brain natriuretic peptide, NYHA functional class, and hemodynamic parameters in 51 children (mean age; 11.6 years) with IPAH. Fifty-one healthy children with comparable demographics served as controls. They found that Tricuspid Em had significant inverse correlations with plasma brain natriuretic peptide levels ($r= -0.60$, $P < 0.001$), right ventricular end-diastolic pressure ($r= -0.79$, $P < 0.001$), and mean PAP ($r=-0.67$, $P < 0.001$). Em, Em/late diastolic myocardial velocity associated with atrial contraction ratio, and systolic myocardial velocity at mitral annulus, septum, and tricuspid annulus in IPAH were significantly reduced compared with controls. Statistically significant differences were observed in tricuspid Em between NYHA functional class II versus combined III and IV (mean and SD; 11.9 ± 4.2 cm/s versus 8.2 ± 3.6 cm/s, respectively, $P= 0.002$). Cumulative event-free survival rate was significantly lower when tricuspid Em was ≤8 cm/s (log-rank test, $P< 0.001$). So they believe Tricuspid Em velocity correlated with NYHA functional class as disease severity and may serve as a useful prognostic marker in children with IPAH. [67].

6.1.1. Right heart catheterization

Right heart catheterization is considered the gold standard for measuring PAP. Evidence of significant RV dysfunction should prompt reevaluation of the need for surgery [68]. All attempts to lower PAP should be done preoperatively. Treatment options include oxygen, bronchodilators, vasodilators and inotropes. In addition to the careful evaluation of the patient's current therapeutic regimen for pulmonary hypertension, all other medications should be reviewed for possible drug-drug interactions. Likewise, it is important to maintain the patient's current therapeutic regimen as discontinuation of medications can potentially lead to rebound or even worsened PH and RV dysfunction. Although medications such as inhaled prostacyclin (epoprostenol or Flolan) are associated with impaired platelet aggregation, they have not been implicated in clinically significant bleeding. Due to the short half-life of this medication, epoprostenol should not be stopped at any time in the perioperative period. The anesthesiologist must ensure preoperative maximization of the patient's therapeutic options being accomplished and coordinated, if needed, a perioperative strategy for continuance of chronic PH therapy [69].

6.1.2. Pulmonary function tests, ventilation/perfusion (V/Q) scanning and pulmonary angiography

Pulmonay function test (PFT) has been used for the assessment of the overall pulmonary function. PFT can help determine patient's tolerability to certain surgical procedures. He *et al* conducted V/Q scanning and computed tomography pulmonary angiography (CTPA) for a total of 114 consecutive patients (49 men and 65 women, average age 43.3 years) suspected of having CTEPH. Interpretation of V/Q images was based on the refined Pulmonary Embolism Diagnosis criteria. For threshold 1, high-probability and intermediate-probability V/Q scan findings were considered to be positive, and low-probability/normal V/Q scan findings were negative. For threshold 2, only a high-probability V/Q scan finding was considered to be positive. And intermediate-probability and low-probability/normal V/Q scan findings were considered to be negative. Their results indicated that 51 patients (44.7%) had a final diagnosis of CTEPH. V/Q scan showed high probability (52 patients), intermediate probability (2 patients), and low probability/normal scan (59 patients) respectively. CTPA revealed 50 patients with CTEPH and 64 patients without CTEPH. The sensitivity, specificity, and accuracy of the V/Q scan were 100, 93.7, and 96.5%, respectively, with threshold 1, and 96.1, 95.2, and 95.6%, respectively, with threshold 2; similarly, the sensitivity, specificity, and accuracy of CTPA were 92.2, 95.2, and 93.9%, respectively. They therefore concluded that both V/Q scanning and CTPA are accurate methods for the detection of CTEPH with excellent diagnostic efficacy [70].

6.1.3. Cardiac Magnetic Resonance Imaging (MRI)

Cardiac magnetic resonance imaging (MRI) has prognostic value in patients with IPAH before starting intravenous prostacyclin [71]. Swift *et al* studied the diagnostic accuracy of MRI derived RV measurements for the detection of pulmonary hypertension (PH) in the assessment of patients with suspected PH. They retrospectively reviewed 233 treatment-naïve patients with suspected PH including 39 patients with no PH who underwent MRI and right heart catheterization (RHC) within 48 hours. The diagnostic accuracy of multiple MRI measurements for the detection of mPAP [greater than or equal to] 25 mmHg was assessed using Fisher's exact test and receiver operating characteristic (ROC) analysis. Ventricular mass index (VMI) was the MRI measurement with the strongest correlation with mPAP (r=0.78) and the highest diagnostic accuracy for the diagnosis of PH (area under the ROC curve of 0.91) compared to an ROC of 0.88 for mPAP measured by echocardiography. Using late gadolinium enhancement, VMI [greater than or equal to] 0.4, retrograde flow [greater than or equal to] 0.3 L/min/m2 and PA relative area change [less than or equal to] 15% predicted the presence of PH with a high degree of diagnostic certainty with a positive predictive value of 98%, 97%, 95% and 94% respectively. No single MRI parameter could definitely exclude the presence of PH. Thus they concluded that MRI is a useful alternative to echocardiography in the evaluation of suspected PH. They support the routine measurement of ventricular mass index, late gadolinium enhancement and the use of phase contrast imaging in addition to right heart functional indices in patients undergoing diagnostic MRI evaluation for suspected pulmonary hypertension [72].

6.1.4. N-Terminal pro-B-type Natriuretic Peptide (NT-proBNP)

Frantz *et al* used N-terminal pro-B-type natriuretic peptide (NT-proBNP) as a biomarker of the disease severity in patients with PAH. They aimed to determine whether baseline NT-proBNP levels correlate with improvement in 6MWD in the pivotal randomized, placebo-controlled, double-blind study of the addition of inhaled treprostinil to oral therapy for PH. They found that baseline NT-proBNP levels demonstrated a strong correlation with treatment in predicting change from baseline for 6MWD ($p < 0.01$), indicating that in the upper quartile (≥1,513.5 pg/ml), patients on inhaled treprostinil had a better response (+64 versus +32 m), whereas patients on placebo fared worse (-13 versus +20 m) when compared with the lower 3 quartiles (<1,513.5 pg/ml). Furthermore, least-squares mean difference in 6MWD between active and placebo groups was +67 and +16 m for the upper and lower 3 quartiles of NT-proBNP, respectively. The investigators concluded that greater improvement in 6MWD in actively treated patients with high levels of NT-proBNP predicts better clinical response to inhaled treprostinil in more advanced disease [73]. Diller *et al* followed up 181 patients (mean follow-up period is 3.3 years, 7 patients with Down syndrome) with 20 deaths. Their results showed that higher BNP concentrations were predictive of all cause mortality on univariate analysis in patients with or without Down syndrome. On multivariable Cox proportional hazard analysis, BNP predicted survival independently of renal function, Down syndrome, or 6MWD (p=0.004). Temporal increases in BNP concentration also predicted mortality in patients with concurrent Eisenmenger syndrome patients. Treatment with disease targeting therapies was associated with a significant reduction in BNP concentrations [74].

Perioperative Risks of PH: The patient with PH is at elevated risk for morbidity and mortality in the perioperative period [5], [76], [77], [78]. There is a relative paucity of literature studying outcomes in this patient population presenting for noncardiac surgery, however, the evidence that does exist points to significantly increased potential for complications in the perioperative period. Ramakrishna *et al* presented the results from an overview of 145 patients with PH presenting for noncardiac surgery. A 42% rate of early (<30 days) morbidity (congestive heart failure, cardiac ischemic event, stroke, respiratory failure, hepatic or renal disfunction, cardiac dysrhythmia) and a 9.7% rate of early mortality in this population have been reported [47]. Ramakrishna *et al* summarized the clinical characteristics associated with early morbidity and mortality in Table-5.

Clinical characteristics prone to early mortality	Clinical characteristics prone to early morbidity
1. Right axis deviation (RAD)	1. NYHA class 2 or higher
2. Right ventricular hypertrophy (RVH)	2. History of pulmonary embolism
3. RVSP/SBP ratio above 0.6	3. Obstructive sleep apnea
4. Intraoperative use of epinephrine or dopamine	4. High-risk surgery
	5. Anesthesia duration 3 hours or longer
	6. Intraoperative use of epinephrine or dopamine

NYHA=New York Heart Association, RVSP=right ventricular systolic pressure, SBP=systolic blood pressure.

Table 5. Clinical characteristics associated with increased morbidity and mortality in PA patients. Modified from reference [47].

Lai *et al*. performed a case-control study examining 67 patients with pulmonary systolic pressures greater than 70 mmHg compared to controls with normal pulmonary pressures [8]. As shown in Table-4, the pulmonary hypertension group developed postoperative heart failure more frequently (9.7 vs. 0%, p =.028), delayed tracheal extubation (21 vs. 0%, p =.004) and greater in hospital mortality (9.7 vs. 0%, p = 0.004). A review of a large U.S. database by Memtsoudis *et al*. estimated the mortality rate in patients undergoing total hip arthroplasty (THA) and total knee arthroplasty (TKA) [7]. The authors identified 1359 THA and 2184 TKA patients with the diagnosis of PH. In comparison to a matched sample without PH, the THA patients had a 4-fold increased adjusted risk of in-hospital mortality and the TKA patients had a 4.5-fold increase (p< 0.001) [7]. Patients with PH are at considerably increased risk in the perioperative period morbidity and mortality. [8].

6.2. Intraoperative considerations

Dependent upon the nature of the scheduled surgical procedure, various anesthesia techniques including general anesthesia, neuraxial anesthesia, peripheral nerve blockade and monitored anesthesia care (MAC) have been reported to be success in the management of patients with PH [45] [79]. Except for few case reports, very little literature exists evaluating the differences of these management strategies for intraoperative and postoperative management of the patient with PH. Furthermore the choice of technique is less important as the ability to adhere to the goals of avoiding elevations in PVR and RHF.

For major procedures in patients with PH, routine ASA standard monitoring should be utilized. The following additional strategies are potentially critical for the appropriate perioperative management of patients with PH:

http://dx.doi.org/10.5772/56056

1. Arterial line for the continuous monitoring of arterial pressure. By using arterial pressure monitoring we can ensure adequate perfusion pressures for all vital organs including heart, lungs and brain. Arterial line can also be used for frequent blood gas analysis.

2. Pulmonary artery catheterization (PAC): PAC can be used for the monitoring of pulmonary artery pressure, for the measurement of CO and for the measurement of mixed venous oxygen saturation. By measuring PCWP, PAC can help determine left ventricular preload in pulmonary hypertensive patients whose cardiac output is limited by right ventricular function. PAP measurement is also critical in determining PH severity, and choice and dosing of therapeutic agents. However, intraoperative PAC placement is controversial in patients with PH because of the potential complications due to PAC placement. Hoeper *et al* performed a multicenter 5-year retrospective and 6-month prospective evaluation of serious adverse events related to right heart catheter procedures in patients with pulmonary hypertension, as defined by a mean pulmonary artery pressure >25 mm Hg. Out of total 7218 PAC procedures, they found the overall number of serious adverse events was 76 (1.1%). The most frequent complications were related to venous access (e.g., hematoma, pneumothorax), followed by arrhythmias and hypotensive episodes related to vagal reactions or pulmonary vasoreactivity testing. The vast majority of these complications were mild to moderate in intensity and resolved either spontaneously or after appropriate intervention. Four fatal events were recorded in association with any of the catheter procedures, resulting in an overall procedure-related mortality of 0.055%. Thus they believe that in experienced centers, right heart catheter procedures in patients with pulmonary hypertension are still safe, only associated with low morbidity and mortality rates [80].

3. Central venous pressure (CVP) may be a more accurate guide for volume administration. Care should be taken in placing PAC and/or CVP catheters as these patients are reliant on sequential atrial-ventricular contraction for adequate preload and cardiac output. Arrhythmias associated with catheter insertion may not be well tolerated by these patients.

4. Non-invasive or minimally invasive CO measurement techniques may also be useful in PH patients undergoing surgical procedures and labor and delivery [81].

5. Bispectral index score (BIS) monitoring helps maintain appropriate depth of anesthesia.

6. Transesophageal echocardiography (TEE): Transesophageal echocardiography can be very useful in assessing the preload, contractility, anatomical irregularities and valvular abnormalities of both right-side and left-side of the heart. TEE can also help evaluate the result of cardiopulmonary surgical procedures [82] [83].

6.3. Strategies of controlling pulmonary arterial pressure

There are multiple methods available to control the increased PAP intraoperatively. These strategies can be categorized into pharmacological and non-pharmacological measures.

Pharmacological management of intraoperative hypertension includes the following:

1. Inhaled nitric oxide: Inhaled nitric oxide (INO) is one of the most potent medications commonly used perioperatively. The usual dose is 20–80 ppm (parts per million). The delivery system is shown in Figure-3. The INO delivery system includes a circuit and a control panel and related tank and tubing. INO can diffuse from the alveoli to the pulmonary capillaries and stimulates guanylate cyclase to increase cyclic guanosine monophosphate (cGMP) which leads to vasodilation. INO does not produce systemic vasodilatation because nitric oxide is inactivated when bound to hemoglobin. It also has the benefit of improving ventilation– perfusion matching by increasing perfusion to areas of the lung that are well ventilated. If the clinical picture is of pulmonary hypertension with systemic hypotension, IV vasodilators may cause worsening of systemic blood pressure, subsequent RV hypoperfusion, ischemia and failure. In this situation, the patient may benefit from therapy selective for the pulmonary vasculature such as inhaled nitric oxide (INO) or prostacyclin. INO has also been shown to improve PH in cardiopulmonary bypass settings [84] [85].

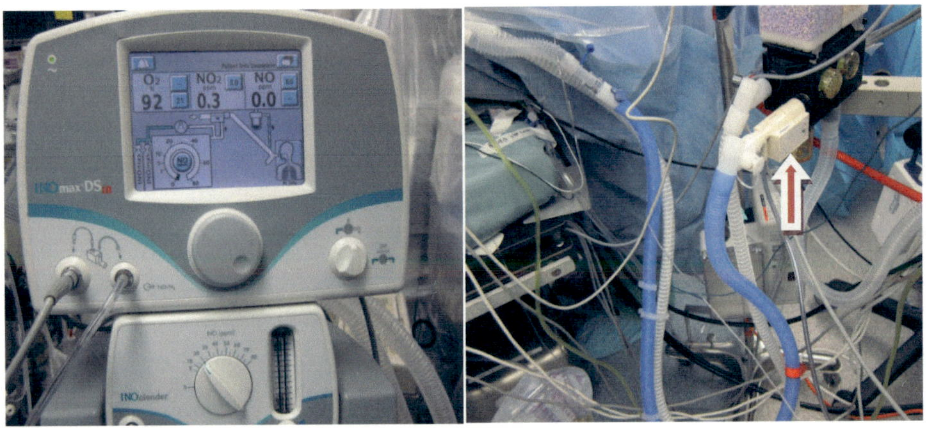

Figure 3. Inhaled nitric oxide delivery system Left: Inhaled nitric oxide delivery system control panel. Right: Inhaled nitric oxide delivery circuit, the arrow indicates the inspiratory limb. (Copyright owned by Henry Liu, MD)

2. Milrinone: Milrinone is a phosphodiesterase-3 inhibitor and prevents the breakdown of cyclic adenosine monophosphate (cAMP). It has shown to reduce both PVR and SVR in addition to causing increases in myocardial contractility [86]. The usual dose of milrinone is 50 mg/kg loading, then 0.5–0.75mg/kg/min for the maintenance.

3. Thromboxane synthase inhibitor: Dipyridamole (tradename: Persantine) can be used intraoperatively in managing PH; its usual dose is 0.2–0.6 mg/kg i.v. over 15 minutes, and it may be repeated after 12 hours. Lepore et al used intravenous dipyridamole combined with INO in 9 patients with congestive heart failure (CHF) and severe PH who were breathing 100% oxygen during right heart catheterization, we administered inhaled NO (80 ppm) alone and in combination with intravenous dipyridamole (0.2-mg/kg bolus, with an infusion of 0.0375 mg/kg/min), and found that Intravenous dipyrida-

http://dx.doi.org/10.5772/56056

mole augments and prolongs the pulmonary vasodilator effects of INO in CHF patients with severe PH [87].

4. Inhaled prostacyclin: Continuous intravenous administration of prostacyclin 50 ng/kg/min after reconstituting prostacyclin in sterile glycine diluent to 30,000 ng/ml (1.5mg of prostacyclin in 50 ml of diluent). For an 80 kg patient, 50 ng/kg/min is 8 ml of this solution per hour. It is nebulized into the inspiratory side of the ventilator circuit; an example of a prostacyclin nebulized delivery system that can be integrated into the anesthesia circuit is shown in Figure-4. Iloprost is a synthetic analogue of prostacyclin PGI_2. Iloprost dilates systemic and pulmonary arterial vascular beds. It also affects platelet aggregation but the relevance of this effect to the treatment of pulmonary hypertension is unknown. The two diastereoisomers of iloprost differ in their potency in dilating blood vessels, with the 4*S* isomer substantially more potent than the 4*R* isomer. Prostacyclin, available in inhaled and intravenous forms, stimulates adenylate cyclase and increases cAMP and release of endothelial NO leading to decreases in PAP, RAP, and increased cardiac output [88]. Combination therapy, with both INO and prostacyclin, has synergistic effects compared to monotherapy [89] [90]. Due to the extremely short half-life of these medications, one should ensure that the medication is delivered continuously without interruption to minimize the risk of rebound PH. Weaning from these medications should be performed gradually with frequent assessment of PAP and RV function. A disadvantage of INO compared to inhaled prostacyclin is its high cost. A recent analysis revealed that INO is approximately 20 times more expensive than prostacyclin ($3000/day vs. $150/day) [91]. Table-6 lists the medical management options, including common doses and common side effects, for intraoperative management of pulmonary hypertension. Lastly, in patients refractory to the above therapies, right ventricular assist device implantation should be considered.

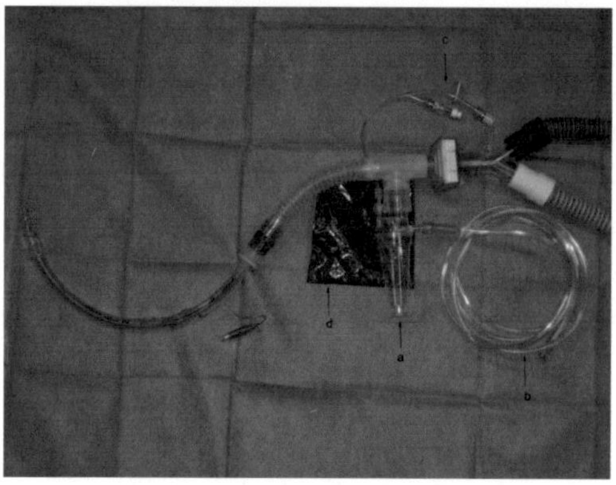

Figure 4. Inhaled prostacyclin delivery system Figure-6: Inhaled prostacyclin delivery system. Reconstituted prostacyclin is delivered by a Lo-Flo Mini Heart nebulizer (a), which is driven by a separate oxygen source at 2 L/min (b). The nebulizer output is 8 mL/h, which allows for 1–3 h of continuous nebulization. The nebulizer should be supported by an IV pole or ventilator side arm to prevent spillage. An IV port (c) allows the chamber to be refilled without disconnecting from the anesthetic circuit. Prostacyclin is photosensitive and requires the nebulizing chamber to be covered from ambient light (d) [88].

5. Intravenous prostacyclin (if inhaled is not available) is 4–10 ng/kg/min. In the U.S., iloprost is inhaled specifically using the I-Neb AAD or Prodose AAD delivery systems. Ventavis is supplied in 1 mL single-use glass ampules containing either 10 mcg/mL or 20 mcg/mL. The 20 mcg/mL concentration is intended for patients who are maintained at the 5 mcg dose and who have repeatedly experienced extended treatment times which could result in incomplete dosing. Transitioning patients to the 20 mcg/mL concentration using the I-neb AAD System will decrease treatment times to help maintain patient compliance. The approved dosing regimen for iloprost is 6 to 9 times daily (no more than every 2 hours) during waking hours, according to individual need and tolerability.

6. Systemic hypotension should be treated according to the potential causes. Phenylephrine and norepinephrine have been used to treat persistent systemic hypotension. Norepinephrine has the advantage of being both a vasoconstrictor and positive inotropic agent. Vasopressin has also been advocated for treatment of hypotension [68] [92]

7. Sildenafil produced significant pulmonary vasodilatory effect relative to placebo in anesthetized cardiac surgical patients with pulmonary hypertension. With respect to the predominant selectivity of sildenafil to pulmonary vasculature shown in this study and other potentially beneficial effects such as myocardial protection, use of sildenafil in the intraoperative period in cardiac surgical patients with pulmonary hypertension should be considered [93]. Sildenafil citrate (INN sildenafil) is a selective phosphodiesterase type 5 inhibitor that is being increasingly recognized as a treatment modality for pulmonary hypertension.

8. Calcium channel blockers have been shown to inhibit the contraction of pulmonary artery smooth muscle cells, reduce right ventricular hypertrophy and improve long-term hemodynamics in PH in a small subset of patients who also show an acute hemodynamic response to calcium channel blockers. An interesting study demonstrated that survival was greatly improved in patients who showed a long-term response to calcium channel blockers; however, in patients that failed on long-term calcium channel blocker therapy, the 5-year survival rate was only 48% [94]. Calcium channel blockers are now only recommended for patients with a positive response during acute vasoreactivity testing and who show sustained hemodynamic improvement [94]. Calcium channel blockers are the only systemic antihypertensive drugs that have been shown to benefit patients with PH. By blocking calcium entry into cells of the pulmonary arterial vasculature, calcium channel blockers can induce vasodilation (or at least prevent vasoconstriction) of pulmonary arteries. In an initial trial in patients who demonstrated a response to calcium channel blockers during acute testing, use of calcium channel blockers led to a significant reduction in mPAP and PVR after 24 hours of treatment. Continued use over 1 year was associated with improvements in symptoms [94].

Non-pharmacological management of pulmonary hypertension is listed in Table-7.

http://dx.doi.org/10.5772/56056

Drug category	Drug name	Delivery pathway/dose	Common side effects
Prostaglandins	Epoprostenol (Tradename:Flolan)	Inhaled 31mcg/kg/min	Occupational health concern
	Iloprost (Ventavis)	Inhaled, 6-9 times/day	Dizziness, headache, flushing, lighheatedness,
	Treprostinil (Tyvaso)	Inhaled, follow doctor's instraction	Cough, headache, throat irritation, pain, flushing
Nitric oxide	Inhaled nitric oxide	Inhaled, 20-50ppm	Methemoglobinemia, Lung toxicity,
Phosphodiesterase Type-5 inhibitors	Milrinone	Intravenous, 50mcg/kg loading, 0.25-0.75 mcg/kg/min maintenance	Ventricular dysrhythmia, tachycardia,
	Sildenafil	Oral, 50 mg preoperatively	hypotension
Endothelin receptor antagonist	Anbrisentan (Letairis in USA, Volibris in EU)	2.5-10mg/day, oral	Birth defects
	Bosentan(Tracleer)	62.5mg twice daily, oral for 4 weeks	Hepatotoxicity Birth defects Anemia
Nitrovasodilator	Nitroglycerin	Intravenous, 0.5 g/kg/min,	Hypotension, headache
Calcium channel blockers	Diltiazem	High oral dose:720mg/day	Constipation, dizziness, flushing, headache
	Nifedipine	Oral 240mg/day	Constipation, cough, flushing, giddiness

Table 6. Pharmacological treatment for pulmonary hypertension [94] [95] [96] [97].

6.4. General anesthesia

Without any doubt, every effort should be made to have a smooth induction of anesthesia and endotracheal intubation which will minimize the hemodynamic instability in highly susceptible patients. Commonly used intravenous anesthetics such as propofol and thiopental are associated with hypotension and myocardial depression. Their use should be very judicious. Etomidate has much fewer effects on SVR, PVR and myocardial contractility and may be a more useful hypnotic for patient with severe PH. Use of volatile anesthetics is associated with decreased SVR, myocardial contractility and potential arrhythmias, all of which can impair right ventricular myocardial perfusion and also right ventricular cardiac output. A balanced technique utilizing high dose narcotics to blunt the sympathetically mediated cardiovascular response to surgical stimulation and minimal volatile anesthetics can limit these adverse effects. Additionally, the anesthesiologist should strive to use basic physiology to her/his advantage. These principles include utilization of 100% oxygen for its pulmonary vasodilator

1. Ensure adequate oxygenation; avoid hypercarbia;
2. Avoidance of acidosis;
3. Avoidance of hypothermia;
4. Whatever medication is used to control PH, wean the medication slowly to prevent rebound pulmonary hypertension;
5. Neuraxial anesthesia, peripheral nerve blockade, and lumbar plexus block can all be used to provide surgical anesthesia for scheduled procedures. But the loading dose should be slow and adjusted according to patient's condition. Epidural anesthesia should be induced slowly. Mixtures of local anesthetics and opioids should be given to reduce the dose of local anesthetics and hypotension;
6. Avoidance of elevating intrapleural pressure which will potentially be transmitted to increased pulmonary arterial pressure.
(Copyright by Henry Liu, MD)

Table 7. Non-Pharmacological management of pulmonary hypertension

effects, and aggressive treatment of hypercarbia, acidosis, and hypothermia as these may cause pulmonary vasoconstriction. Certain anesthetic agents such as nitrous oxide and ketamine have been associated with increases in PVR and should be used with caution [98] [99]. Uncompensated vasodilatation or myocardial depression induced by anesthetics and mechanical ventilation may be responsible for acute RV dysfunction associated with low systemic blood pressure. Cardiovascular collapse can develop after institution of one-lung ventilation and pulmonary artery clamping during thoracotomy. An acute increase in pulmonary pressure results in a decrease in RV ejection fraction and then acute RV failure. Interdependence of the right and left ventricles occurs such that RV function can alter LV function. Early detection of impending circulatory and/or respiratory deterioration is warranted to prevent an irreversible decline in cardiac output. Inhaled nitric oxide represents the first choice for treatment of PH and RV failure associated with systemic hypotension during lung transplantation. Intraoperative situations requiring CPB must be identified before development of systemic shock, which represents a late ominous sign of RV failure [61].

The anesthetic goals of intraoperative management include optimizing PAP, RV preload and avoiding RV ischemia and failure. Intraoperatively, often times there are significant alterations in all above parameters and appropriate vigilance and monitoring are paramount. Intraoperative management of the RV can be made on the presence of RV failure and the presence of systemic hyper- or hypotension. Initially, one should ensure that oxygenation, ventilation, and acid/base status are optimized. Treatment options for PH include both intravenous and inhaled agents. Intravenous vasodilators, such as nitroglycerin, sodium nitroprusside, beta blockers, calcium channel blockers, and certain prostaglandin preparations will cause dilation of both the pulmonary and systemic vascular beds and can be useful in the setting of PH with systemic hypertension. The advantages to intravenous preparations are the relative decreased cost, easier availability of medications, and longer duration of action and ease of administration in comparison to inhaled agents.

http://dx.doi.org/10.5772/56056

6.5. Regional anesthesia

Regional anesthetic techniques, including neuraxial blockade (epidural, spinal anesthesia, or combined epidural and spinal anesthesia) and peripheral nerve blockade (cervical plexus, auxillary plexus, sciatic nerve, femoral, etc), have all been successfully used in surgical procedures in patients with severe pulmonary hypertension [100]. Among the benefits of regional anesthesia are potential minimization of the stimulation-related (direct laryngoscopy, endotracheal intubation, etc) sympathetic activation. Even with adequate intravenous anesthetic induction agents, opioids and neuromuscular blockade, it is difficult to avoid increases in sympathetic nervous system activity due to laryngoscopy and induction. These sympathetic responses include tachycardia, systemic hypertension and increased myocardial oxygen consumption, which could lead to increases in PVR and potential acute right heart failure. During surgery and general anesthesia, due to various surgery-related (incision, surgical dissection, blood loss etc) or other surgical environment-related stimulations (hypothermia, psychological stress etc), the anesthesiologist has to continually balance excessive sympathetic outflow, increased PVR and potential acute right heart failure on one hand and excessive depth of anesthesia, low cardiac output, low coronary perfusion and cardiovascular collapse on the other hand [101]. A healthier patient tolerates these variations well, but the patient with severe PH has limited reserve to compensate for acute increases in PVR or decreased coronary perfusion. A peripheral nerve block technique could potentially limit anesthesia to the specific location of the surgery and avoid the need for the stimulation of intubation and reduced likelihood of sympathectomy and low blood pressure as one would achieve with general anesthesia. An important distinction is that a sympathectomy is still possible when utilizing a regional anesthesia technique such as epidural or spinal anesthesia. This may lead to arterial and venous dilatation and reduced preload and cardiac output compromising coronary perfusion. When utilizing neuraxial or peripheral nerve block techniques, it is important to ensure adequate ventilation and oxygenation to prevent increases in PVR due to hypoxemia. For example, sedation provided to allow the patient to tolerate placement of a peripheral nerve block or to tolerate lying on the narrow, stiff operating table may lead to hypoxemia and hypercarbia secondary to hypoventilation. On the other hand, lack of adequate sedation can promote anxiety, pain and sympathetic stimulation. Achieving the delicate balance can be a daunting task for anesthesia providers.

For those patients with PH to undergo minor surgical procedures with only monitored anesthesia care (MAC), special attention should be paid to provide adequate sedation to minimize patients' anxiety, which can be harmful because it may lead to increased sympathetic outflow as we discussed previously. Over-sedation should be avoided to prevent respiratory suppression and subsequent hypoventilation and hypoxemia which may induce hypoxic vasoconstriction and elevated PAP.

6.6. Postoperative management

These patients with moderate to severe PH warrant intensive care monitoring in the postoperative period by experienced critical care personnel. As the analgesic and sympathetic nervous system effects of opioids, volatile anesthetics, and regional anesthetics disappear, the patient can develop sudden worsening of PH and RV ischemia. Thus weaning from the ventilatory support and endotracheal extubation should be done gradually with close attention to adequate oxygenation, ventilation and analgesia. Even routine events such as bucking on the ventilator due to tracheal stimulation, while tolerated by the average patient, can lead to acute rises in PVR and RV failure in patient with severe PH [78]. Postoperative pain management of patients with PH warrants special attention, because in clinical practice, the most commonly used analgesic agents are opioids which are potent respiratory depressants also. Depression of respiratory drive will likely cause hypoventilation which leads to increased PAP. Thus using multimodal analgesic strategy is critical in minimizing the side effect of respiratory inhibition by opioids and avoiding hypoventilation-associated increase of PAP.

7. Special populations potentially with pulmonary hypertension

7.1. Pediatrics

Pediatric patients with PH have some unique clinical features comparing with adult PH patients. Genetic factors seem to play a more important role in the pathogenesis of PH. Chida *et al* studied fifty-four patients with IPAH or HPAH whose disease was diagnosed at <16 years of age. Functional characteristics, hemodynamic parameters, and clinical outcomes were compared in BMPR2 and ALK1 mutation carriers and noncarriers. Overall 5-year survival for all patients was 76%. Eighteen BMPR2 mutation carriers and 7 ALK1 mutation carriers were detected in the 54 patients with childhood IPAH or HPAH. Five-year survival was lower in BMPR2 mutation carriers than mutation noncarriers (55% vs 90%, hazard ratio 12.54, $p = 0.0003$). ALK1 mutation carriers also had a tendency to have worse outcome than mutation noncarriers (5-year survival rate 64%, hazard ratio 5.14, $p=0.1205$). These indicated that patients with childhood IPAH or HPAH with BMPR2 mutation have the poorest clinical outcomes. ALK1 mutation carriers tended to have worse outcomes than mutation non-carriers. It is important to consider aggressive treatment for BMPR2 or ALK1 mutation carriers [102]. Carmosino *et al* retrospectively studied 156 children with PH with median age 4.0 years who underwent anesthesia or sedation for noncardiac surgical procedures or cardiac catheterizations from 1999 to 2004. PH etiology was 56% idiopathic (primary), 21% AHD, 14% chronic lung disease, 4% chronic airway obstruction, and 4% chronic liver disease. Baseline PAP was subsystemic in 68% patients, systemic in 19%, and suprasystemic in 13%. The anesthetic techniques were 22% sedation, 58% general inhaled, 20% general IV. Minor complications occurred in eight patients (5.1% of patients, 3.1% of procedures). Major complications including cardiac arrest and pulmonary hypertensive crisis, occurred in seven patients during cardiac catheterization procedures (4.5% of patients, 5.0% of cardiac catheterization procedures, 2.7% of all procedures). There were two deaths associated with pulmonary hypertensive crisis (1.3% of patients, 0.8% of procedures). Based on their observation, they believe baseline suprasystemic PH was a significant predictor of major complications by multivariate logistic regression analysis ($OR = 8.1$, $P = 0.02$) and complications were not significantly associated with age, etiology of PH, type of anesthetic, or airway management. Children with suprasystemic PH have a significant risk of major perioperative complications, including cardiac arrest and pulmonary hypertensive crisis [103]. Management of pediatric patients with PH poses unique challenges to pediatric anesthesiologists: PAC may not be available for many smaller pediatric patients due to the small sizes of their cardiac chamber and blood vessels. TEE may not be available to some pediatric patients due to lack of suitable size of TEE probe. So transthoracic or epicardial echocardiography will play a much more important role for those pediatric patients without TEE and PAC. Minimally invasive/non-invasive monitoring of MAP, CO/CI, SVV may play some role intraoperatively, however these current technologies may not work as well in children as in adults [104]. And information from randomized controlled clinical studies on the treatment of pediatric PH is currently very limited, unanimous opinions are to refer to the guidelines and treatment strategies for the treatment of adult PH. Therefore, the recommended treatment for children is only grade IIa with the level of evidence class C.

7.2. Obstetrics

Curry *et al* reported two maternal deaths out of 12 pregnancies in 9 patients. One of the two deaths was related to pre-eclampsia and the other related to cardiac arrhythmia. Maternal morbidity included postpartum hemorrhage (five cases), and one post-caesarean evacuation of a wound hematoma. There were no perinatal death, nine live births and three first-trimester miscarriages. Mean birthweight was 2197 grams, mean gestational age was 34 weeks (range 26-39), and mean birthweight percentile was 36 (range 5-60). Five babies required admission to the neonatal intensive care unit, but were all eventually discharged home. All women were delivered by caesarean section (seven elective and two emergency deliveries), under general anesthesia except for one emergency and one elective caesarean performed under regional block [105]. Maternal and fetal outcomes for women with PH has improved; however, the risk of maternal mortality remains significant, so that early and effective counseling about contraceptive options and pregnancy risks should continue to play a major role in the management of such women when they reach reproductive maturity.

8. Summary

We have gained better understanding of PH and have significantly more sophisticated management strategies now compared with two decades ago. PH can develop due to pulmonary vascular remodeling (cellular proliferation), abnormal vasoconstriction, mechanical obstruction (chronic thromboembolic events, interstitial lung diseases) or left-side heart diseases. Thorough preoperative evaluation is mandatory. A clear understanding of the etiology of pulmonary hypertension is extremely important to understand how to optimally manage these patients in the operating room. Echocardiography plays a key role in preliminary screening, monitoring the progress and evolution of PH, and intraoperative monitoring and treatment. Right heart catheterization remains the gold standard for the diagnosis of PH. Evaluation of the overall pulmonary functional status is also important in assessing patients' tolerability to the planned surgical procedure. Perioperatively these patients can present very challenging clinical scenarios due to the complexity of their PH and increased risks for significant complications with elevated morbidity and mortality. Several clinical characteristics predict early mortality: right axis deviation, right ventricular hypertrophy, RVSP/SBP ratio above 0.6, and intraoperative use of epinephrine or dopamine. Intraoperative control of elevated pulmonary pressure can be achieved with inhaled nitric oxide or prostacyclin, PDE inhibitors (milrinone, sildenafil), calcium channel blockers, nitrodilators and adequate oxygenation. The ideal perioperative care of these patients requires a multidisciplinary approach with appropriate planning for pre-procedural optimization, comprehensive intraoperative monitoring and delicate management of PAP as well as intensive care unit monitoring in the postoperative period. This approach will test the expertise and resources of medical institutions. Anesthesiologists will require a thorough understanding of the current treatment options, pathophysiology of the disease, and the implications of various anesthetic agents and techniques to provide the highest level of patient safety and care to the patients with PH.

Author details

Henry Liu*, Philip L. Kalarickal, Yiru Tong, Daisuke Inui, Michael J. Yarborough, Kavitha A. Mathew, Amanda Gelineau, Alan D. Kaye and Charles Fox

*Address all correspondence to: henryliula@gmail.com

Department of Anesthesiology, Tulane University Medical Center, New Orleans, Louisiana, USA

References

[1] Simonneau G, Robbins I, Beghetti M, et al. Updated clinical classification of pulmonary hypertension. J Am Coll Cardiol. 2009;54:43-54.

[2] Gaine S. Pulmonary hypertension. (2000). JAMA. Vol. 284, No. 24, (December, 2000), pp. 3160–3168, ISSN: 0098-7484

[3] Runo JR, Loyd JE. Primary pulmonary hypertension. Lancet 2003; 361:1533-44.

[4] Murali S, Benza RL. Pulmonary hypertension. Heart Fail Clin. 2012 Jul;8(3):xxi-xxii.

[5] Galiè N, Hoeper MM, Humbert M, Torbicki A, Vachiery JL, Barbera JA, Beghetti M, Corris P, Gaine S, Gibbs JS, Gomez-Sanchez MA, Jondeau G, Klepetko W, Opitz C, Peacock A, Rubin L, Zellweger M, Simonneau G; ESC Committee for Practice Guidelines (CPG). Guidelines for the diagnosis and treatment of pulmonary hypertension: the Task Force for the Diagnosis and Treatment of Pulmonary Hypertension of the European Society of Cardiology (ESC) and the European Respiratory Society (ERS), endorsed by the International Society of Heart and Lung Transplantation (ISHLT). Eur Heart J. 2009 Oct;30(20):2493-537. Epub 2009 Aug 27.

[6] Nef HM, Möllmann H, Hamm C, Grimminger F, Ghofrani HA. Pulmonary hypertension: updated classification and management of pulmonary hypertension. Heart. 2010 Apr; 96(7):552-9.

[7] Memtsoudis, SG, Ma Y, Chiu, YL et al. Perioperative Mortality in Patients with Pulmonary Hypertension Undergoing Major Joint Replacement. (2010). Anesthesia and Analgesia. Vol. 111, No. 5, (November, 2010), pp. 1110-6, ISSN: 0003-2999

[8] Lai HC, Lai HC, Wang KY et al. Severe pulmonary hypertension complicates postoperative outcome of non-cardiac surgery. (2007). British Journal of Anesthesia. Vol. 99, No. 2, (August, 2007), pp. 184-90, ISSN: 1471-6771

[9] Strange G, Playford D, Stewart S, Deague JA, Nelson H, Kent A, Gabbay E. Pulmonary hypertension: prevalence and mortality in the Armadale echocardiography cohort. Heart. 2012 Jul 3.

[10] Savale L, Maitre B, Bachir D, Galactéros F, Simonneau G, Parent F. Pulmonary arterial hypertension and sickle cell disease. Presse Med. 2012 Jun 26.

[11] Rose M, Strange G, King I, Arnup S, Vidmar S, Kermeen F, Grigg L, Weintraub R, Celermajer D. Congenital Heart Disease Associated Pulmonary Arterial Hypertension: Preliminary Results From a Novel Registry. Intern Med J. 2011 Dec 29. doi: 10.1111/j.1445-5994.2011.02708

[12] Andersen CU, Mellemkjær S, Hilberg O, Nielsen-Kudsk JE, Simonsen U, Bendstrup E. Pulmonary hypertension in interstitial lung disease: prevalence, prognosis and 6 min walk test. Respir Med. 2012 Jun;106(6):875-82.

[13] http://www.livestrong.com/article/281048-otc-drugs-that-increase-pulmonary-pressure/

[14] Loyd JE, Butler MG, Foroud TM, et al. Genetic anticipation and abnormal gender ratio at birth in familial primary pulmonary hypertension. (1995). American Journal of Respiratory and Critical Care Medicine. Vol. 152, No. 1, (July, 1995), pp. 93–97, ISSN: 1073-449X

[15] Phillips BG, Norkiewk K, Perck CA, et al. Effects of obstructive sleep apnea onendothelin-1 and blood pressure. (1999). Journal of Hypertension.Vol. 17,No. 1, (January, 1999), pp. 61–66. ISSN: 0263-6352

[16] MacLean MR. Endothelin-1 and serotonin: mediators of primary and secondary pulmonary hypertension? (1999). Journal of Laboratory and Clinical Medicine. Vol.134, No. 2. (August 1999), pp. 105–144, ISSN: 0022-2143

[17] Tuder RM, Cool CD, Yeager M, et al. The pathobiology of pulmonary hypertension: endothelium.(2001). Clinics in Chest Medicine. Vol. 22, No. 3, (September, 2001), pp. 405–418, ISSN: 0272-5231

[18] Nicolls MR, Taraseviciene-Stewart L, Rai PR, Badesch DB, Voelkel NF. Autoimmunity and pulmonary hypertension: a perspective. Eur Respir J. 2005 Dec.;26(6):1110–1118.

[19] Tamosiuniene R, Nicolls MR. Regulatory T cells and pulmonary hypertension. Trends Cardiovasc Med. 2011 Aug;21(6):166-71.

[20] Dhala A. Pulmonary arterial hypertension in systemic lupus erythematosus: current status and future direction. Clin Dev Immunol. 2012;2012:854941. Epub 2012 Mar 22. PMID:22489252

[21] Sanchez O, Sitbon O, Jaïs X, Simonneau G, Humbert M. Immunosuppressive therapy in connective tissue diseases-associated pulmonary arterial hypertension. Chest. 2006 Jul;130(1):182-9

[22] Medoff BD. Fat, Fire and muscle - The role of adiponectin in pulmonary vascular inflammation and remodeling. Pulm Pharmacol Ther. 2012 Jun 26.

[23] Guglin M, Kolli S, Chen R. Determinants of pulmonary hypertension in young adults. Int J Clin Pract Suppl. 2012 Oct;(177):13-9. doi: 10.1111/ijcp.12008.

[24] Voelkel NF, Gomez-Arroyo JG, Abbate A, Bogaard HJ, Nicolls MR. Pathobiology of pulmonary arterial hypertension and right ventricular failure. Eur Respir J. 2012 Jun 27.

[25] Buehler PW, Baek JH, Lisk C, Connor I, Sullivan T, Kominsky DJ, Majka SM, Stenmark KR, Nozik-Grayck E, Bonaventura J, Irwin DC. Free hemoglobin induction of pulmonary vascular disease:Evidence for an inflammatory mechanism. Am J Physiol Lung Cell Mol Physiol. 2012 Jun 22.

[26] Xing AP, Hu XY, Shi YW, Du YC. Implication of PDGF signaling in cigarette smoke-induced pulmonary arterial hypertension in rat. Inhal Toxicol. 2012 Jul;24(8):468-75.

[27] Panzhinskiy E, Zawada WM, Stenmark KR, Das M. Hypoxia induces unique proliferative response in adventitial fibroblasts by activating PDGFβ receptor-JNK1 signalling. Cardiovasc Res. 2012 Aug 1;95(3):356-65.

[28] Zhang L, Ma J, Shen T, Wang S, Ma C, Liu Y, Ran Y, Wang L, Liu L, Zhu D. Platelet-derived growth factor (PDGF) induces pulmonary vascular remodeling through 15-LO/15-HETE pathway under hypoxic condition. Cell Signal. 2012 Oct;24(10):1931-9. Epub 2012 Jun 23.

[29] Ruggiero RM, Bartolome S, Torres F. Pulmonary hypertension in parenchymal lung disease. Heart Fail Clin. 2012 Jul;8(3):461-74.

[30] Wang D, Prakash J, Nguyen P, Davis-Dusenbery BN, Hill NS, Layne MD, Hata A, Lagna G. Bone Morphogenetic Protein signaling in vascular disease: anti-inflammatory action through Myocardin-related transcription factor A. J Biol Chem. 2012 Jun 20.

[31] Nasim MT, Ogo T, Chowdhury HM, Zhao L, Chen CN, Rhodes C, Trembath RC. BMPR-II deficiency elicits pro-proliferative and anti-apoptotic responses through the activation of TGFβ-TAK1-MAPK pathways in PAH. Hum Mol Genet. 2012 Jun 1;21(11):2548-58.

[32] Shiraishi I. Mutations in bone morphogenetic protein receptor genes in pulmonary arterial hypertension patients. Circ J. 2012 May 25;76(6):1329-30.

[33] Pfarr N, Szamalek-Hoegel J, Fischer C, Hinderhofer K, Nagel C, Ehlken N, Tiede H, Olschewski H, Reichenberger F, Ghofrani AH, Seeger W, Grünig E. Hemodynamic and clinical onset in patients with hereditary pulmonary arterial hypertension and BMPR2 mutations. Respir Res. 2011th ed. 2011;12:99.

[34] Machado RD, Eickelberg O, Elliott CG, Geraci MW, Hanaoka M, Loyd JE, Newman JH, Phillips JA, Soubrier F, Trembath RC, Chung WK. Genetics and genomics of pulmonary arterial hypertension. Journal of the American College of Cardiology. 2009 Jun. 30;54(1 Suppl):S32–42.

[35] Pullamsetti SS, Doebele C, Fischer A, Savai R, Kojonazarov B, Dahal BK, Ghofrani HA, Weissmann N, Grimminger F, Bonauer A, Seeger W, Zeiher AM, Dimmeler S, Schermuly RT. Inhibition of microRNA-17 improves lung and heart function in experimental pulmonary hypertension. Am J Respir Crit Care Med. 2012 Feb 15;185(4): 409-19.

[36] Brock M, Trenkmann M, Gay RE, Michel BA, Gay S, Fischler M, Ulrich S, Speich R, Huber LC. Interleukin-6 modulates the expression of the bone morphogenic protein receptor type II through a novel STAT3-microRNA cluster 17/92 pathway. Circ Res. 2009 May 22;104(10):1184-91.

[37] Bockmeyer CL, Maegel L, Janciauskiene S, Rische J, Lehmann U, Maus UA, Nickel N, Haverich A, Hoeper MM, Golpon HA, Kreipe H, Laenger F, Jonigk D. Plexiform vasculopathy of severe pulmonary arterial hypertension and microRNA expression. J Heart Lung Transplant. 2012 Jul;31(7):764-72.

[38] Dempsie Y, Nilsen M, White K, Mair KM, Loughlin L, Ambartsumian N, Rabinovitch M, Maclean MR. Development of pulmonary arterial hypertension in mice over-expressing S100A4/Mts1 is specific to females. Respir Res. 2011 Dec 20;12:159.

[39] Moraca RJ, Kanwar M. Chronic thromboembolic pulmonary hypertension. Heart Fail Clin. 2012 Jul;8(3):475-83.

[40] Bossone E, Naeije R. Exercise-induced pulmonary hypertension. Heart Fail Clin. 2012 Jul;8(3):485-95.

[41] Argiento P, Chesler N, Mulè M, D'Alto M, Bossone E, Unger P, Naeije R. Exercise stress echocardiography for the study of the pulmonary circulation. Eur Respir J. 2010 Jun;35(6):1273-8.

[42] Cahill E, Costello CM, Rowan SC, Harkin S, Howell K, Leonard MO, Southwood M, Cummins EP, Fitzpatrick SF, Taylor CT, Morrell NW, Martin F, McLoughlin P.

Gremlin plays a key role in the pathogenesis of pulmonary hypertension. Circulation. 2012 Feb 21;125(7):920-30.

[43] Abud EM, Maylor J, Undem C, Punjabi A, Zaiman AL, Myers AC, Sylvester JT, Semenza GL, Shimoda LA. Digoxin inhibits development of hypoxic pulmonary hypertension in mice. Proc Natl Acad Sci U S A. 2012 Jan 24;109(4):1239-44.

[44] Krowka MJ, Mandell MS, Ramsay MA, et al. Hepatopulmonary syndrome and portopulmonary hypertension: a report of the multicenter liver transplant database. (2004). Liver Transplantation. Vol. 10, No. 2, (February, 2004), pp. 174–182, ISSN: 1527-6465

[45] Martin JT, Tautz TJ, Antognini JF. Safety of regional anesthesia in Eisenmenger's syndrome. (2002). Regional Anesthesia and Pain Medicine. Vol. 27, No. 5, (September, 2002), pp. 509–513, ISSN:1098-7339

[46] Roberts NV, Keast PJ. Pulmonary hypertension and pregnancy: a lethal combination. (1993). Anaesth Intensive Care.Vol. 18, No. 3, (August, 1993), pp. 366–374, ISSN: 1472-0299

[47] Ramakrishna G, Sprung J, Ravi BS, et al. Impact of pulmonary hypertension on the outcomes of noncardiac surgery: predictors of perioperative morbidity and mortality. (2005). Journal of the American College of Cardiology. Vol. 45, No. 10, (May, 2005), pp. 1691–1699, ISSSN: 0735-1097

[48] Tan HP, Markowitz JS, Montgomery RA, et al. Liver transplantation in patients with severe portopulmonary hypertension treated with preoperative chronic intravenous epoprostenol. (2001). Liver Transplantation. Vol. 7, No. 8, (August, 2001), pp. 745–749, ISSN: 1527-6465

[49] Weiss BM, Atanassoff PG. Cyanotic congenital heart disease and pregnancy: natural selection, pulmonary hypertension, and anesthesia. (1993). Journal of Clinical Anesthesia. Vol. 5, No. 4, (July, 1993), pp. 332–341, ISSN: 0952-8180

[50] Kahn ML. Eisenmenger's syndrome in pregnancy. (1993). New England Journal of Medicine. Vol. 329, No. 12, (September, 1993), p. 887, ISSN: 0028-4793

[51] Ross AF, Ueda K. Pulmonary hypertension in thoracic surgical patients. (2010). Current Opinion in Anaesthesiolology. Vol. 23, No. 1, (February, 2010), pp. 25–33, ISSN: 0952-7907

[52] Blaise G, Langleben D, Hubert B. Pulmonary arterial hypertension: pathophysiology and anesthetic approach. (2003). Anesthesiology. Vol. 99, No. 6, (December, 2003), pp. 1415–1432, ISSN: 0003-3022

[53] Ahearn GS, Tapson VF, Rebeiz A, Greenfield JC Jr. Electrocardiography to define clinical status in primary pulmonary hypertension and pulmonary hypertension secondary to collagen vascular disease. (2002). Chest. Vol. 122, No. 2, (August, 2002), pp. 524–527, ISSN: 0012-3692

[54] Bossone E, Paciacco G, Iarussi D, et al. The prognostic role of the ECG in primary pulmonary hypertension. (2002). Chest. Vol. 121, No. 2, (February, 2002), pp. 513–518, ISSN: 0012-3692

[55] Nauser TD, Stites SW. Diagnosis and treatment of pulmonary hypertension. (2001). American Family Physician. Vol. 63, No. 9, (May, 2001), pp. 1789–1798, ISSN: 0002-838X

[56] Ramos RP, Arakaki JS, Barbosa P, Treptow E, Valois FM, Ferreira EV, Nery LE, Neder JA. Heart rate recovery in pulmonary arterial hypertension: relationship with exercise capacity and prognosis. Am Heart J. 2012 Apr;163(4):580-8.

[57] Minai OA, Gudavalli R, Mummadi S, Liu X, McCarthy K, Dweik RA. Heart rate recovery predicts clinical worsening in patients with pulmonary arterial hypertension. Am J Respir Crit Care Med. 2012 Feb 15;185(4):400-8.

[58] Bossone E, Bodini BD, Mazza A, Allegra L. Pulmonary Arterial Hypertension, The Key Role of Echocardiography. (2005). CHEST. Vol. 127, No. 5, (May, 2005), pp. 1836-1843, ISSN: 0012-3692

[59] Mookadam F, Jiamsripong P, Goel R, Warsame TA, Emani UR, Khandheria BK. Critical Appraisal on the Utility of Echocardiography in the Management of Acute Pulmonary Embolism. (2010). Cardiology in Review. Vol. 18, No. 1, (January, 2010), pp. 29-37, ISSN: 1061-5377

[60] Morikawa T, Murata M, Okuda S, et al. Quantitative Analysis of Right Ventricular Function in Patients with Pulmonary Hypertension Using Three-Dimensional Echocardiography and a Two-Dimensional Summation Method Compared to Magnetic Resonance Imaging. (2011). American Journal of Cardiology. Vol. 107, No. 3, (February, 2011), pp. 484-89, ISSN: 0002-9149

[61] Feltracco P, Serra E, Barbieri S, Salvaterra F, Rizzi S, Furnari M, Brezzi M, Rea F, Ori C. Anesthetic concerns in lung transplantation for severe pulmonary hypertension. Transplant Proc. 2007 Jul-Aug;39(6):1976-80.

[62] Janda S, Shahidi N, Gin K, Swiston J. Diagnostic accuracy of echocardiography for pulmonary hypertension: a systematic review and meta-analysis. (2011). Heart. Vol. 97, No. 8, (April, 2011), pp. 612-622, ISSN: 1355-6037

[63] Sciomer S, Magri D, Badagliacca R. Non-invasive assessment of pulmonary hypertension: Doppler-echocardiography. (2007). Pulmonary Pharmacology and Therapeutics. Vol. 20, No. 2, pp. 135-40, ISSN: 1522-9629.

[64] Fisher MR, Forfia PR, Chamera E, et al. Accuracy of Doppler Echocardiography in the Hemodynamic Assessment of Pulmonary Hypertension. (2009). American Journal of Respiratory and Critical Care Medicine. Vol. 179, No. 7, (April, 2009), pp. 615-21, ISSN: 1073-449X

[65] Pedoto A and Amar D. Right heart function in thoracic surgery: role of echocardiography. (2009). Current Opinion in Anaesthesiology. Vol. 22, No. 1, (Februar,y 2009). pp. 44-49, ISSN: 0952-7907

[66] McLaughlin VV, Archer SL, Badesch DB, et al. ACCF/AHA 2009 expert consensus document on pulmonary hypertension: a report of the American College of Cardiology Foundation Task Force on Expert Consensus Documents and the American Heart Association: developed in collaboration with the American College of Chest Physicians, American Thoracic Society, Inc., and the Pulmonary Hypertension Association. Circulation. Vol. 119, No. 16, (April, 2009), pp. 2250-94, ISSN: 0009-7322

[67] Takatsuki S, Nakayama T, Jone PN, Wagner BD, Naoi K, Ivy DD, Saji T. Tissue Doppler Imaging Predicts Adverse Outcome in Children with Idiopathic Pulmonary Arterial Hypertension. J Pediatr. 2012 Jun 28.

[68] Pearl RG. Perioperative management of PH: covering all aspects from risk assessment to postoperative considerations. (2005). Advances in Pulmonary Hypertension. Vol. 4, No. 4, (Winter, 2005), pp. 6–15, ISSN: 1933-088X

[69] Brown AT, Gillespie JV, Miquel-Verges F, Holmes K, Ravekes W, Spevak P, Brady K, Easley RB, Golden WC, McNamara L, Veltri MA, Lehmann CU, McMillan KN, Schwartz JM, Romer LH. Inhaled epoprostenol therapy for pulmonary hypertension: Improves oxygenation index more consistently in neonates than in older children. Pulm Circ. 2012 Jan;2(1):61-6.

[70] He J, Fang W, Lu B, He JG, Xiong CM, Liu ZH, He ZX. Diagnosis of chronic thromboembolic pulmonary hypertension: comparison of ventilation/perfusion scanning and multidetector computed tomography pulmonary angiography with pulmonary angiography. Nucl Med Commun. 2012 May;33(5):459-63.

[71] Yamada Y, Okuda S, Kataoka M, Tanimoto A, Tamura Y, Abe T, Okamura T, Fukuda K, Satoh T, Kuribayashi S. Prognostic value of cardiac magnetic resonance imaging for idiopathic pulmonary arterial hypertension before initiating intravenous prostacyclin therapy. Circ J. 2012 Jun 25;76(7):1737-43.

[72] Swift AJ, Rajaram S, Condliffe R, Capener D, Hurdman J, Elliot CA, Wild JM, Kiely DG. Diagnostic accuracy of cardiovascular magnetic resonance of right ventricular morphology and function in the assessment of suspected pulmonary hypertension. J Cardiovasc Magn Reson. 2012 Jun 21;14(1):40.

[73] Frantz RP, McDevitt S, Walker S. Baseline NT-proBNP correlates with change in 6-minute walk distance in patients with pulmonary arterial hypertension in the pivotal inhaled treprostinil study TRIUMPH-1. J Heart Lung Transplant. 2012 Aug;31(8): 811-6.

[74] Diller GP, Alonso-Gonzalez R, Kempny A, Dimopoulos K, Inuzuka R, Giannakoulas G, Castle L, Lammers AE, Hooper J, Uebing A, Swan L, Gatzoulis M, Wort SJ. B-type natriuretic peptide concentrations in contemporary Eisenmenger syndrome patients:

predictive value and response to disease targeting therapy. Heart. 2012 May;98(9): 736-42.

[75] Cuenco J, Tzeng G, Wittels B. Anesthetic management of the parturient with system iclupus erythematosus, pulmonary hypertension, a nd pulmonary edema. (1999). Anesthesiology. Vol. 91, No. 1, (August, 1999), pp. 568–570, ISSN: 0003-3022

[76] Kuralay E, Demirkilic U, Oz BS, et al. Primary pulmonary hypertension and coronaryartery bypass surgery. (2002). Journal of Cardiac Surgergy. Vol. 17, No. 1, (January, 2002), pp. 79–80, ISSN: 0886-0440

[77] Tay SM, Ong BC, Tan SA. Cesarean section in a mother with uncorrected congenital coronary to pulmonary artery fistula. (1999). Canandian Journal of Anaesthesia. Vol. 46, No. 4, (April, 1999), pp. 368–371, ISSN: 0832-610X

[78] Rodriguez RM, Pearl RG. Pulmonary hypertension and major surgery. (1998). Anesthesia and Analgesia. Vol. 87, No. 4, (October, 1998), pp. 812–815, ISSN: 0003-2999

[79] Armstrong P. Thoracic epidural anaesthesia and primary pulmonary hypertension. (1992). Anaesthesia. Vol. 47, No. 6, (June, 1992), pp. 496–499, ISSN: 0003-2409

[80] Hoeper MM, Lee SH, Voswinckel R, Palazzini M, Jais X, Marinelli A, Barst RJ, Ghofrani HA, Jing ZC, Opitz C, Seyfarth HJ, Halank M, McLaughlin V, Oudiz RJ,Ewert R, Wilkens H, Kluge S, Bremer HC, Baroke E, Rubin LJ. Complications of right heart catheterization procedures in patients with pulmonary hypertension in experienced centers. J Am Coll Cardiol. 2006 Dec 19;48(12):2546-52.

[81] Baron CM, Swedlo D, Funk DJ. Minimally invasive cardiac output monitoring for a parturient with pulmonary hypertension. Int J Obstet Anesth. 2012 Oct 30.

[82] Neema PK, Singha SK, Manikandan S, Rathod RC. Transesophageal echocardiography and intraoperative phlebotomy during surgical repair of coarctation of aorta in a patient with atrial septal defect, moderately severe mitral regurgitation and severe pulmonary hypertension. J Clin Monit Comput. 2012 Jun;26(3):217-21.

[83] Kandachar S, Chakravarthy M, Krishnamoorthy J, Suryaprakash S, Muniappa G, Pandey S, Jawali V, Xavier J. Unmasking of patent ductus arteriosus on cardiopulmonary bypass: role of intraoperative transesophageal echocardiography in a patient with severe pulmonary hypertension due topulmonary vein stenosis and cor triatriatum. Ann Card Anaesth. 2011 May-Aug;14(2):152-3.

[84] Ichinose F, Roberts JD, Zapol WM. Inhaled nitric oxide: a selective pulmonaryvasodilator – current uses and therapeutic potential. (2004). Circulation. Vol. 109, No. 25, (June, 2004), pp. 3106–3111, ISSN: 0009-7322

[85] Kavanaugh BP, Pearl RG. Inhaled nitric oxide in anesthesia and critical care medicine. (1995). International Anesthesiology Clinics. Vol. 33, No.1, (Winter, 1995), pp. 181–210, ISSN: 0020-5907

[86] Tanake H, Tajimi K, Moritsune O, et al. Effects of milrinone on pulmonary vasculaturein normal dogs and dogs with pulmonary hypertension. (1991). Critial Care Medicine. Vol 19, No. 1, (January 1991), pp. 68–74, ISSN: 0090-3493

[87] Lepore JJ, Dec GW, Zapol WM, Bloch KD, Semigran MJ. Combined administration of intravenous dipyridamole and inhaled nitric oxide to assess reversibility of pulmonary arterial hypertension in potential cardiac transplant recipients. J Heart Lung Transplant. 2005 Nov;24(11):1950-6.

[88] Jerath A, Srinivas C, Vegas A, Brister S. The successful management of severe protamine-induced pulmonary hypertension using inhaled prostacyclin. Anesth Analg. 2010 Feb 1;110(2):365-9.

[89] Atz AM, Lefler AK, Fairbrother DL, et al. Sildenafil augments the effect of inhaled nitric oxide for postoperative pulmonary hypertensive crises. (2002). Journal of Thoracic and Cardiovascular Surgery. Vol. 124, No. 3, (September, 2002), pp. 628–629, ISSN: 0022-5223

[90] Petros AJ, Turner SC, Nunn AJ. Cost implications of using inhaled nitric oxide compared with epoprostenol for pulmonary hypertension. (1995). Journal of Pharmacy Technology. Vol. 11, No. 4, (July, 1995), pp. 163–166, ISSN: 8755-1225

[91] De Wet CJ, Affleck DJ, Jacobsohn E, Avidan MS, Tymkew H, Hill ll, Zanaboni PB, Moazami N, Smith JR. Inhaled prostacyclin is safe, effective, and affordable in patients with pulmonary hypertension, right heart dysfunction,and refractory hypoxemia after cardiothoracic surgery. (2004). The Journal of Thoracic and Cardiovascular Surgery. Vol 127, No. 4, (Aril 2004), pp. 1058-67, ISSN: 0022-5223

[92] Subramaniam K, Yared JP. Management of pulmonary hypertension in the operating room. (2007). Seminars in Cardiothoracic and Vascular Anesthesia. Vol. 11, No. 2, (June, 2007), pp. 119–136, ISSN: 1089-2532

[93] Shim JK, Choi YS, Oh YJ, Kim DH, Hong YW, Kwak YL. Effect of oral sildenafil citrate on intraoperative hemodynamics in patients with pulmonary hypertension undergoing valvular heart surgery. J Thorac Cardiovasc Surg. 2006 Dec;132(6):1420-5.

[94] Rich S, Brundage BH. High-dose calcium channel-blocking therapy for primary pulmonary hypertension: evidence for long-term reduction in pulmonary arterial pressure and regression of right ventricular hypertrophy. Circulation 1987;76: 135–41.

[95] http://www.empr.com/cardiovascular-system/pulmonary-hypertension/pnote/149/

[96] http://www.4ventavis.com/?s_kwcid=TC|6584|iloprost||S|e|12604955101

[97] http://www.drugs.com/sfx/nifedipine-side-effects.html

[98] Rich GF, Roos CM, Anderson SM, et al. Direct effects of intravenous anesthetics on pulmonary vascular resistance in the isolated rat lung. (1994). Anesthesia and Analgesia. Vol. 78, No. 5, (May,1994):961–966, ISSN: 0003-2999

[99] Schulte-Sasse U, Hess W, Tarnow J. Pulmonary vascular responses to nitrous oxide in patients with normal and high pulmonary vascular resistance. (1982). Anesthesiology. Vol. 57, No. 1, (July, 1982), pp. 9–13, ISSN: 0003-3022

[100] Davies MJ, Beavis RE. Epidural anaesthesia for vascular surgery in a patient with primary pulmonary hypertension. (1984). Anaesthesia and Intensive Care. Vol. 12, No. 2, (May, 1984), pp. 115–117, ISSN: 0310-057X

[101] Höhn L, Schweizer A, Morel DR, Spiliopoulos A, Licker M. Circulatory failure after anesthesia induction in a patient with severe primarypulmonary hypertension. Anesthesiology. 1999 Dec;91(6):1943-5.

[102] Chida A, Shintani M, Yagi H, Fujiwara M, Kojima Y, Sato H, Imamura S, Yokozawa M, Onodera N, Horigome H, Kobayashi T, Hatai Y, Nakayama T, Fukushima H, Nishiyama M, Doi S, Ono Y, Yasukouchi S, Ichida F, Fujimoto K, Ohtsuki S, Teshima H, Kawano T, Nomura Y, Gu H, Ishiwata T, Furutani Y, Inai K, Saji T, Matsuoka R, Nonoyama S, Nakanishi T. Outcomes of Childhood Pulmonary Arterial Hypertension in BMPR2 and ALK1 Mutation Carriers. Am J Cardiol. 2012 May 25.

[103] Carmosino MJ, Friesen RH, Doran A, Ivy DD. Perioperative complications in children with pulmonary hypertension undergoing noncardiac surgery or cardiac catheterization. (2007). Anesthesia and Analgesia. Vol. 104, No. 3, (March, 2007), pp. 521–527, ISSN: 0003-2999

[104] Teng S, Kaufman J, Pan Z, Czaja A, Shockley H, da Cruz E. Continuous arterial pressure waveform monitoring in pediatric cardiac transplant, cardiomyopathy andpulmonary hypertension patients. Intensive Care Med. 2011 Aug;37(8):1297-301.

[105] Curry RA, Fletcher C, Gelson E, Gatzoulis MA, Woolnough M, Richards N, Swan L. BJOG. 2012 May; 119(6):752-61. doi: 10.1111/j.1471-0528.2012.03295.x.